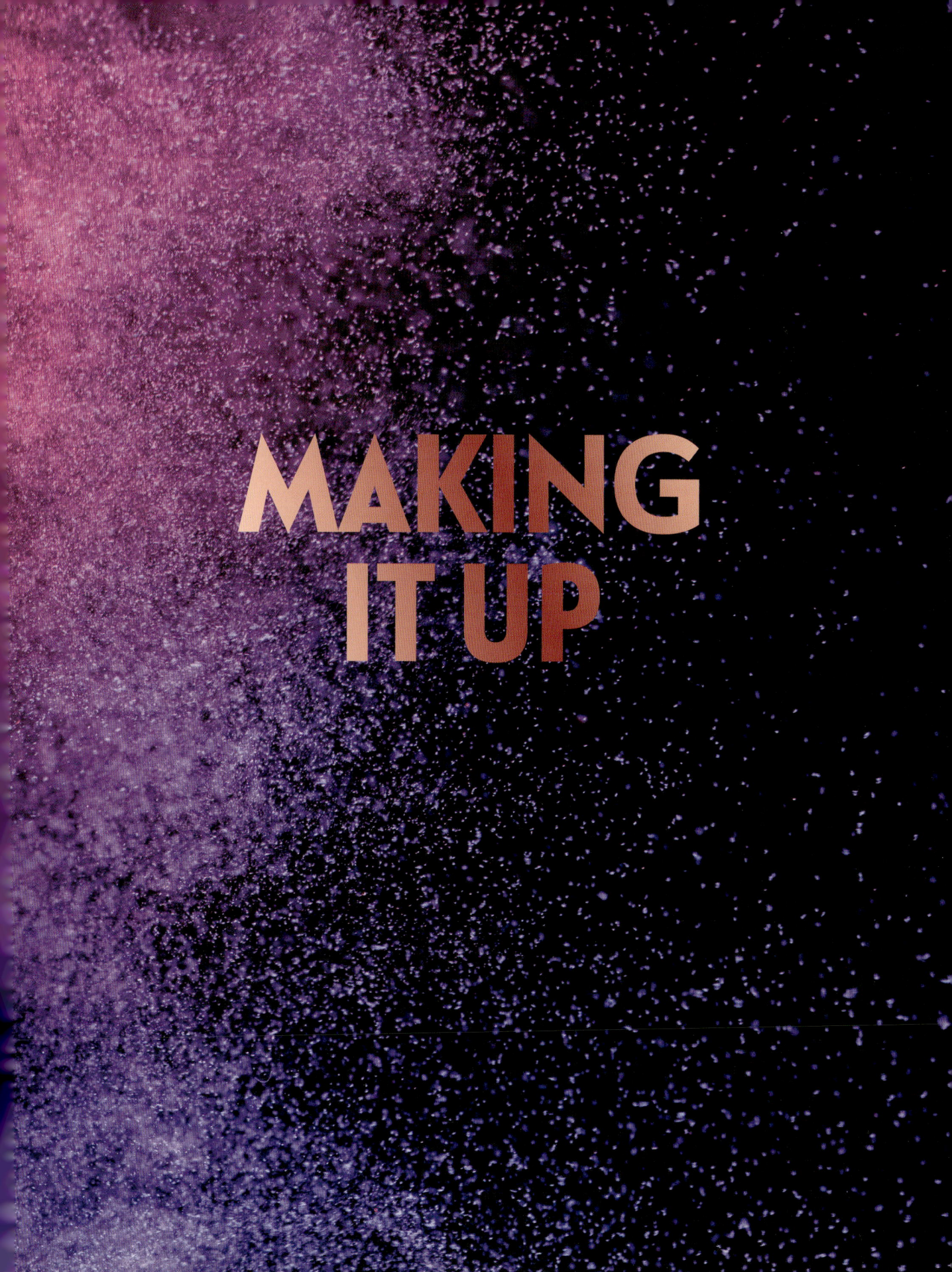

to my Frenchie

True beauty is a feeling inside, but there is nothing wrong with sprinkling glitter on it. Be your best YOU. I am your biggest cheerleader xxx

MAKING IT UP

Makeup Minus the Rules

NICOLE THOMPSON

Photography by Steven Popovich

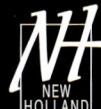

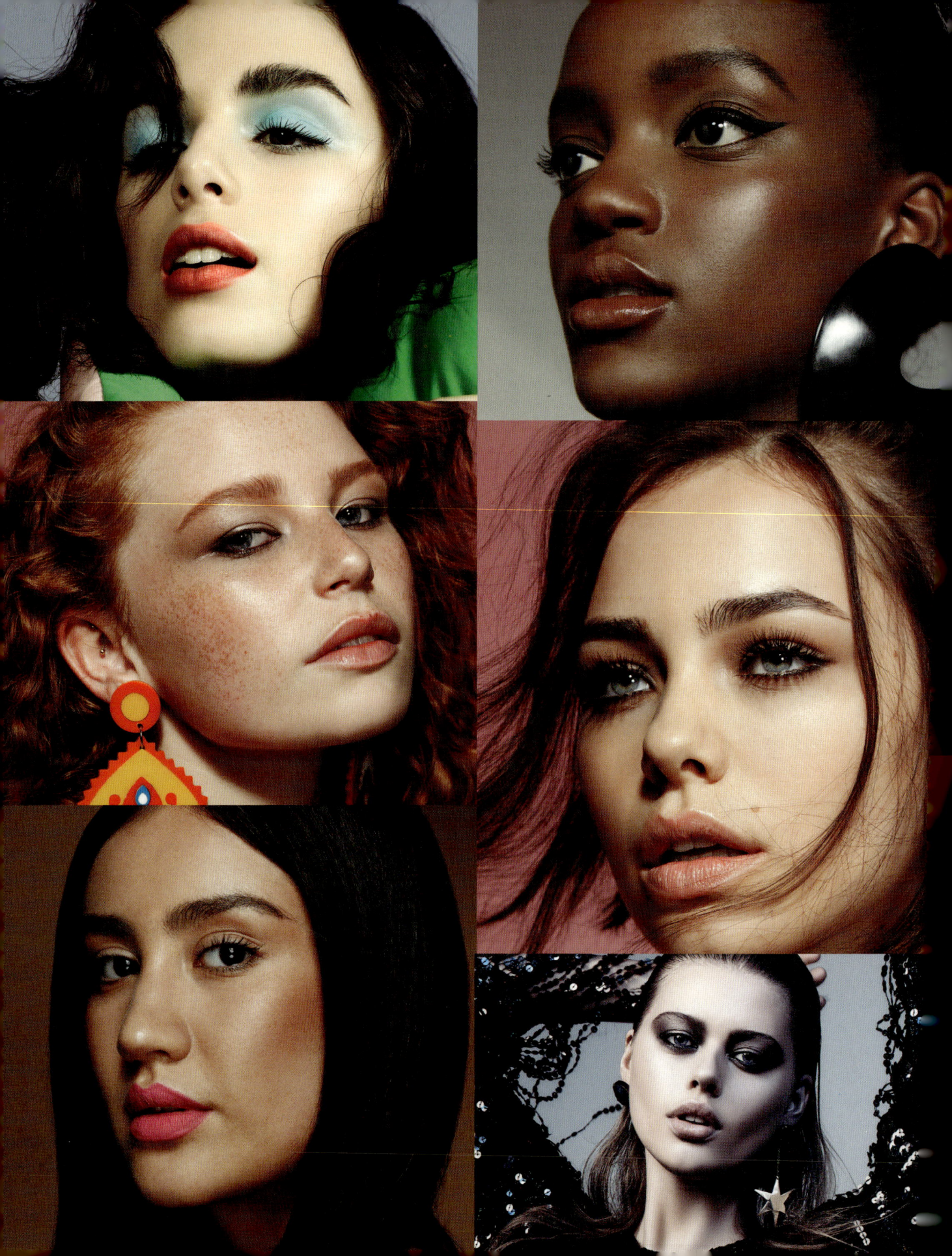

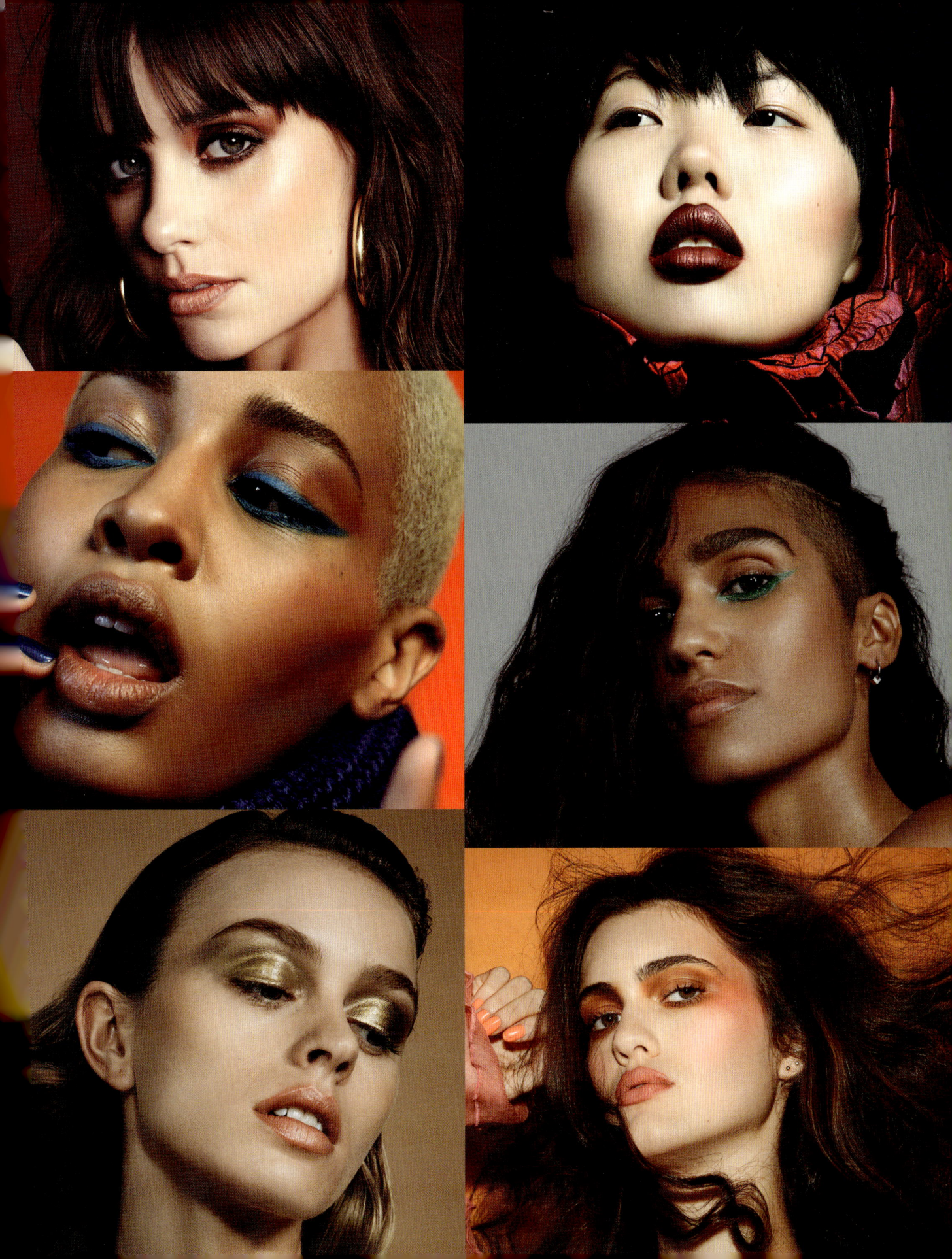

Contents

THE PATH TO PINKY — 11

SKIN IS A THING — 17
The Four Basic Skin Types — 20
Cleansing — 21
Polishing — 24
Moisturizing — 28
Primer — 39

ALL ABOUT THAT BASE — 45
Finding Your Color in the Wall — 47
Where to Contour — 48
Highlighting — 49
Sheer and glowing — 50
Creamy coverage — 58
Velvet matte with highlights — 66

A BODY OF WORK — 73
Exfoliation — 75
Moisturizing — 76
Foundation — 77
Bronzing — 78
Highlighting — 79
Keep It Consistent — 81

BROWS LIKE A BOSS — 83
Shape — 85
Color Choice — 87
My Favorite Brow Tools! — 89
Brows from Nothing — 90
Power Brow — 102

EYE SPY WITH MY SMOKY EYE — 109
Nude Contoured Eye — 112
The Not-So-Smoky Eye — 118
Metallic Eye — 124
What Are You Using as a Base to Your Metallic Eye? — 127
What Are You Mixing It With? — 128
Pastel Lavender Glossed Eyes — 132
Glitter Eyes — 136

LOOKING FINE MS EYELINE — 143
Black Flick Liner — 144
Pop Color Liner — 150
The Perfect Smudge — 154

LASHES GET PASHES — 159

Mascara Types	160
Naturally Defined (Epic) Lashes	162
Chunky Lashes	168
False Lashes	172

POWER OF THE POUT — 179

Exfoliation Is the Key	181
Nude Full Lips	182
The Art of the Stain	188
Bold Matte Lip	192
Dark Lip	196
Metallic Lips	202

CHEEKS ON FLEEK — 207

Bronzing	209
Blush	209
Bronzing	210
Placement of Color	212
Color Choice	213
Tools	213
Blend	214
Which Texture Is the One for You?	214
Cream Blush	218
Powder Blush	222

MAMA DIDN'T RAISE NO TOOL — 227

Brushes	228
Sponges and Puffs	234
Keep 'em Clean!	236

YOU COMPLETE ME — 239

A Rose Has Thorns	244
Boys Will Be Boys	246
Bronze in Bohemia	250
Cindy with the Blue Jeans	254
Color Is the Kee	257
Friday Night Lights	258
Metallic in the Moonlight	263
Pastel on Porcelain	268
Pop Sugar	271
Read My Lips	276
Shiny Disco Balls	281

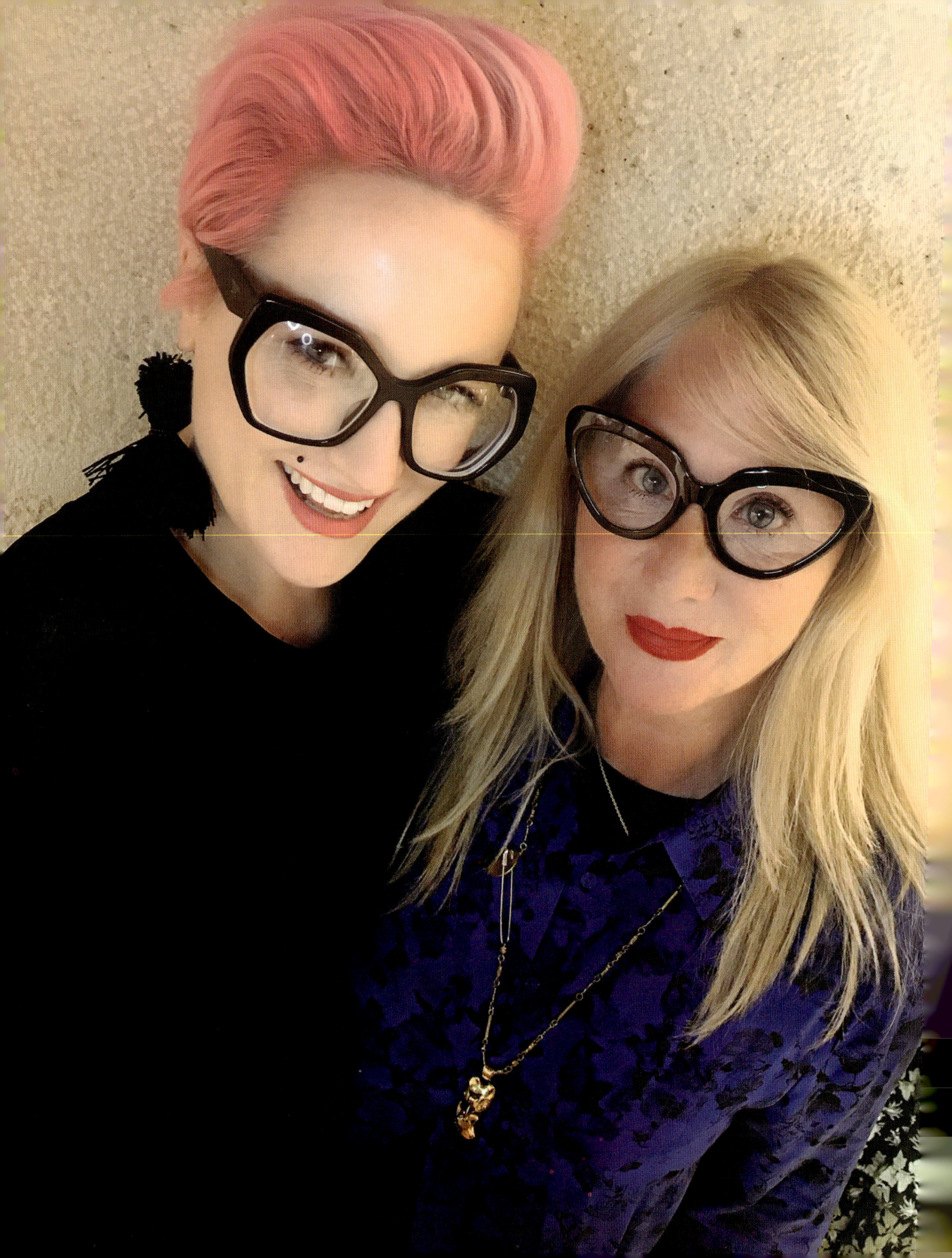

Foreword

Our diverse individuality is what sets each and every one of us apart as humans. We must embrace our own uniqueness.

The concept of beautification in the form of makeup is its power to be transformative. We are emotive beings, that's why art, music, nature and our environment are crucial to us as a community. Popping on a lippy is the first step to your own personal empowerment. Makeup is a tool to express one's individuality, whether a little or a lot. Makeup is the magic wand of confidence. Own it!

In the midst of what is real and what is virtual, the only way to sustain the human race is to keep thinking, keep creating. Never conform, never compromise, be the person you want to be.

Pinky, as I know her, has been in my life for the past ten years and from the moment we were introduced at one of the many fashion shows we have done together, I knew I was in the presence of greatness. The innate positivity that is Pinky ensures that the moment she walks into a room we are all immediately transported to a very happy place.

Oh! Did I fail to mention that when I think of Pinky, the possibility of kaleidoscopic color exciting the senses is an imminent thrill when looking at her work? Her sense of challenge and commitment to adventure has truly led us all into a wonderful pageant of beatious bliss!

VAL GARLAND

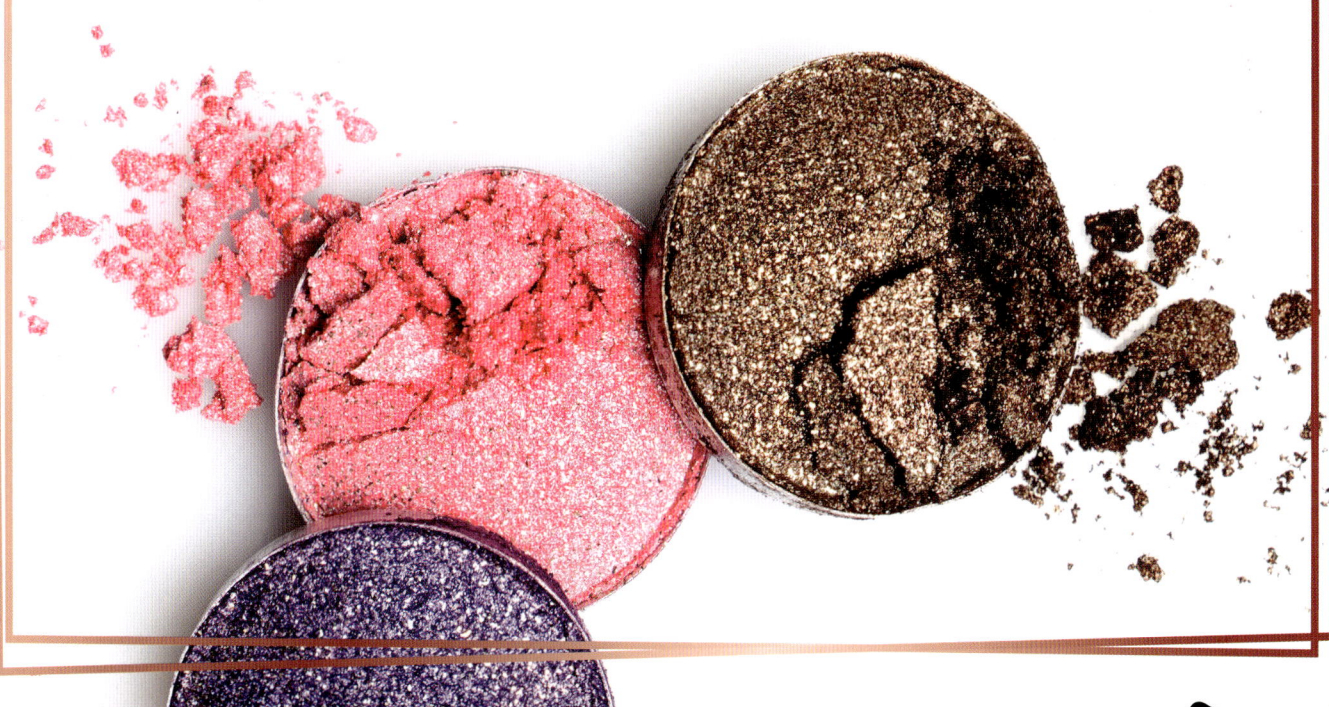

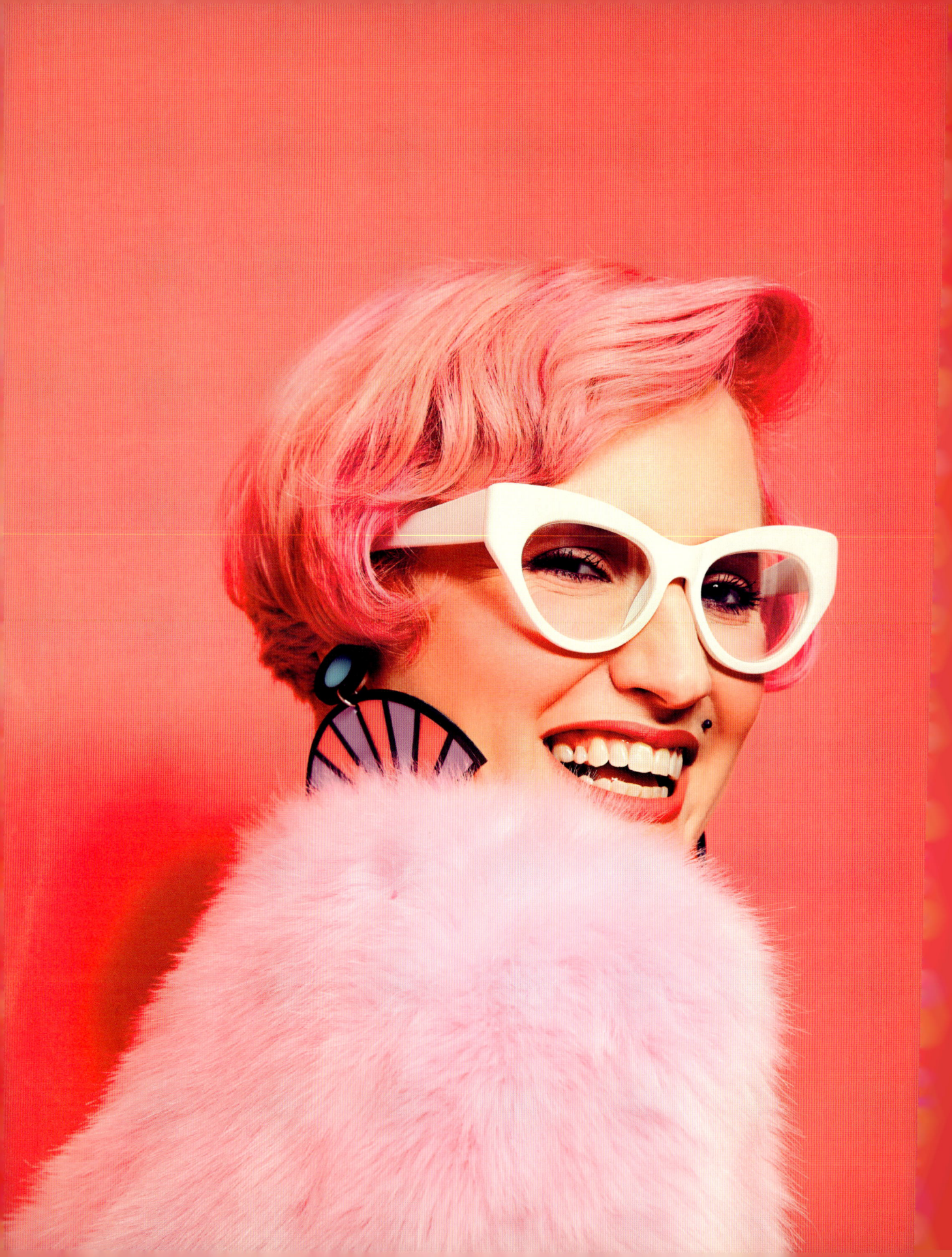

The path to Pinky

My first memory of makeup was my grandmother Ruth's collection of lipsticks. In her bathroom, she had all her Estée Lauder lipsticks (it was the only makeup brand she ever purchased) standing up like little red and pink soldiers. Whenever we would visit I would sneak in there, lock the door and try them on. I'm assuming it was a secret, but I am sure she probably knew.

Neither of my grandmas ever left the house without lipstick on, and both loved a brow. I am obsessed with the beauty trends of the forties and fifties and it started with them. Even my mum and my sister have been influenced by my grandmothers' beauty rituals, even if not to the extent that I was. Mum still doesn't leave the house without some lippy on and my sister Danielle, a successful marketing executive, will always tackle a big day in the corporate jungle with a full, fierce face of makeup.

By the time I had reached high school, the beauty bug had definitely hit. It was the nineties and I was obsessed with Poppy lipsticks, it was how I expressed myself. I was constantly getting in trouble for touching up in class, when I should have been getting reprimanded for wearing strictly matte products, all the time. My teenage years were summed up at our Year 12 review where my art teacher played the role of me in a comedy skit by school staff. She was basically in a world of her own, doing her makeup, which is essentially right on the money.

When I left school I never considered a career in cosmetics; I didn't know there was one, to be fair, and began study and work as an interior decorator and merchandiser. It is still something that I love but moving furniture around each and every day is not my idea of fun. Then there was a game changer.

In 2002, I started dating a boy named Adam. At the time, he was working as a DJ and karaoke host and actually scored his first date with me serenading me and giving me a rose at the local bar, but that's a story for another day. After a few months together, I mentioned to him that I was getting very bored and tired of the work I was doing. His response was pretty succinct.

'Why don't you do something else?'

Adam made the suggestion that since I loved art and was obsessed with makeup (both on myself and my girlfriends), why don't I study to become a makeup artist. It was the light-bulb moment I had been waiting for as I wandered aimlessly into a degree through my early twenties. I enrolled to commence my studies not long after at the Australian College of Make Up and Special Effects in Sydney, and instantly felt at home.

I studied through 2003 and then worked at a cafe in 2004 while I assisted any makeup artist who would have me. I worked on short films, TV commercials, test shoots – basically if the work was going I was taking it. I didn't always get to do makeup either, some of my early jobs I was cleaning brushes, fetching products and setting up stations. It was mostly for free but I loved it, and as they say, when you are doing something for love, you don't work a day in your life.

Watching how great makeup artists work was hugely important in my development. Assisting artists like Liz Kelsh and Linda Jefferyes taught me how to conduct myself on set, work with

stylists and photographers, when to take control and when to allow others to take the wheel. While many of my early days as an assistant were spent standing around watching someone else do makeup, I learnt as much then as I did during any part of my career.

By 2005, I was done serving cappuccinos and wanted the chance to work full-time in makeup, and beyond that, fashion. At that time, there was only one brand that provided a clear pathway to working on the big shows both in Australia and abroad and that was MAC Cosmetics.

I scored a job working part-time behind a MAC counter, continuing to balance that with my assisting work. I quickly discovered that this would be more than a security gig so that I could pay my rent. I had found a company where I could find myself. It was all about self-expression and individuality, it embraced diversity and couldn't care less about the status quo. This was me, or at least the person I aspired to be, and now I was with a group of awesome people who wanted the same thing.

Within a year I had worked at Australian Fashion Week and within three I had traveled to New Zealand, China and Japan doing a job that I loved. By 2009, I was elevated to the Global Senior Artist team, becoming the Brand Ambassador for MAC Cosmetics here in Australia. Life was everything I had dreamed it could be at this point, but my journey of self-discovery as a makeup artist was far from complete.

My next seminal moment came at my first international fashion week in Milan. On the advice of Oprah (because, obviously) I had a scrapbook with all my dreams and goals, and featuring heavily was the opportunity to work at the big shows in Europe and New York. I was beyond excited but the reality of some corners of our industry whacked me in the face like a truck.

I felt so judged by some of the older makeup artists back stage for being excited and expressing myself through my look. I returned home in tears, consoled by my now husband Adam, feeling like I was Lindsay Lohan in *Mean Girls,* before she joined the bullies. Six months later I returned to Milan, I had dyed my hair brown and turned the dial right down on my makeup. I was determined to do anything I could to blend into the background; it would be safe there.

> **"MY AIM IS TO BE A PERSON WHO IS HAPPY...CREATIVE...EXCITED AND TO MAKE MY MARK ON THE WORLD.
> I WANT TO MAKE PEOPLE FEEL SPECIAL, HAPPY, BEAUTIFUL AND INSPIRED TO BE DIFFERENT.**

That same season, I worked in Paris for the first time. This was surreal as more than anything else working here was my mecca. I remember calling Adam in tears again (yes, I cry a lot), this time swept up in complete happiness that I was finally living my dream of working on Paris Fashion Week and was about to work on one of the most iconic shows in all of fashion – Vivienne Westwood, with my makeup idol Val Garland.

Watching Val wielding her mighty makeup brush was something of pure beauty.

As I snapped myself out of being in awe, Val gave us her instructions.

'That's the feeling of the look now go away and do your own version.'

Put simply, I shat myself. I was tense and clammy and more concerned about getting it wrong than I was about getting it right. I was trying too hard and I knew it and when Val came by to check on how I was progressing she asked how I thought I was going. My trepidation was enough for her to encourage me to do whatever I thought I should to make it look good to me. She was telling me to express myself, something I had been avoiding for the previous few weeks whilst working backstage. That show I found myself again and it finished with a high five from my hero, Val Garland. I always loved Val's makeup but I loved the way she inspired me to embrace my artistry even more.

Returning from Europe, I was determined to not only express my true self through my artistry but also help others do the same. Today I proudly embody my nickname Pinky, but it wasn't always that way. The reality was it took some time for people in the industry, even in Australia, to see past my look and simply judge me for my work. The difference was that I was determined to not get caught in the trap of blending in, because that wasn't me. Not everyone is going to like me and that's okay, their judgment doesn't matter because I can only control what I can control. I decided to be myself because everyone else was taken.

I was now in a position where young artists were assisting me, which outside of having energetic and passionate people around me, was giving me a passion for teaching and passing on knowledge. I was presented an opportunity to embrace this newfound passion, at the most extreme level, traveling to Japan to spend five weeks teaching the cast of Cirque du Soleil how to do their own makeup. I would do group lessons that would span about five hours before doing one-on-one sessions. The best part was the majority of the people I was working with did not understand a word of English. I was teaching makeup through feelings not instructions. It reminded me that beauty is not about how you look, it is actually about how you feel.

On the last page of my before mentioned Oprah-inspired scrap book I wrote a mission statement.

There have been times during my career, where I have forgotten this statement, but it absolutely still rings true. It is why I have written this book.

In the age of social media where every expression has become an opportunity for judgment and bullying, I'm going to choose to look through a different lens. Since having my daughter Frenchie, she has taught me to see the wonder and beauty in everything. Watching her sense of discovery and exploration looking at some of the simplest things has rekindled that light in me. I want to have new experiences, I want to learn and I want to challenge myself to look outside the square.

It is said that there is no such thing as a bad idea, and while I will stop short of saying there is no such thing as bad makeup, you should feel empowered to experiment with different looks, colors and techniques. When I say there are no rules, I mean it. Trust your instincts, because more often than not they are right.

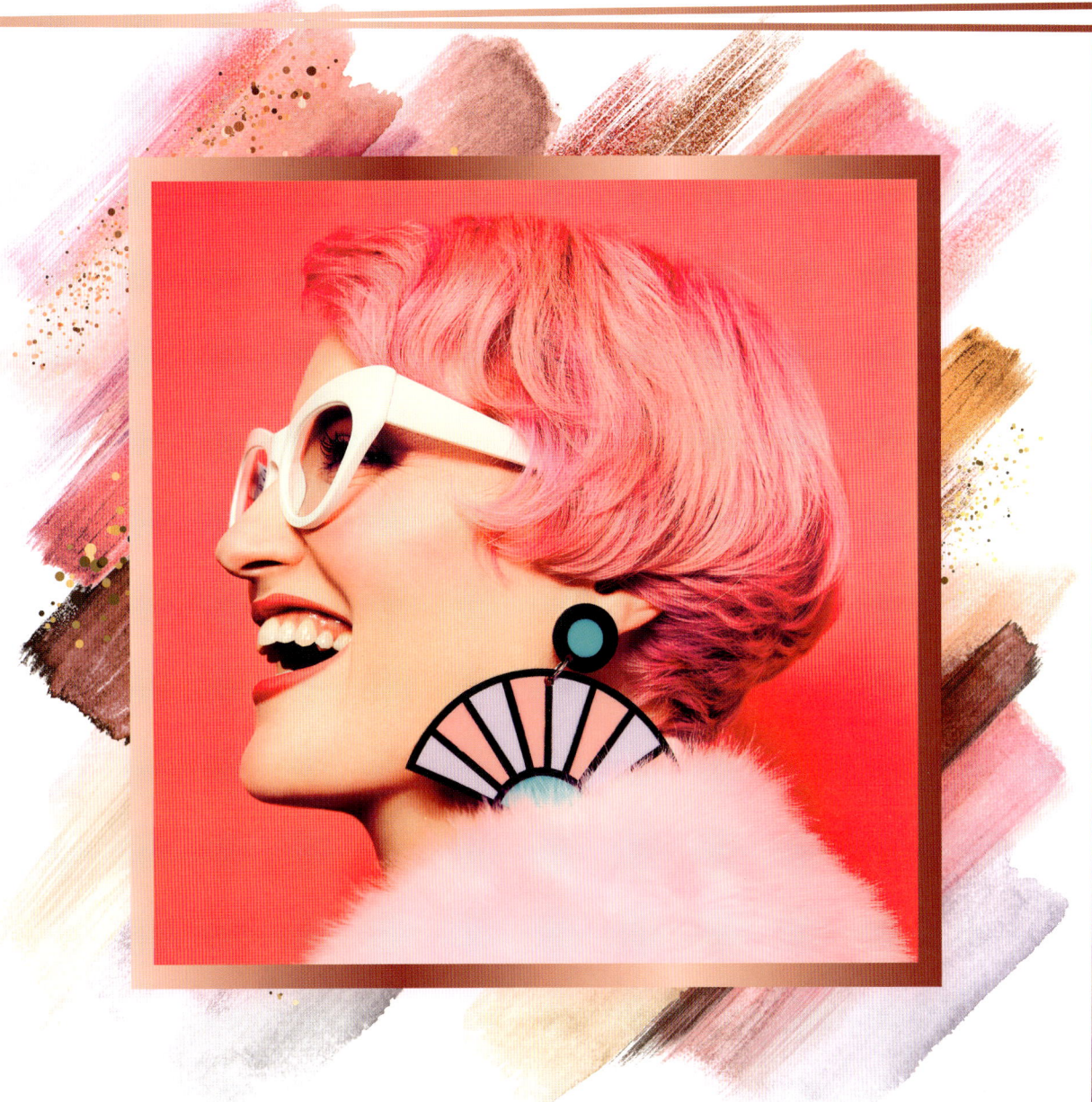

PINK JACKET TRELISE COOPER, EARRING DOODAD AND FANDANGO, POLKA DOT BLOUSE ROMANCE WAS BORN

Makeup is and should always be an accessible form of expression, regardless of your budget, gender, age or race. Like all makeup artists, I have my favorite products, but products don't make the look, you do. Be led by how it makes you feel. Putting on powder should rarely be about covering up and more about sharing with the world how you are feeling on the inside.

This is not some kind of makeup bible or rules book – I hate rules and when it comes to makeup you should to! The purpose of this book is to provide you with a makeup wardrobe, where you can whip out different techniques and tips on any given day. What I hope you do next is tweak, twist and put your own individual spin on everything in here.

'Learn the rules like a pro, so you can break them like an artist.' — Pablo Picasso

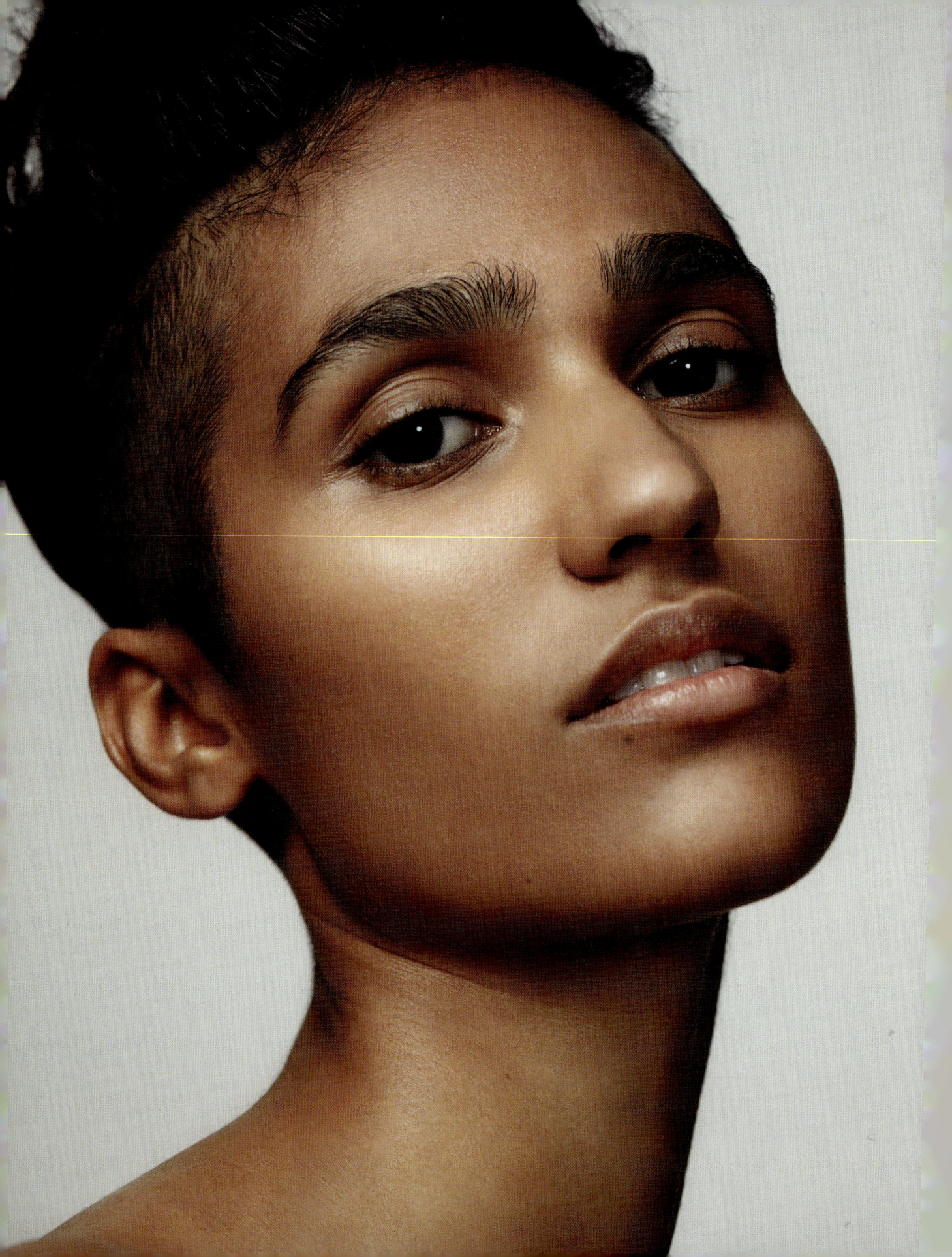

Skin is a thing

TIARE FROM BELLA MODEL MANAGEMENT

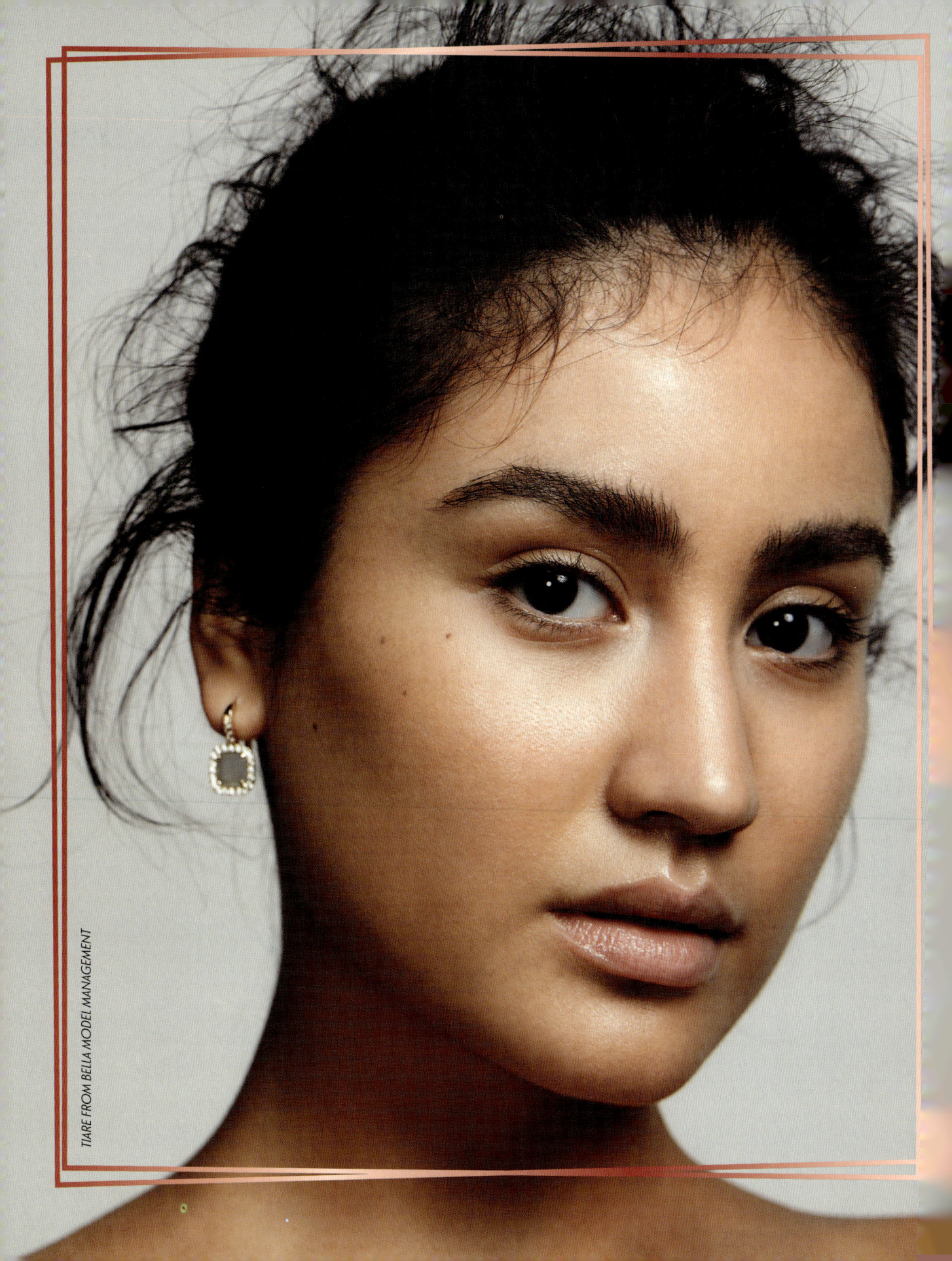

'Oh you work on models, it must be so much easier doing makeup on perfect skin.'

Sure, I do work on models, but what you see in the pages of the magazines is more often than not a far cry from the person who sits down in my makeup chair. They are very much normal, and like us are not immune to blemishes, dryness or oiliness. What models do have is people like me to polish their look. I have seen with my own eyes a once sculpted, plumped, naturally luminous *angel* return to my chair, weeks since leaving a lasting impression, only to see her immaculate skin be ruined by bad skincare and makeup!

We are all different and there is certainly something beautiful and special about that. But it can be a total bitch when it comes to beauty routines, and in particular skincare. You can't just do the same thing you saw someone else do and expect the same results. You need to have your own unique skincare technique that works for you.

The moral of the story here is listen to your skin. So many factors can affect your complexion, some you can control and some you cannot. For instance, your skin loves the sun about as much as my husband likes watching *Sex and the City* re-runs, which for the record is not very much at all. Hormones, which I wish as a woman we had a little more influence over, can impact our skin through acne and breakouts, and while there isn't a cream on the supermarket shelf that can get them (completely) under control, medical intervention early may save you a bunch of money later on trying to fix that permanent skin discoloration.

I learned quickly as a makeup artist that if I can transform my clients' skin in my chair, I have made a friend for life. Two key lessons I learned early in my career have got me a long way to achieving this almost all the time. Firstly, foundation alone cannot correct bad skin and secondly, customizing the skincare and prep work to the skin type and the final look I want, rather than just throwing the same tube of god knows what on everyone in my chair will get me a long way towards skin that delivers a win!

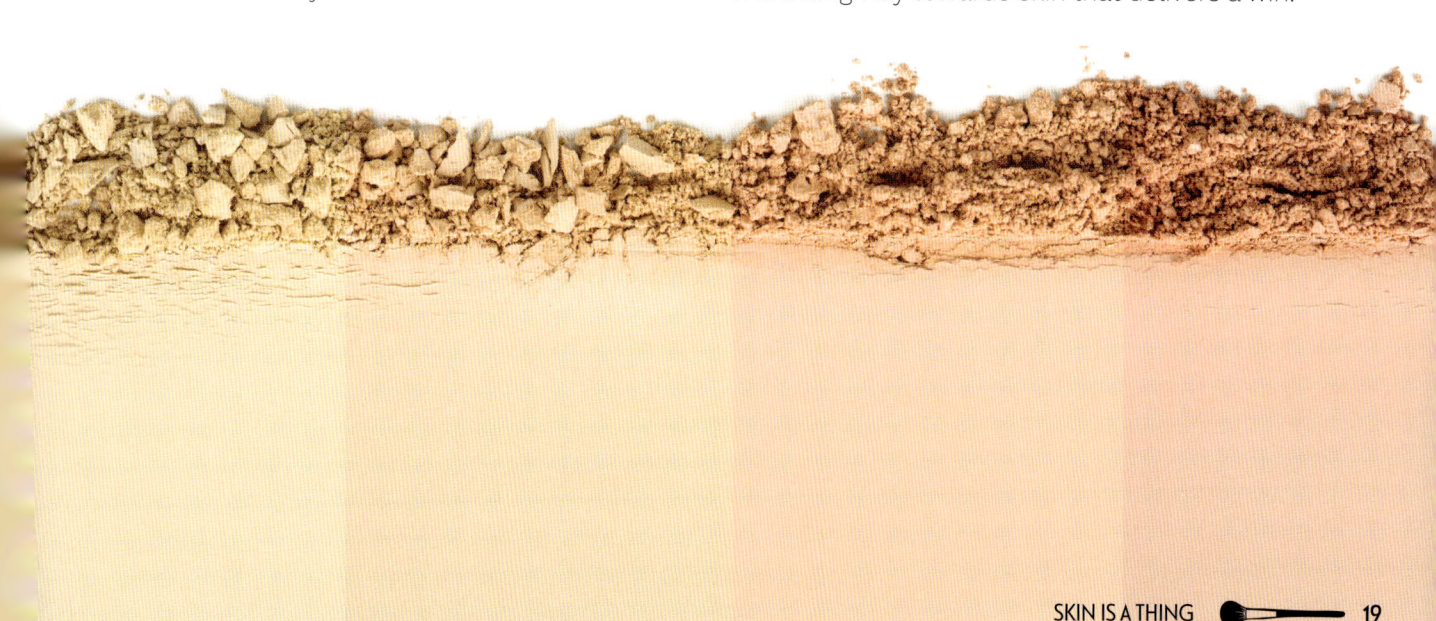

The Four Basic Skin Types

There are four basic skin-type categories. A bit like my personality your skin can change from time to time so it is good to be across all of them.

Normal skin
You are pretty balanced, you don't find that your skin gets either too oily or too dry, your pores don't tend to bother you too much and you get occasional blemishes. You are lucky. All other skin types hate you.

Oily skin
Your skin is producing sebum (an oily substance created by the body to lubricate the skin) like there is no tomorrow! Most of the time your pores will be showing, your skin will constantly be shiny and your makeup slides around. You probably suffer from mild to more extreme acne. There is a cherry on this cupcake though, many people believe that oily skin stays looking younger for longer! Glass half full, right?

Dry/dehydrated skin
Your skin hates producing sebum, doesn't want any part of it. So that means that your skin doesn't have the lipids (your skin's natural fats) it needs to hold that moisture in. Your skin can build a cloak of armor for all the pesky outside elements, which will often lead to dry and sensitive skin. There are very different levels of dry skin, from patchy surface dryness to your skin feeling quite tight, which may cause your wrinkles to be more pronounced. Isn't this fun?

Combination skin (oily T-zone)
The name says it all! You got some mixed up skin! Generally you will have an oily T-zone (nose, chin and forehead) while your cheeks will be normal to dry.

If you have *zero* idea which group you fall into, or perhaps it's changed over time, I would suggest heading straight to a dermatologist or skin specialist so they can poke, prod and figure you out!

Cleansing

Righto, I even need to make note of this myself as I am guilty of sleeping in my makeup if I am super tired. Gasp! I know! I'm normal! But you (and I) must cleanse, twice a day! In the morning to get rid of that excess oil and get the best possible start to your makeup routine and then at night to wash that makeup mask off. Cleansing is super-important to keep those open pores at bay; you can cover them all you want with layers on top, but cleansing them is the magic trick here.

Micellar water

AKA Magic Water. This original French cleansing water started its own trend – now every brand out there has one! I trust a French woman when she says she won't use anything else – I mean have you *seen* how beautiful French women are?? Backstage at fashion week this is a model favorite, which speaks volumes, as they have to remove their makeup up to five times daily during fashion week.

Micellar water looks just like plain old water but is far from it! Put simply, it has teeny tiny oil molecules called micelles floating in softened water that stick to all the gunk on your face and dissolve it. The magic part is, it removes the bad stuff without stripping away the natural oils on your complexion! People have found that this cleanser actually improves the skins texture. It will remove *almost* all makeup – you will need something a little more hard core for waterproof makeup.

Bioderma Micellar Water, La Mer Cleansing Micellar Water

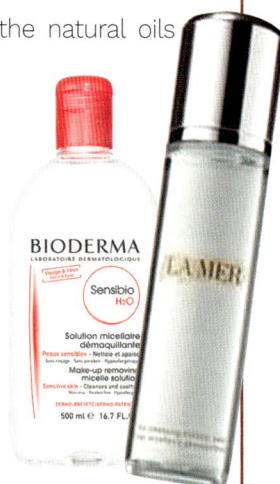

Oil cleansers

Hello hero! Don't let the name fool you, whether you are normal, dry or have oily skin, this remover will work for you to completely dissolve any ingredient on the skin, even heavy-duty waterproof makeup and lashes, in half the time!

I do like to give a quick rinse afterwards so there is no residue on the skin before I go in with any other skin care.

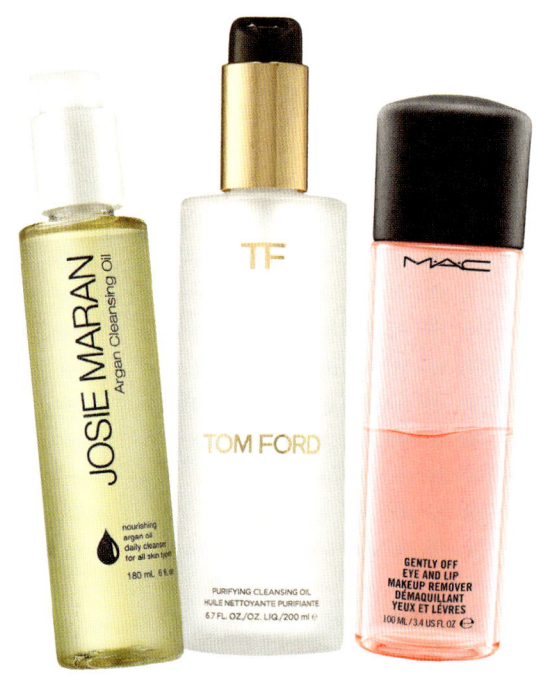

Josie Maran Cosmetics Argan Cleansing Oil, Tom Ford Purifying Cleansing Oil, MAC Gently Off Eye And Lip Makeup Remover

SKIN IS A THING

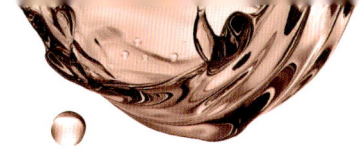

Silicone-based removers

A dual-phase remover, and as the name suggests, it replaces the oil components of other cleansers with silicone. Shake the bottle and use on eyes and lips. This powerful one-swipe remover is for those people who want it all gone but prefer not to use oil on their skin.

Clinique Take The Day Off Makeup Remover For Lids, Lashes & Lips

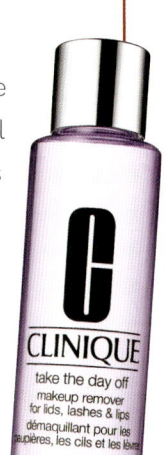

Double the cleanse

I believe in this! Tried, tested and approved. Now it doesn't have to mean twice the product! 'OMG, how annoying, I don't have time,' but cleansing takes about 30 seconds so doubling it would mean…well you can do the maths. I reckon you could spare a whole minute each night so you get the entire day off you. Think about how many layers are often in people's makeup application these days; do you really think one cleanse will get it *all* off? Me thinks not. Go, forth and cleanse.

Cleansing balms

I love these as a gentle option to use in the shower. A balm is just that, a salve for the skin – it's perfect for those who suffer from dryness and sensitivity, yet also want to remove *everything* from their skin. Scoop onto a cotton pad or onto your finger, rub together to activate it into a silky sheer cleanser and take all over the face. Leaves you feeling clean and moisturized in one!

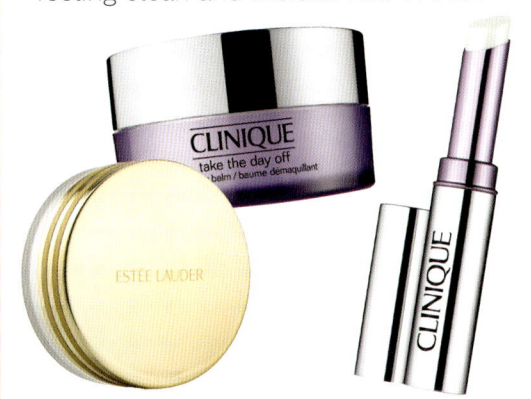

Estée Lauder Advanced Night Micro Cleansing Balm, Clinique Take The Day Off Makeup Remover For Lids, Lashes & Lips, Clinique Take The Day Off Remover Stick

Cleansing wipes

A lazy person's best friend (my hand is up!). We are spoiled for choice out there with removing wipes, yay! Fast, effective, easy. If you have sensitive, dry skin go for non-fragranced wipes so you don't regret it later – leave the other wipes to the chicks with the normal to oily skin and a hectic schedule. These aren't an everyday affair though. Even the 'sensitive' ones can be a little rough on the skin and they will not give you that good deep clean you need on a day-to-day basis.

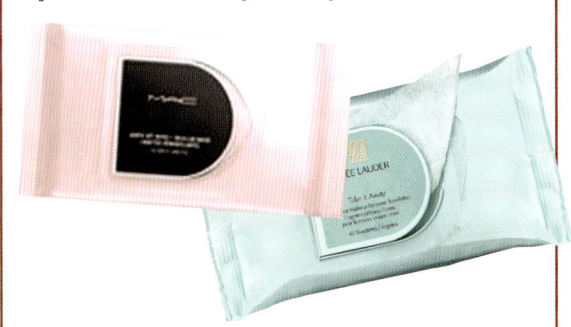

MAC Gently Off Wipes + Micellar Water, Estée Lauder Double Wear Long-Wear Makeup Remover Wipes

SKIN IS A THING

Color removes color

If you are trying to remove stubborn colors from near your eye or lip area (I'm talking to you red eye shadow wearers!) don't underestimate the power of massage when it comes to getting rid of the product. Rather than just vigorously wiping, take your time to massage a well-lubricated cotton pad over the area. Then keep massaging. Even if the cotton pad is covered in the product, keep massaging the cleanser in to really melt the color away. Finish with a fresh soaked cotton pad to smooth away the residue.

Be gentle!

I have seen people rub their eyes with their cotton pads of remover so hard I was surprised they still had eyeballs! Woah, slow down. I know we are all in a hurry but speed doesn't mean efficiency when it comes to makeup removal. Drench your cotton pad in remover and SLOWLY move it across the area. When you move slower you are allowing the remover to do its job and melt away the product, and you keep your skin intact at the same time.

Try some mechanics

There is simply not one solution for every face, so let's get technical. Just like some people like the feeling of an electric toothbrush and believe it gives that extra deep clean, the same can be said for face cleansing brushes. Some come with both cleansing brush heads and massage heads to use for a more thorough treatment application. Many makeup artists carry a version in their kits and start their beauty application by really polishing the skin with one of these – the results are incredible. I tell you, when I have given my face a car wash with one of these my skin feels cleaner than ever and is visibly more supple!

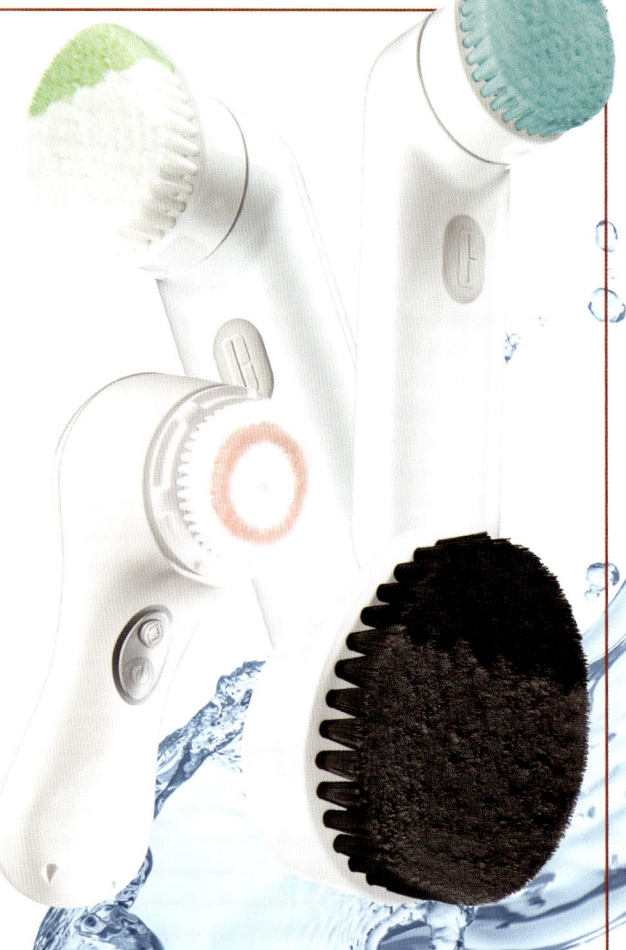

Clarisonic Cleansing Brush, Clinique Sonic System Brush, Clinique Sonic System Charcoal Cleansing Brush, Clinique Anti-Blemish Solutions Deep Cleansing Brush

Polishing

Polishing is really about preparing a surface that is devoid of any superficial imperfections and is in the best possible condition to absorb moisture. We achieve this by toning and exfoliating, which will restore the skin after cleansing and smooth the skin to give you an even canvas to work with for the remainder of your beauty routine.

TONING

Ah toning, so eighties. And just like the music and fashion from the decade of my birth, toning has made a comeback.

Using a toner is the step a lot of people drop off the routine, but this step restores your PH balance that was lost during cleansing. It will tighten pores and brighten and refresh the skin in preparation for treatment products or moisturizing! Even when I feel squeaky clean, when I do this step I'm surprised by the makeup that is still being removed by the toner that the cleanser missed! I mean, WHERE DOES IT ALL COME FROM?!

Seal It with a cold water fresh shock!

Cold water stimulates fresh blood flow and circulation, which can boost tired skin. Cold water will tighten pores. Cold water will shock you awake so it's also a brilliant boost for a hangover!

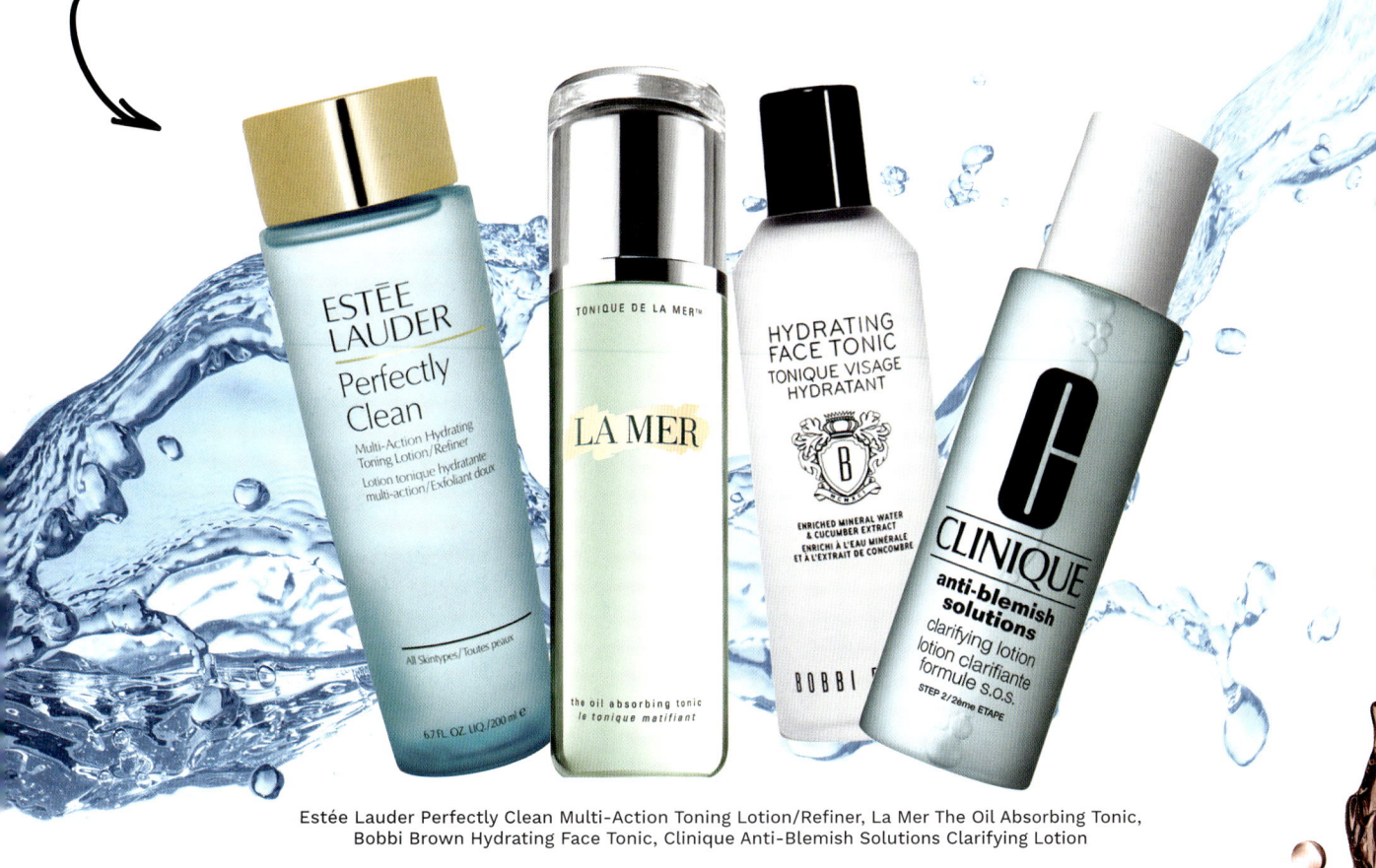

Estée Lauder Perfectly Clean Multi-Action Toning Lotion/Refiner, La Mer The Oil Absorbing Tonic, Bobbi Brown Hydrating Face Tonic, Clinique Anti-Blemish Solutions Clarifying Lotion

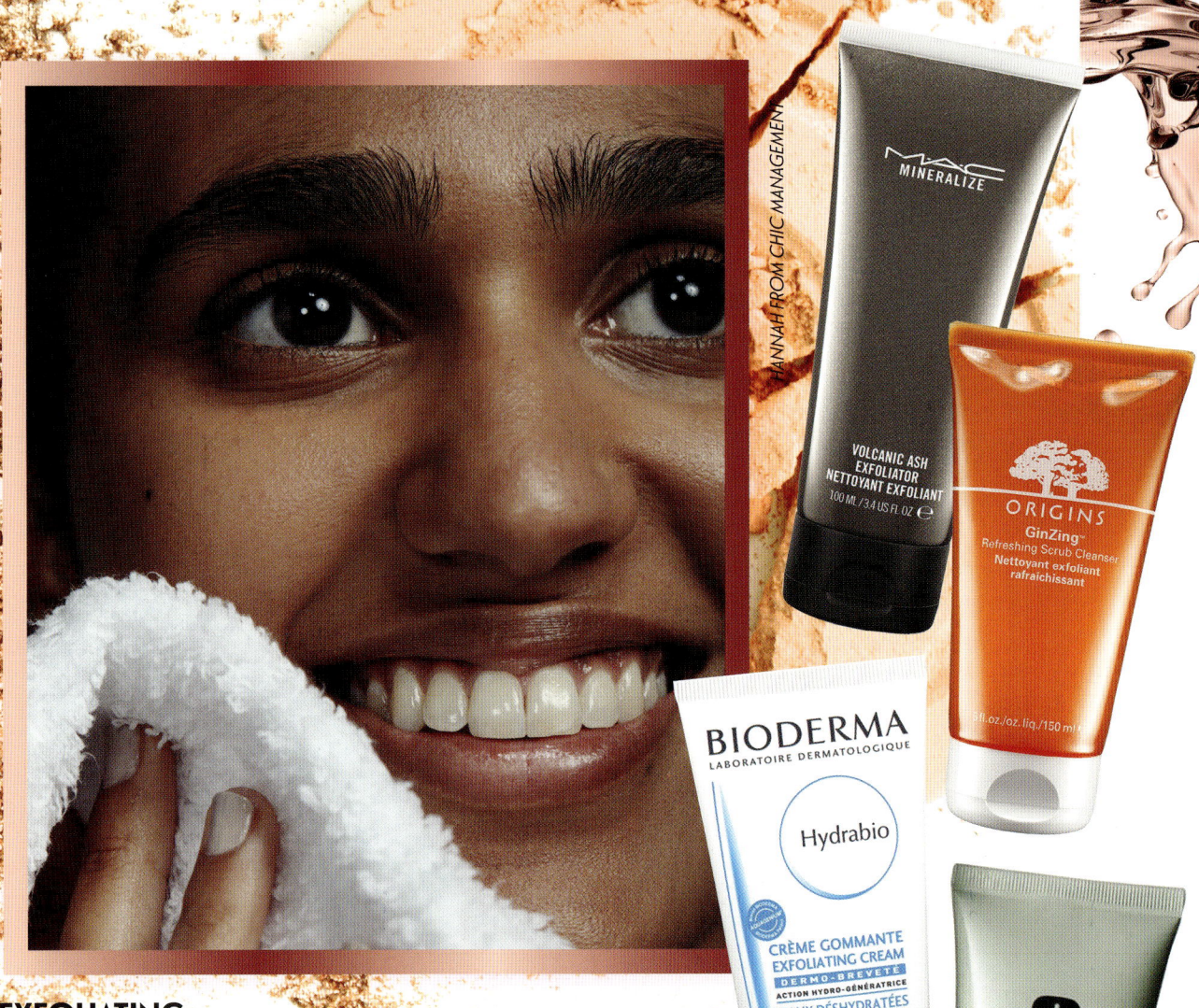

EXFOLIATING

The ultimate skin polisher, this bad boy should come out a couple of times a week to shed the old layers of skin that are dulling us down, holding us back and making us look older. Without exfoliating your skin it will not absorb the moisturizer as well as it could, and your makeup will not apply evenly. Exfoliate to polish your complexion which will let serums and moisturizers *really* soak into the skin and do their job!

If you have sensitive skin, you may want to exfoliate a little less, perhaps once a week, as your skin may get irritated. If you get oily, or live somewhere humid, you increase to once every two days to refresh.

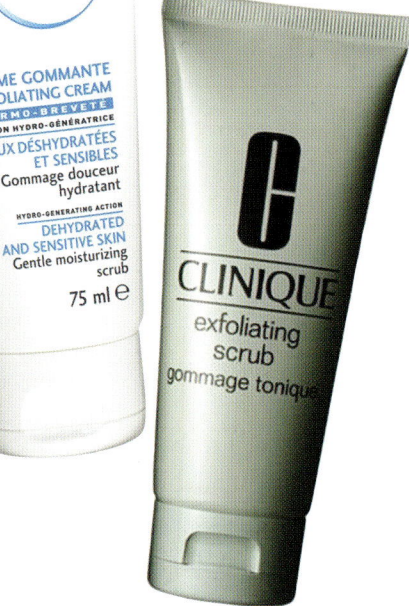

MAC Mineralize Volcanic Ash Exfoliator, Origins GinZing Refreshing Scrub Cleanser, Bioderma Exfoliating Cream, Clinique Exfoliating Scrub

HANNAH FROM CHIC MANAGEMENT

SKIN IS A THING

Exfoliating wipes

I love an exfoliating wipes\ for flaky noses and dry lips in particular. They are fast and user friendly, perfect for scrubbing away the rough skin before you pucker up!

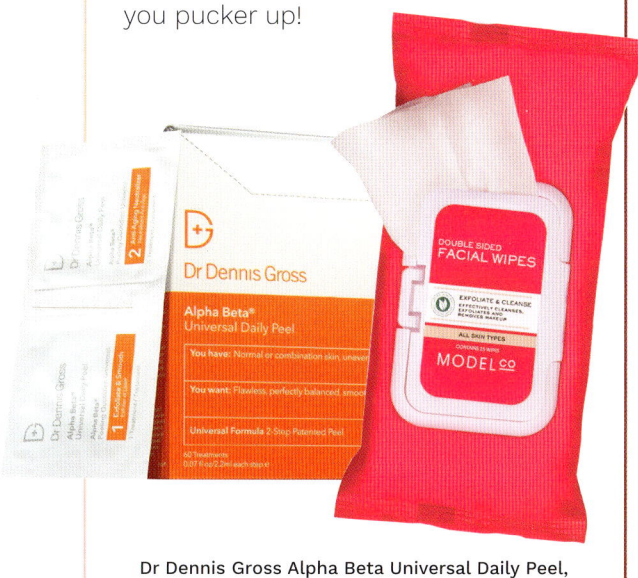

Dr Dennis Gross Alpha Beta Universal Daily Peel, ModelCo Double Sided Cleansing & Exfoliating Face Wipes

Not too wet!

Give your face a light splash prior to using an exfoliating cream to assist in its movement over your skin. You do not want to water it down too much as it needs to be thick and grainy to do its job. Start on the forehead, work in a circular motion down over the nose and chin before finishing on the cheeks.

Go natural

If you don't have an exfoliating cream handy, mix some brown sugar into coconut or olive oil, or even your facial cleanser, and use that over your skin to smooth it out.

Don't forget your neck, shoulders & hands

These areas are the telltale signs of aging and we never pay them enough attention! If you want to keep getting asked for ID, don't forget them. When was the last time you exfoliated your hands? That's right, never. Man it feels and looks good. And the same applies for cleansing, exfoliating and moisturizing! If that skin is showing you should polish it.

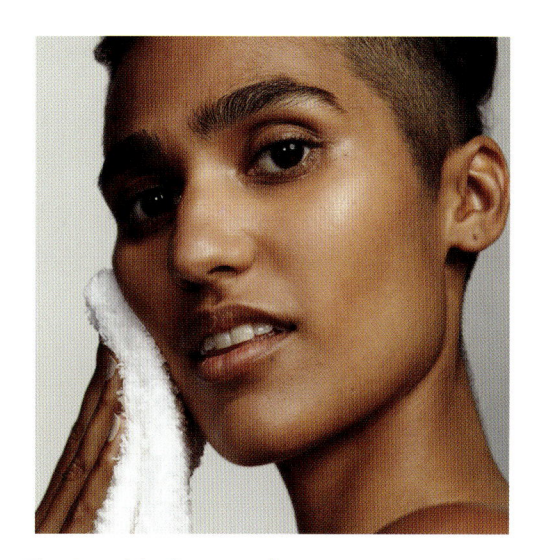

The humble face washer

This guy gets the gold medal in my book of cleansing and exfoliating. Do you use one? You MUST! Nothing will make your skin feel cleaner than a steaming hot face washer gliding over your skin. I have found that even on my toughest makeup applications, the winner has been the simple combination of heat and texture of the cloth to get right into every crevice and pore and give a mild exfoliation as well. Sometimes I start a makeup application with it on my client. What a perfect, refreshing start to makeup!

TIARE FROM BELLA MODEL MANAGEMENT

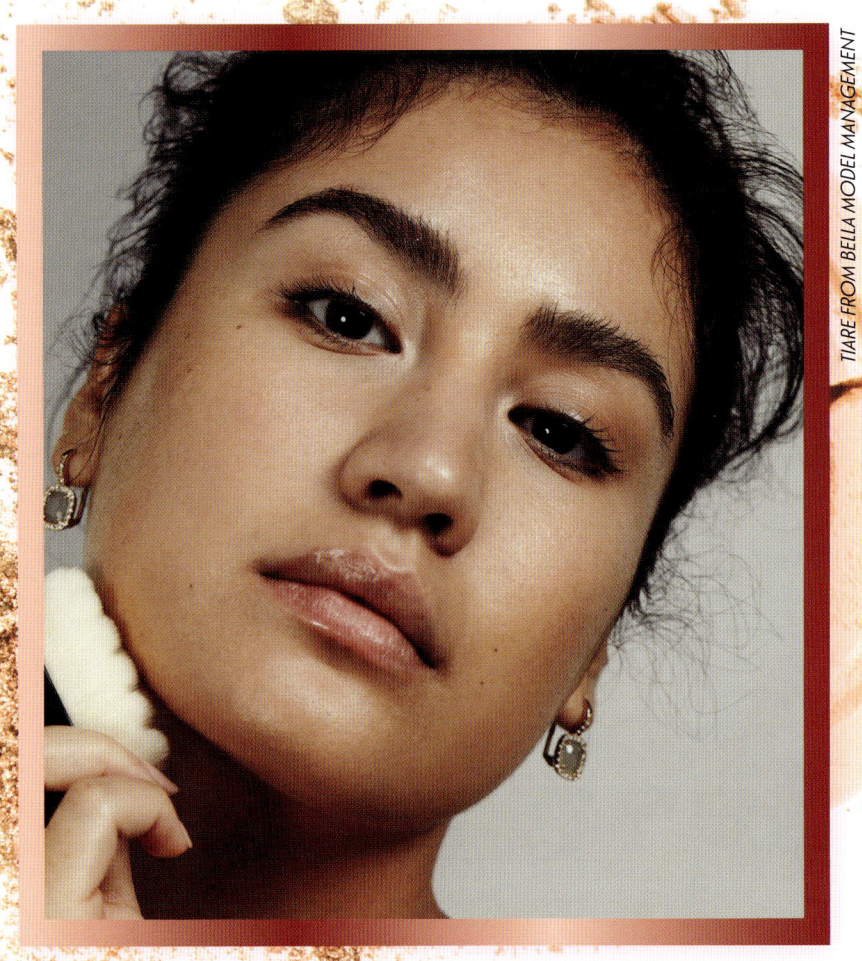

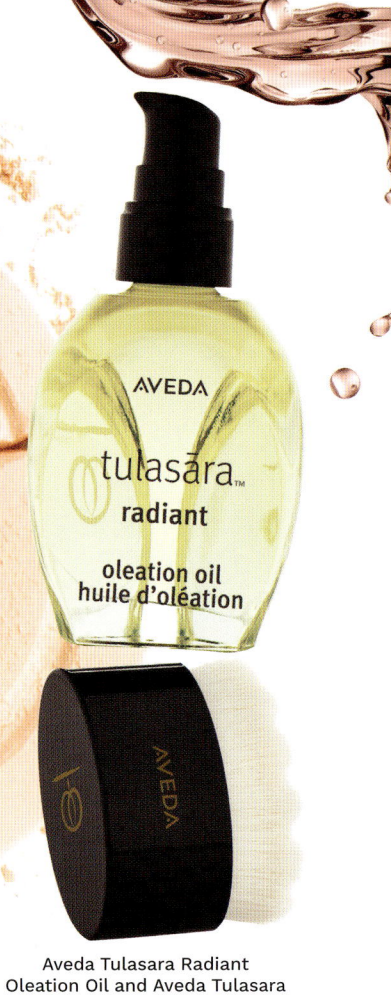

Aveda Tulasara Radiant Oleation Oil and Aveda Tulasara Radiant Facial Dry Brush

DRY BRUSHING

I am such a fan of body and face dry brushing – these brushes are great tools to do what a topical product cannot. Dry brushing is a fast track to seriously luminous skin. Use a dry brush on cleansed skin all over the face and neck to speed up the rejuvenation process, supporting skin cell turn over. Brush in circular motions over dry skin, then apply an oil to the skin and repeat. Radiance ahoy.

Don't overdo it on oily areas

Beware of over exfoliating acne-prone skin or specific oily areas on the skin. Scrubbing does not make spots and oiliness go away; in fact, it does the opposite! Exfoliating too hard will strip the skin of its natural oils and encourage your body to produce more oil where you may not have had a problem! A more fierce scrubbing action does not mean a better exfoliation. You don't get any more skin given to you so be kind to it! YOLO!

Good morning exfoliation

Your skin tends to repair itself overnight, so do your exfoliating in the morning and you will feel beyond fresh.

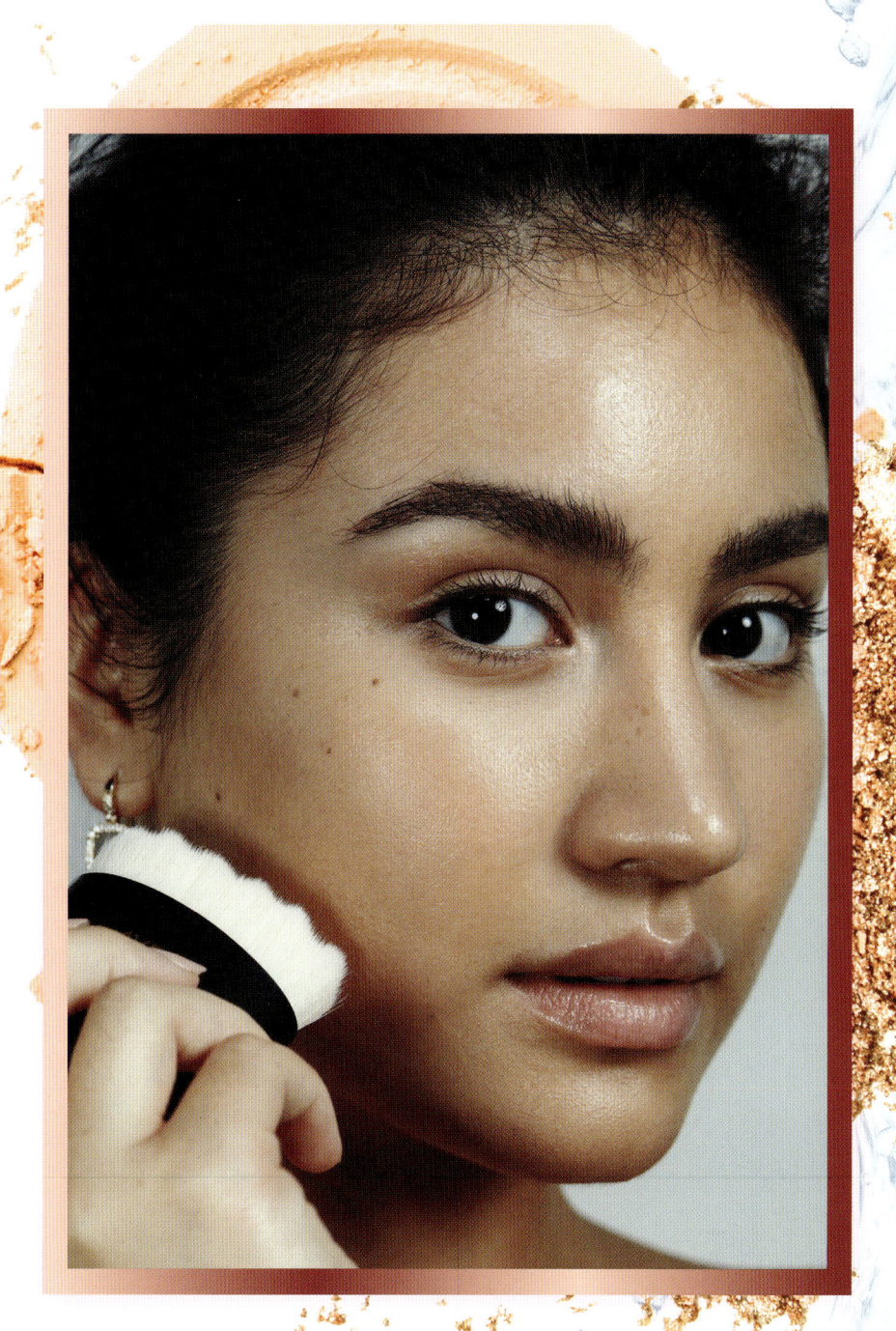

Moisturizing

Anyone else confused about the order in which your moisturizers should go on? Let me break down my order for you.

1. Facial mist
2. Serum
3. Moisturizer
4. Oils

BAM. You can of course add/subtract/substitute but that is a general guide.

Get mist-ical

Enter one of the most-used products in my makeup kit, both personally and professionally – the hydrating facial mist. If you have heard of a facial mist, yet you do not own one, stop. Put the book down, go and purchase. I'll be here when you get back. Why am I, and others, so obsessed with drowning the skin before every makeup? The results are *instant*. You know you have a goodie when the skin feels supple, bouncy and soft to the touch.

My all-time favorite mist is MAC Fix+, with over 15 years of experience with it on all different skin types. I first fell in love with it during fashion week. With models needing to remove makeup looks multiple times a day, it is my job as a makeup artist to not only give the skin a service, I need to make it *glow*.

One spray is simply not enough. Put your snorkel on and soak your skin. Then massage it into the skin with your hands or with a brush to soothe. Work specifically on dry areas on the skin, working the spray in with your fingertips. It has 101 uses, which you will see throughout the book. Best thing about it? All skin types can use a hydrating mist! It will only do good things.

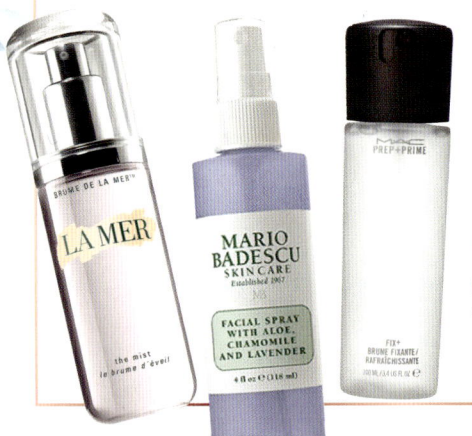

La Mer The Mist, Mario Badescu Facial Spray with Aloe, Chamomile and Lavender, MAC Prep + Prime Fix+

Serums

Don't worry, you aren't alone if you are completely confused as to what a serum is. Let's simplify it. Serums are thin and quickly absorbed into the skin, penetrating deeply with ease. The active ingredients in serums are super helpful in targeting specific skin concerns. Serums which include retinol (a form of vitamin A) are great to increase radiance by removing dead skin cells and minimizing pores. This, along with aloe vera, will calm redness in the skin, and peptides, as well as Vitamin C, help to reduce wrinkles and boost collagen. Vitamin E, glycolic and hyaluronic acid are also ingredients you want to see for *major* plumping and hydration action.

Beware of the power! Because the ingredients are so potent in serums don't overload it on the skin. Sensitive skin can react to robust ingredients, so make sure you test a little out first.

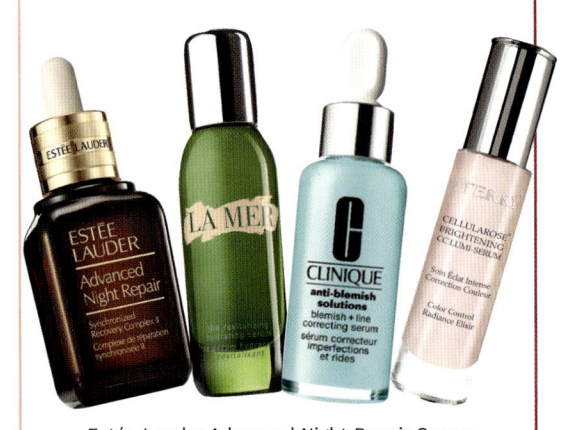

Estée Lauder Advanced Night Repair Serum, La Mer The Revitalizing Hydrating Serum, Clinique Anti-Blemish Solutions Blemish + Line Correcting Serum, By Terry umi Serum

SKIN IS A THING

MARLO FROM CHADWICK MODELS

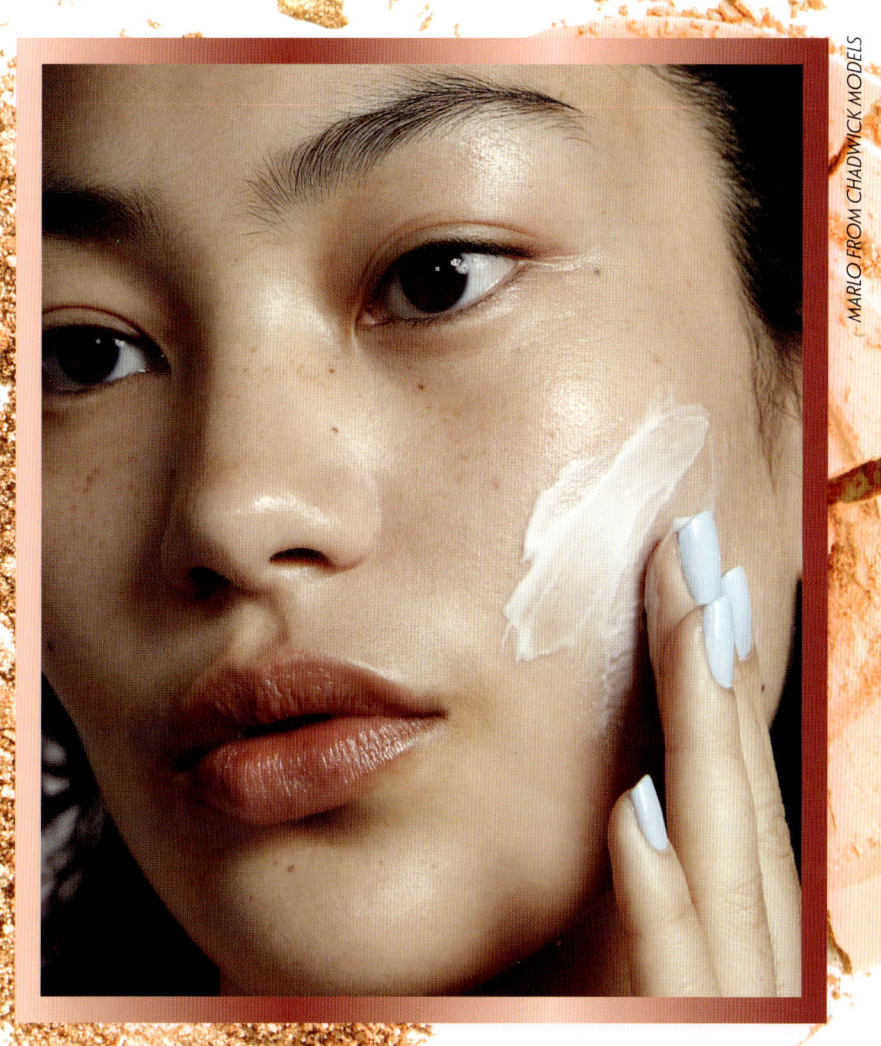

MOISTURE CREAMS

These guys seal the serum into the skin by creating a protective barrier to hold all that good moisture in. This is the one step you should never miss. Moisture is the key to fighting the aging process and also assists in the day to day battle against blemishes. Plus the added bonus that well moisturized skin needs less makeup!

Normal skin

Yummy ingredients like green tea, chamomile, pomegranate, or licorice root extract and that old favorite humectant hyaluronic acid are faves to keep normal skin radiant and youthful.

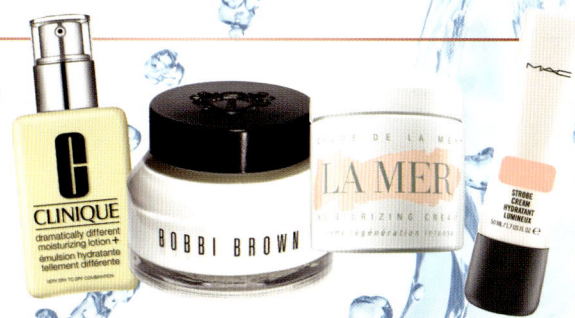

Clinique Dramatically Different Moisturizing Lotion, Bobbi Brown Hydrating Face Cream, La Mer Crème De La Mer, MAC Strobe Cream

SKIN IS A THING

Dry skin

Your thirsty skin is looking for rich creams that include ingredients like shea butter hyaluronic acid, glycerin and lanolin. Go for a day and night cream for the ultimate hydration! If you fall into the sensitive category, you want to stick with calming creams that are fragrance free – and testing it out is a must!

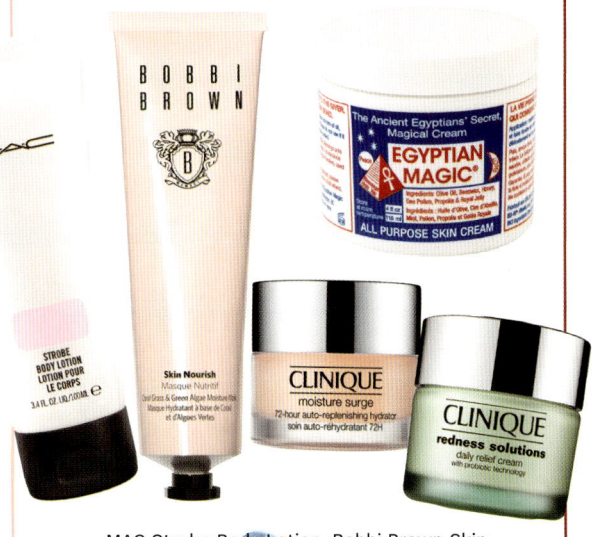

MAC Strobe Body Lotion, Bobbi Brown Skin Nourish Mask, Bobbi Brown Egyptian Magic All Purpose Skin Cream, Clinique Moisture Surge 72-hour Auto-Replenishing Hydrator, Clinique Redness Solutions Daily Relief Cream

Oily skin

People with oily skin are often scared of using moisturizer as they think it will worsen the situation, but fear not, this is just a myth. Avoiding moisturizing will leave your skin dehydrated resulting in the production of extra oil, which is far from what you want! Control the oil in your skin by using oil-free lotions and lightweight creams that contain hyaluronic acid. Lotions and gel formulas help you hold your moisture while stamping out the grease factor.

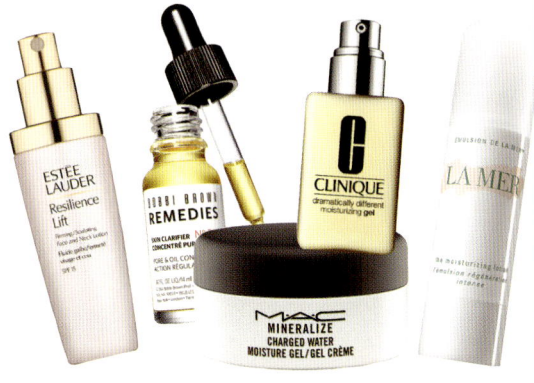

Estée Lauder Resilience Lift Firming/Sculpting Face and Neck Lotion, Bobbi Brown Remedies Skin Clarifier Pore & Oil Control, MAC Mineralize Charged Water Moisture Gel, Clinique Dramatically Different Moisturizing Gel, La Mer The Moisturizing Soft Lotion

Combination

Target your different areas with special treatment. Keep the moisturizer to the dryer areas of the face, traditionally around the outside of the face, and either apply with a lighter touch through the oily T-zone or just rely on an extra hydrating facial mist, like a softening lotion, through that area so the shine does not take over.

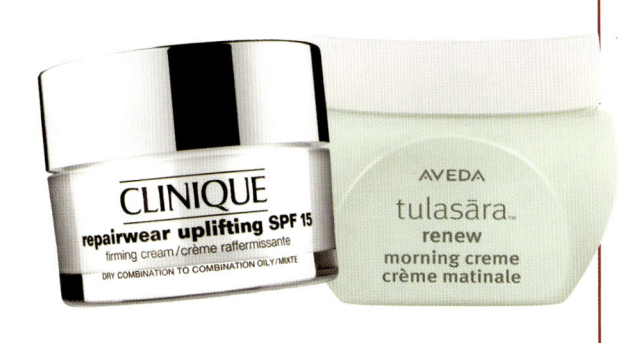

Clinique Repairwear Uplifting Firming Cream, Aveda Tulasara Renew Morning Creme

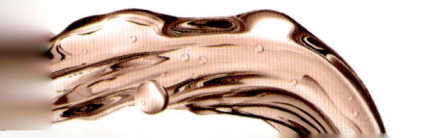

SKIN IS A THING

FACIAL OILS

YouTube is inundated with videos of people dripping oils down their cheeks before buffing a full coverage foundation over the top. Whether you are tapping it, dripping it or even pouring it, this is more than just a trend. The feeling of a beautiful face oil on your skin is becoming an addiction, but what exactly do they do?

Oils provide superficial hydration just below the surface of the skin, providing an instant soft and lush texture which provides smooth and silky makeup application. Your moisturizing creams go deeper into the skin with long-lasting hydration. Face oils look and feel silky on the surface which is why people love to mix them into their moisturizers for an extra boost, or mix with their foundations for extra luminosity.

For people with dry skin, using oils on the skin provides a seal to keep that moisturized feeling throughout the day. When you have dry skin you can keep pressing oils or crème oils onto the skin to refresh it and the skin will happily drink it up without your makeup slipping out of place. Using oils is not limited to people with dry skin but if your skin is naturally well hydrated don't be too heavy-handed during your application process.

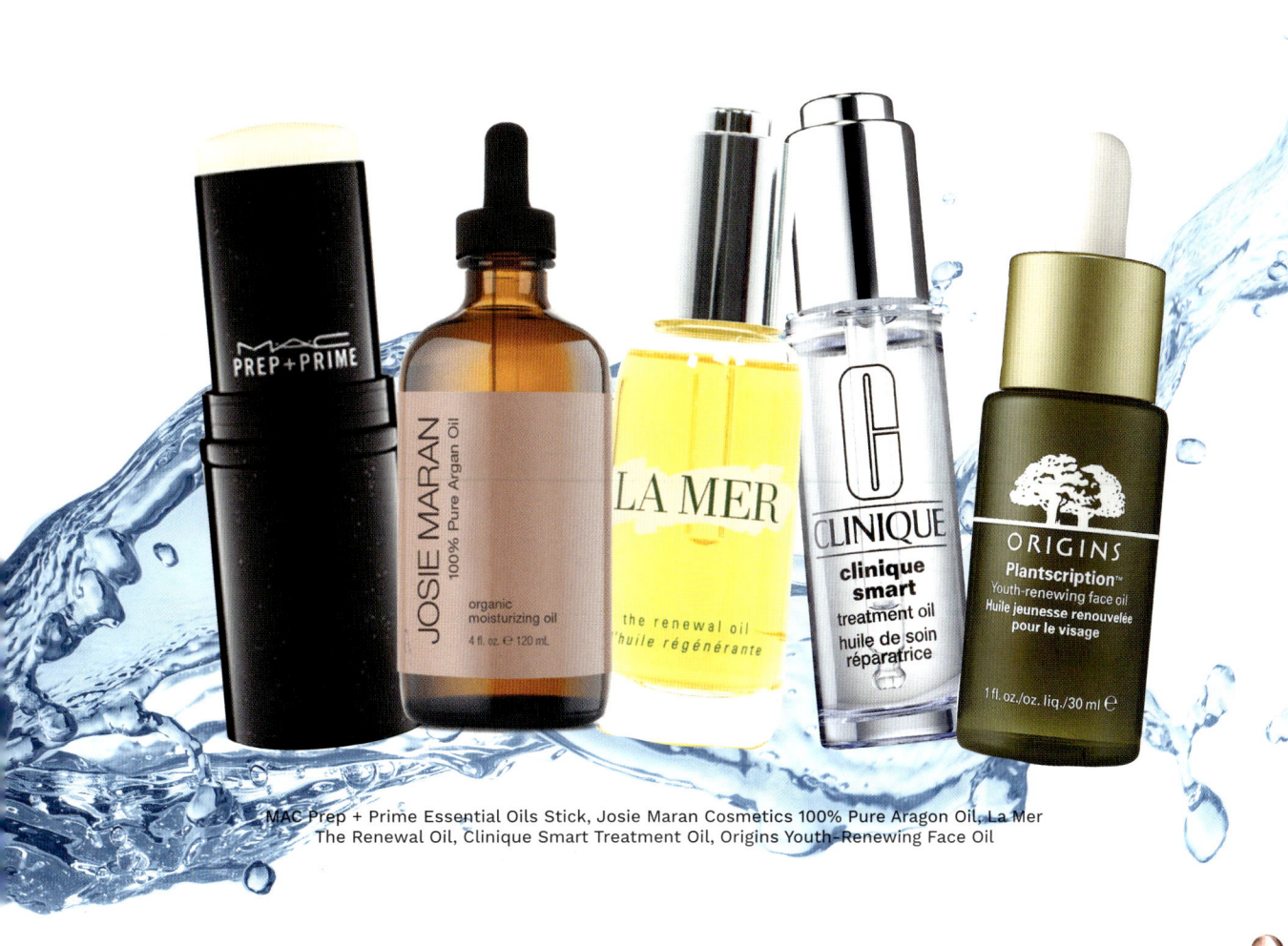

MAC Prep + Prime Essential Oils Stick, Josie Maran Cosmetics 100% Pure Aragon Oil, La Mer The Renewal Oil, Clinique Smart Treatment Oil, Origins Youth-Renewing Face Oil

SKIN IS A THING

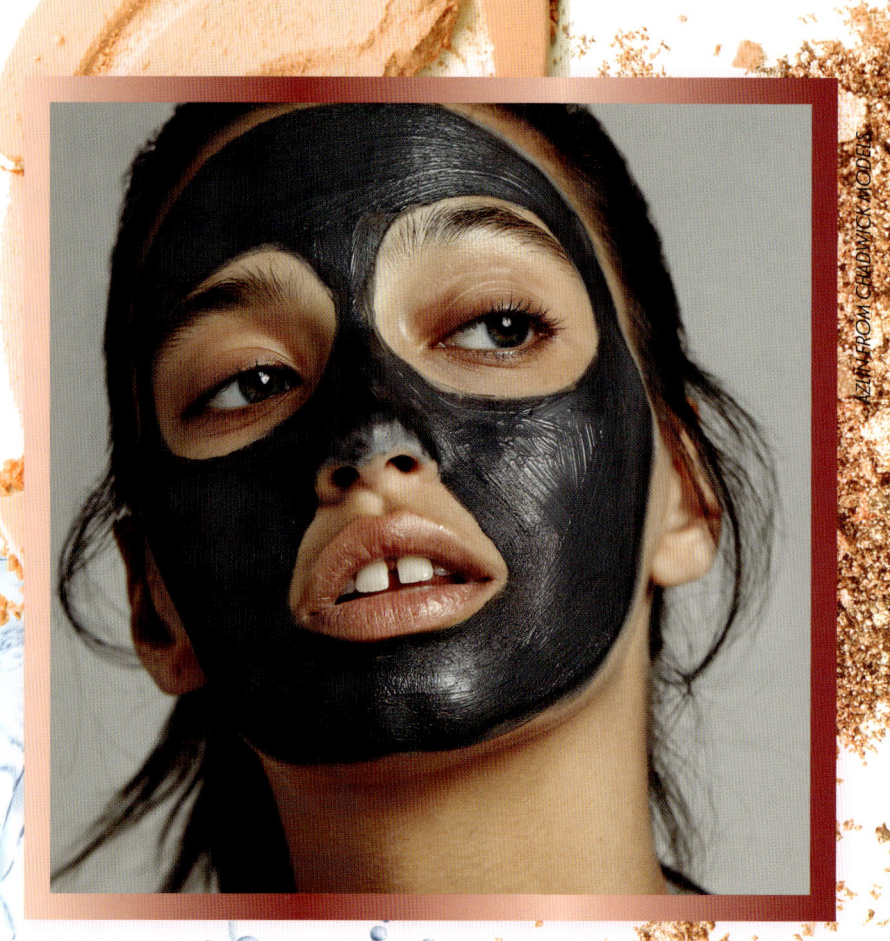

FACE MASKS

A few girlfriends, wine, cheese and a rom-com is my idea of a Friday night, but it wouldn't be complete without a face mask. We all find so much satisfaction after wearing one, so why don't we do it more often than once in a blue moon.

From $2 to $200 the choice is yours

Face masks used to be reserved for rare occasions, as an indulgence, but these days the products are as readily available as the results are instantly addictive. Women and men in equal measure are injecting them into their weekly and even daily routines, and feeling much better for it.

Who has gone to pick up a few eye masks and been confronted with a *wall* of masks staring back at you? You then picked up a few, reading the back like you would a packet of gluten-free chips at the supermarket, all the while pretending to know what you are looking for. After much contemplation, you end up walking out with the ones with the prettiest packets. Well if you are like me and your eyes have been crossed trying to figure it out, the ingredients are the things to understand.

Tighten it up

Vitamin C can replenish collagen and beat fatigue and stressed out skin. You could even go gold! Some great masks out there contain gold which can increase luster and luminosity while softening age spots, wrinkles and fine lines!

SKIN IS A THING

SAMEERAH FROM CHIC

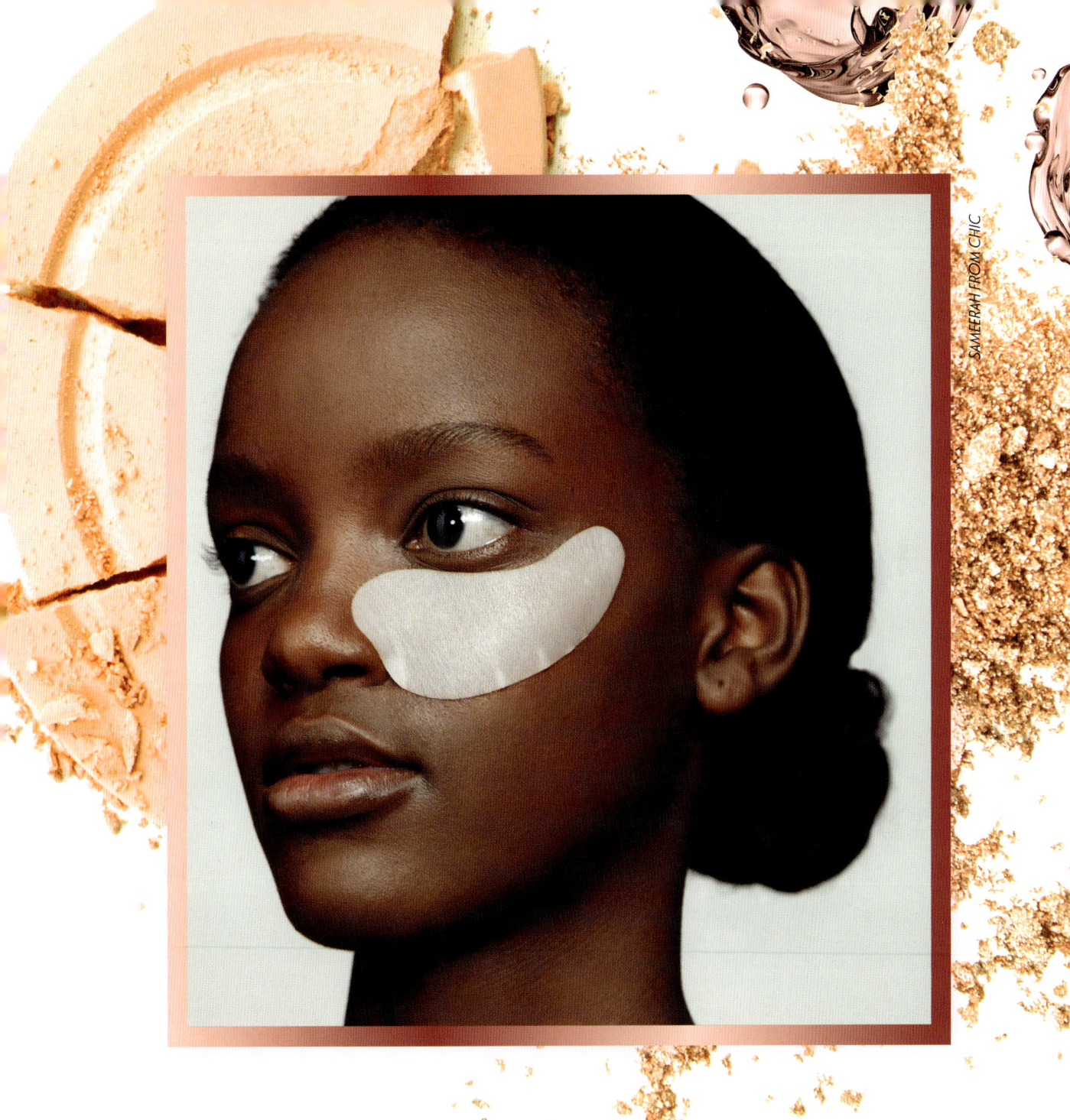

Unclog pores and detox

Green tea is amazing for detoxing and purifying – so sip a tea and look for it in your mask. This is also where our old mates charcoal and clay come in – a savior for oily skin, and an enemy to toxins and redness. These masks will purify and brighten skin while absorbing excess oil. Don't let it completely dry though! If you do, by this stage in the mask process it will be drawing ALL the moisture from your skin and you will end up feeling dry. Wash it off before it cracks.

SKIN IS A THING

See ya blemishes
Keep an eye out for masks with salicylic acid, which is oil-soluble and well suited to treat acne in oily skin. It does this by getting rid of excess oils as well as exfoliating dead skin cells and shrinking your pore size. If your skin is quite sensitive try alpha hydroxy acids like glycolic and lactic acid for less irritation on the surface of the skin.

Light and bright
Look for masks that have exfoliating qualities to give you a brighter complexion. Go for lactic acid, glycolic acid to brighten things up, as will retinols and vitamin A and C while also assisting in the reduction of fine lines. Masks that include edible ingredients like extracts from papaya, orange, lemon and ginseng will take the fight to dull skin and generally smell good too!

Drench your desert face
Hydration is immediate with a mask. Look for hyaluronic acid, aloe vera, glycerin, avocado oils and honey for a much needed moisture boost

Sheets masks and rubber masks are great when you are focused on giving your skin a good drink. You may look like an ax murderer for 3–20 minutes, but for those minutes that sheet is delivering intensive ingredients and hydration deep into your skin. Peel it off and rub the excess product into your skin for super luminosity.

You need to calm the farm
Ingredients such as oatmeal, aloe vera, vitamin E and chamomile are the warm cuddle that our skin needs from time to time. This type of mask is just the tonic to calm your irritated skin, oatmeal especially will work to protect and soothe. Vitamin B3 is a bonus for its anti-aging capabilities, and who doesn't want that.

Eye masks
The poor sensitive, thin skin under our eyes needs love too. Whether you are puffy or dry throw on an eye mask while you are doing your brows and eyes. By the time you have finished those you will really see what moisture and a little bit of attention to this area can do to lift your entire look.

SPF SHOULD ALWAYS BE THERE
Whether it be in your skincare, primer, foundation, or you might like to include an actual sunscreen into your routine – there are *no* excuses for not having sunscreen on your skin in this day and age. A must do.

THE IMPORTANCE OF MASSAGE IN APPLICATION
There is a reason why when you get a facial, so much of the time is spent massaging the product into the skin. Massage improves blood circulation, helps the skin breath, retains elasticity and creates firmness! You can spend all your hard-earned money on incredible skincare, but massage is going to amplify the moisturizing qualities of what you have applied way beyond the price point.

Massage in upward motion. Period. The only way is up when it comes to your facial features! Every cream, liquid or oil should be pressed and worked in – upwards.

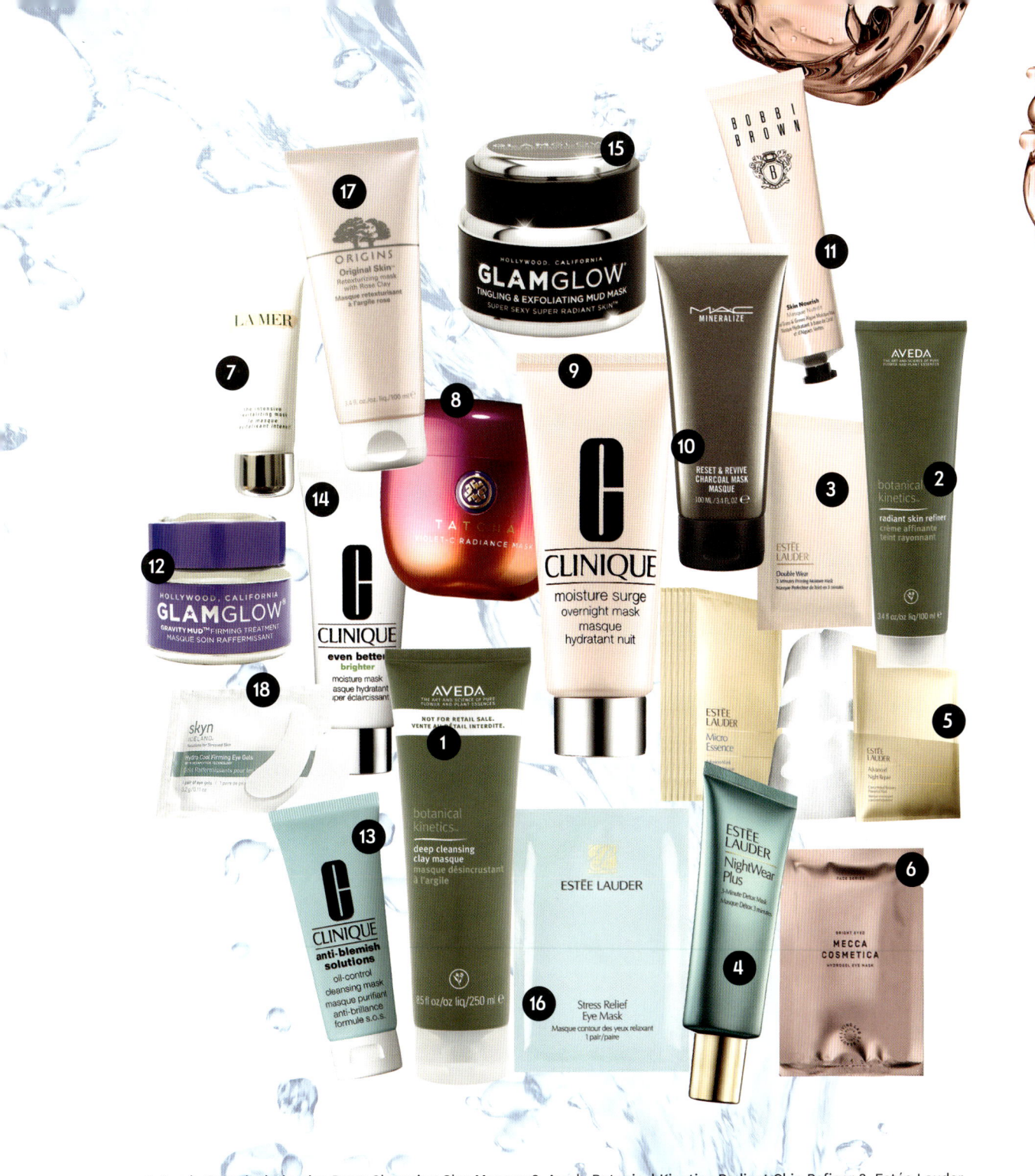

1. Aveda Botanical Kinetics Deep Cleansing Clay Masque 2. Aveda Botanical Kinetics Radiant Skin Refiner 3. Estée Lauder Double Wear 3 Minute Moisture Priming Mask 4. Estée Lauder NightWear Plus 3 Minute Detox Mask, 5. Estée Lauder Advanced Night Repair Concentrated Recovery Powerful Mask 6. MECCA Cosmetica Bright Eyed Eye Mask 7. La Mer The Intensive Hydrating Mask 8. Tatcha Violet-C Radiance Mask 9. Clinique Moisture Surge Overnight Mask 10. MAC Mineralize Reset & Revive Charcoal Mask 11. Bobbi Brown Skin Nourish Mask 12. GlamGlow Gravity Mud Firming Treatment 13. Clinique Anti-Blemish Solutions Oil-Control Cleansing Mask 14. Clinique Even Better Brightening Moisture Mask 15. GlamGlow TingleExfoliate Treatment 16. Estée Lauder Stress Relief Eye Mask 17. Origins Drink Up Intensive Overnight Mask 18. Origins Original Skin Retexturizing Mask with RoseClay 19. Skyn Iceland Hydro Cool Firming Eye Gels

SKIN IS A THING

AZLIN FROM CHADWICK MODELS

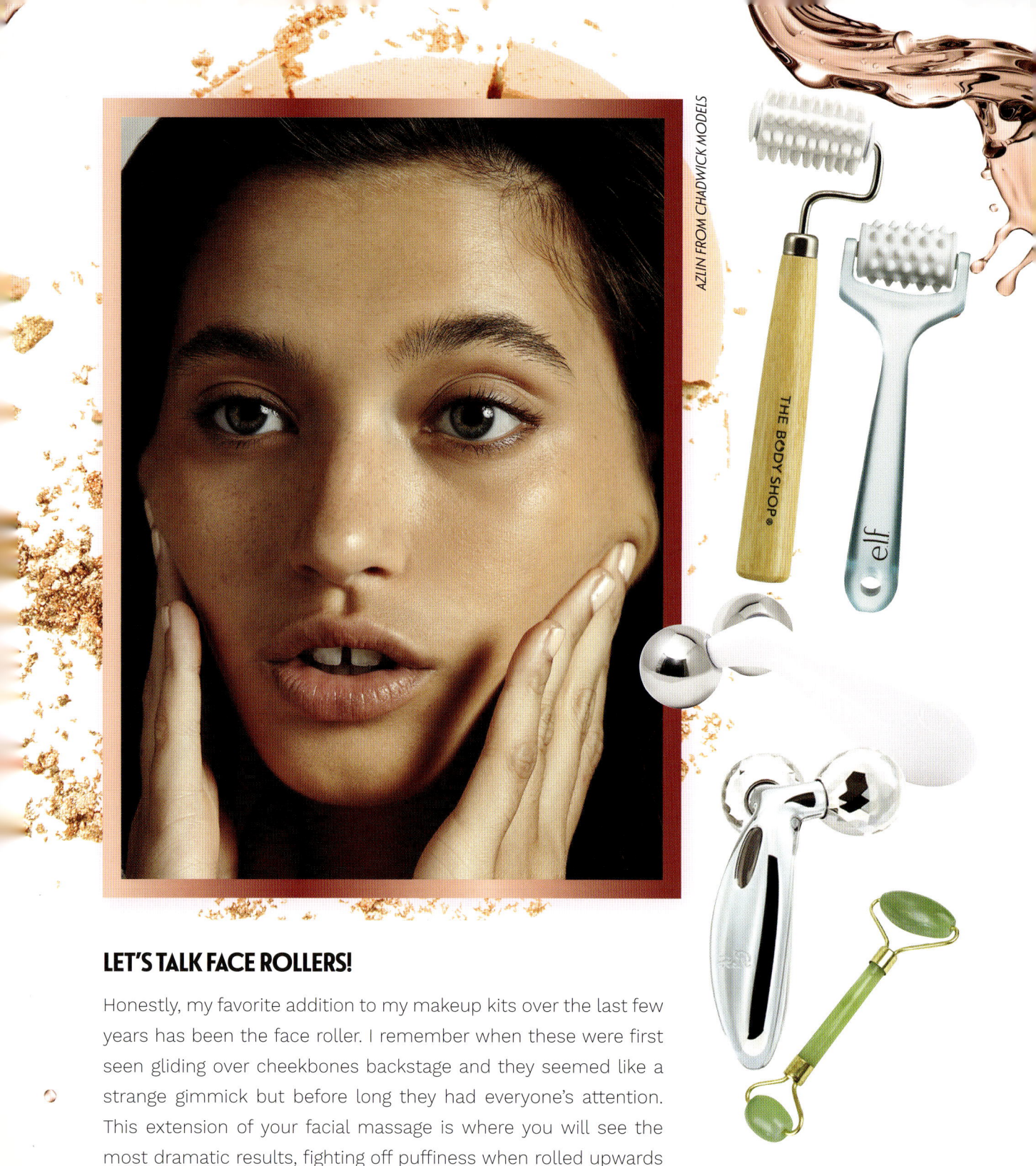

LET'S TALK FACE ROLLERS!

Honestly, my favorite addition to my makeup kits over the last few years has been the face roller. I remember when these were first seen gliding over cheekbones backstage and they seemed like a strange gimmick but before long they had everyone's attention. This extension of your facial massage is where you will see the most dramatic results, fighting off puffiness when rolled upwards and over cheekbones, jawlines and temples – this is the kickstart to your contouring!

The Body Shop Facial Massager, e.l.f. Cosmetics Facial Massager, The Body Shop Twin-Ball Revitalising Facial Massager, ReFa Carat Platinum Massage Roller, jade roller

SKIN IS A THING

GEE GEE FROM KULT

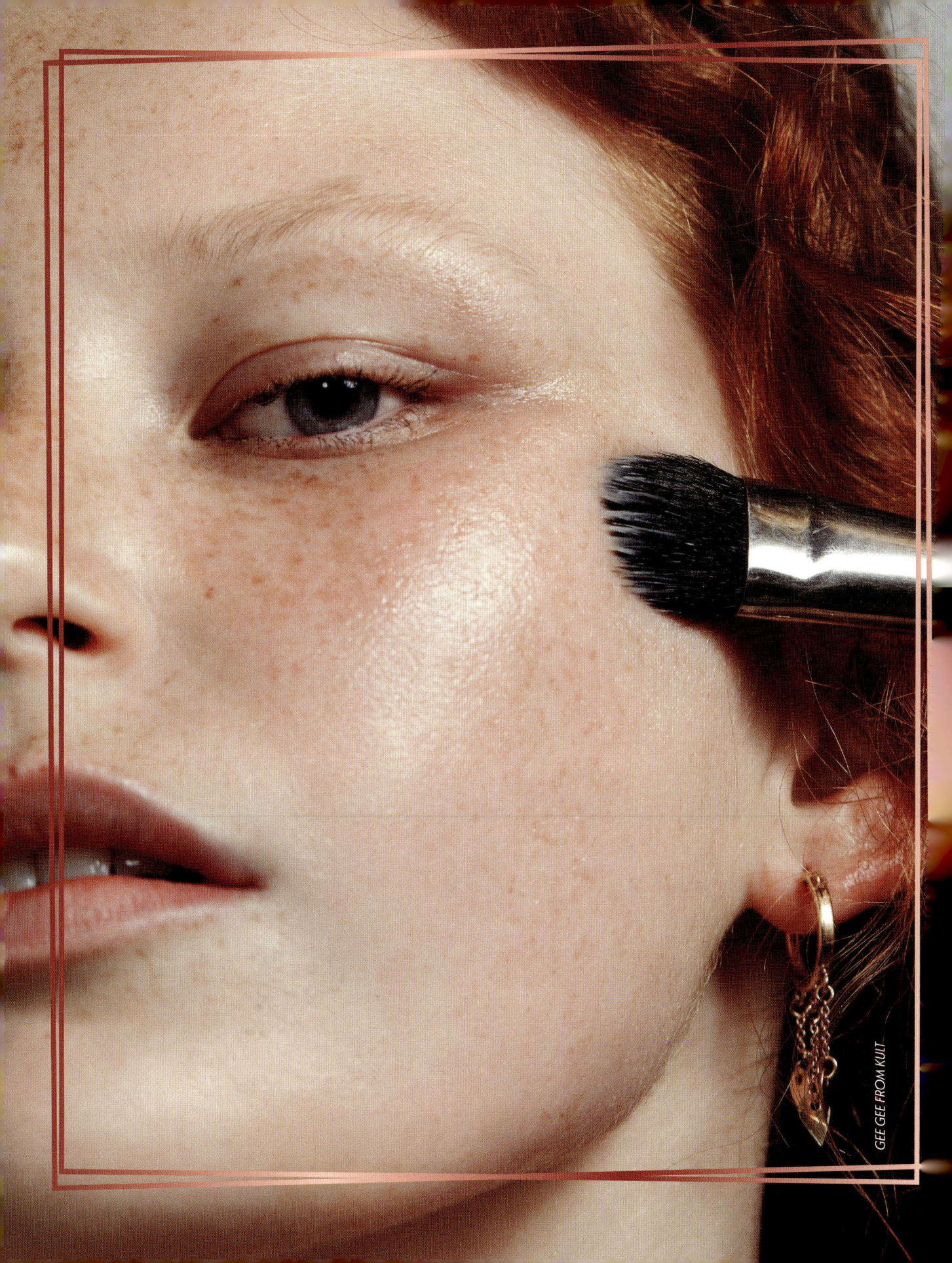

Primer

If you haven't been using primer you have been majorly missing out. In the beginning it was easy to put them down to a passing trend we didn't have time for. Did they really do anything anyway? The answer is YES!

Why do we use primer?

- Do you want your makeup to last all day and in some cases all night? Yah.
- Do you want your skin and pores to appear smoother? Yah.
- Do you want that magic glow you apply to still be magic later in the day? Yah.
- Do you want eye shadow not to crease and move during the day and again at night? Yah.
- Do you get crazy shiny during the day and you would like to stop that affecting your makeup? Yah.
- Do you want that overdrawn lip to stay in perfect shape and not end up dry or fuzzy around the edges? Yah.
- Do you live in an extremely hot or humid climate? Yah. (That isn't a makeup question, you now just need a primer!)
- Do you hate bleeding, blotching and fading of color? Yah. Okay, well this is kind of a repeat for dramatic effect.

I feel like you are picking up what I am putting down here. By adding an additional 30 seconds to your beauty routine you can now see the benefits. It used to be a one primer fits all situation, now there is something for every concern and need.

Primer is the Spanx of the makeup world. Holds everything in place on your face and we look better for longer. There is a reason why when you have your makeup professionally done it looks smoother, you look younger and it magically stays in place for such a long time. They have buffed and puffed you with the right skincare, the right tools and importantly, undercoated you with a suitable P-R-I-M-E-R.

TIP!

Less is more! A statement you don't often hear come out of my mouth, but it really is true when it comes to primer. Primer is a product that locks in place, so if you do too many layers it will set on top of product instead of beneath it, resulting in the 'balling' of the primer on your skin. I hear many people complain about this; it's not the primer's fault, you are simply using too much. A small amount on your fingertips and worked from the T-zone outwards will work wonders!

HANNAH FROM CHIC MANAGEMENT

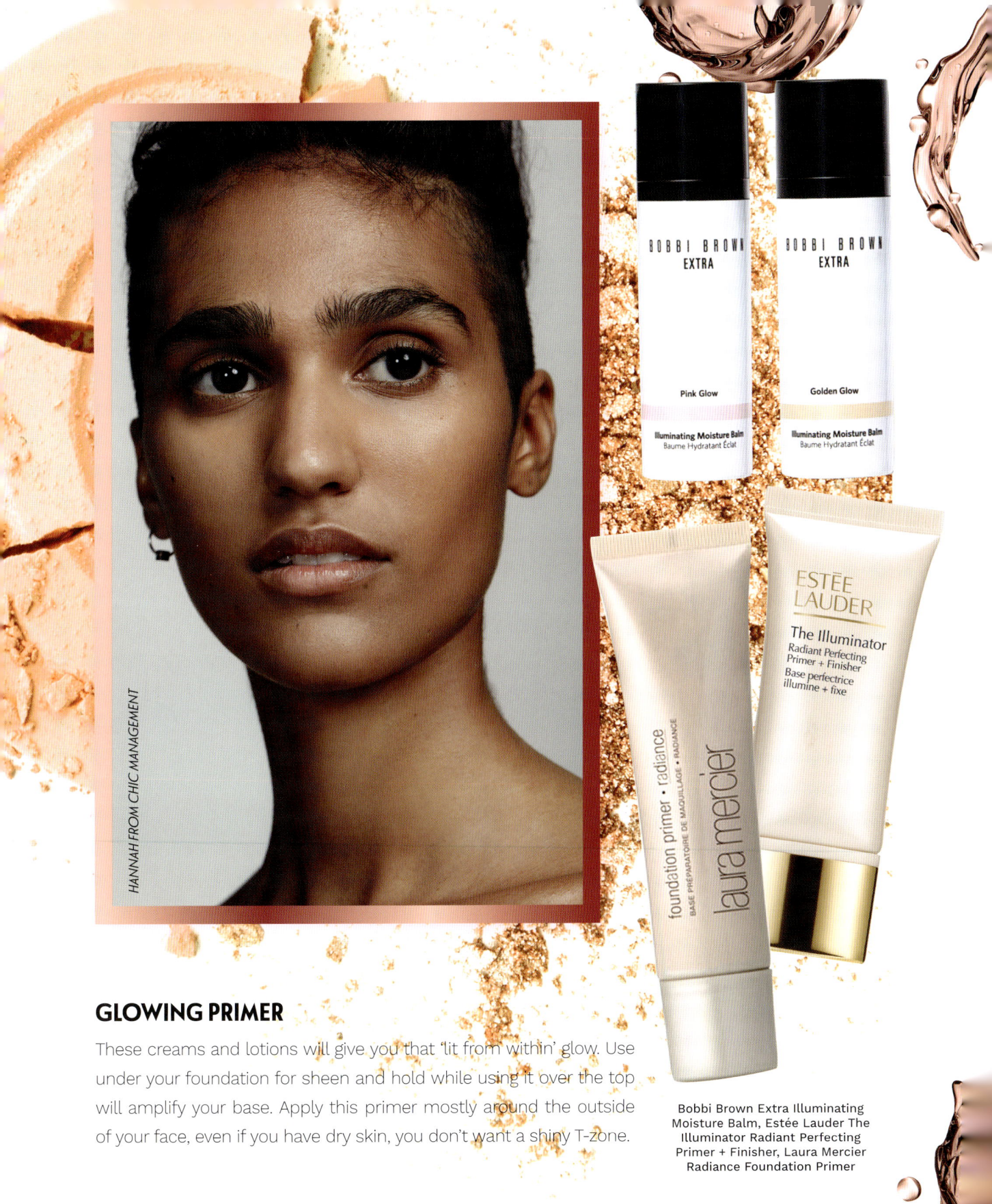

GLOWING PRIMER

These creams and lotions will give you that 'lit from within' glow. Use under your foundation for sheen and hold while using it over the top will amplify your base. Apply this primer mostly around the outside of your face, even if you have dry skin, you don't want a shiny T-zone.

Bobbi Brown Extra Illuminating Moisture Balm, Estée Lauder The Illuminator Radiant Perfecting Primer + Finisher, Laura Mercier Radiance Foundation Primer

SKIN IS A THING

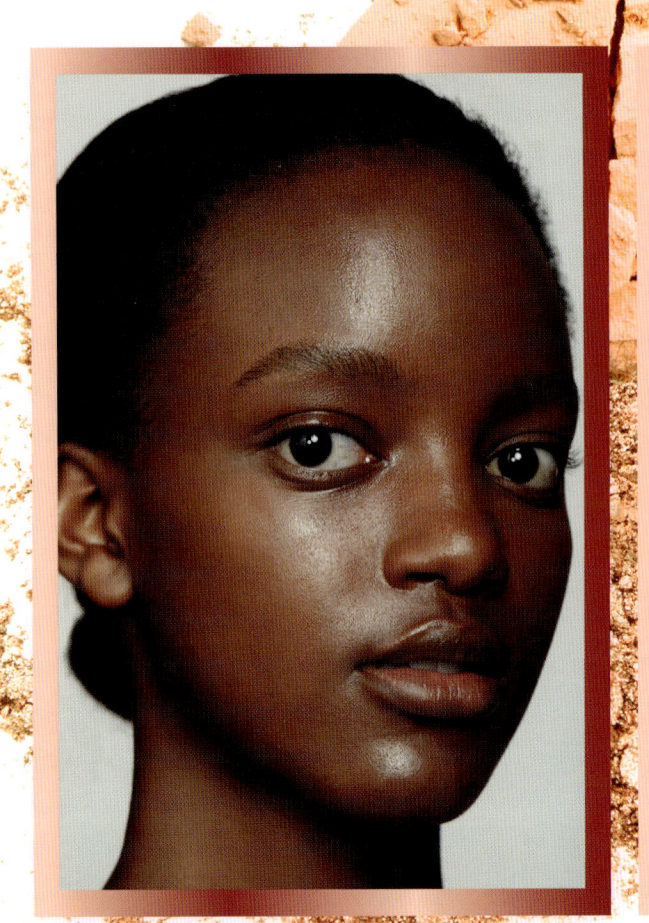

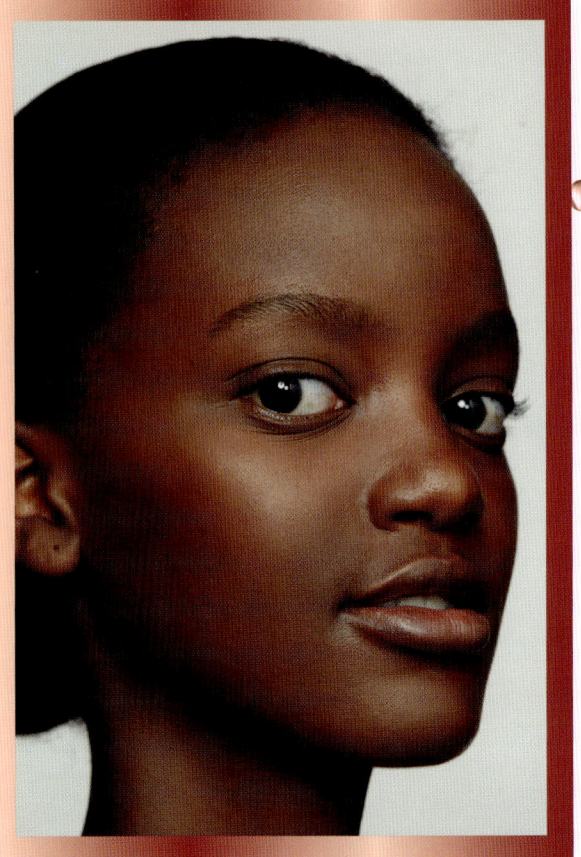

MATTIFYING AND OIL CONTROLLING

These oil-free primers will help to control shine on the spot and throughout the day for a flawless complexion all over the face and down the neck.

    These fantastic little numbers are great for targeted oil control and can be applied on top of your makeup during the day. I really like using these in the T-zone only in combination with a glowing primer around the outside of the face – for those who want the glow in only the flattering areas!

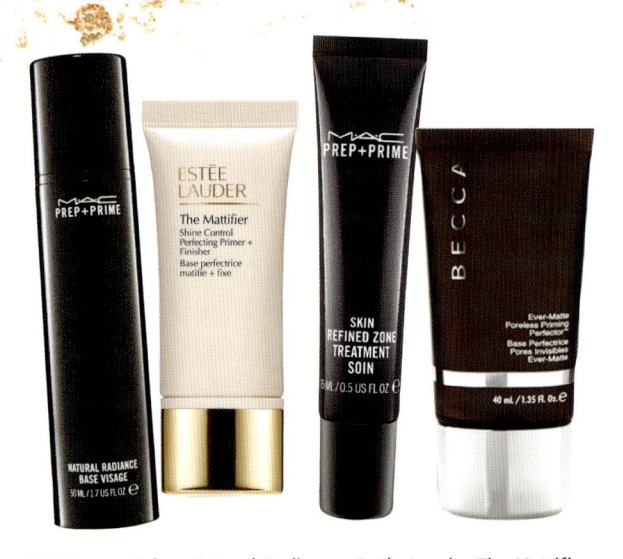

MAC Prep + Prime Natural Radiance, Estée Lauder The Mattifier Shine Control Perfecting Primer + Finisher, MAC Prep + Prime Skin Refined Zone, BECCA Ever-Matte Poreless Priming Perfector

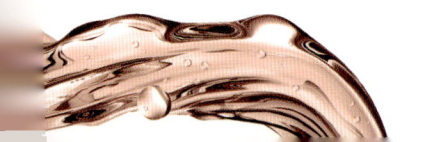

SKIN IS A THING

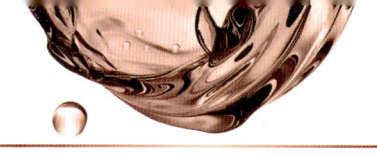

SMOOTHING

Smooth beyond belief, the trick to minimizing wrinkles and pores effectively is to use a soft brush or fingertips to really push this product into the skin, so it is not sitting on top.

The bottom two are face filters in real life: a blurring stick for easy, targeted smoothing control and the compact smoother to sneak right into your bag and touch-up with during the day instead of a powder!

ALL-ROUNDERS

These guys will do it all, softening fine lines, subtly smoothing your complexion and giving your skin the binding qualities to hold your makeup in place. This is your quick go-to when you haven't got any pressing skin worries, need some radiance and require the time-saving properties of a multitasker.

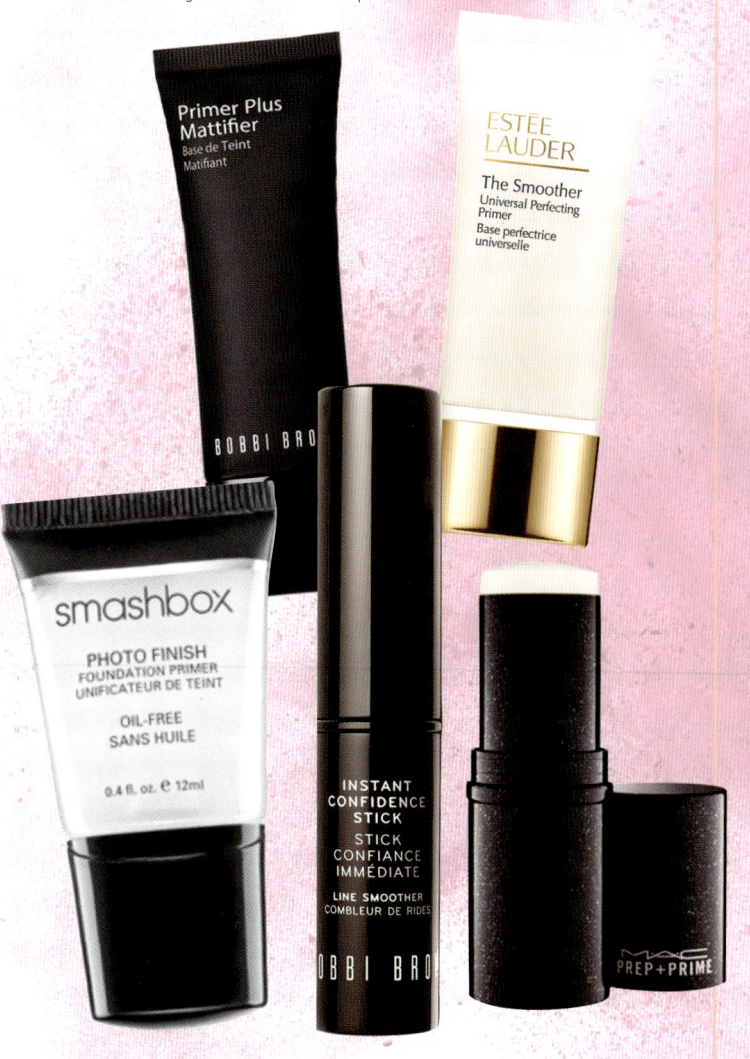

Bobbi Brown Primer Plus Mattifier, Estée Lauder The Smoother Universal Perfecting Primer, Smashbox Photo Finish Foundation Primer, Bobbi Brown Instant Confidence Stick, MAC Prep + Prime Pore Refiner Stick

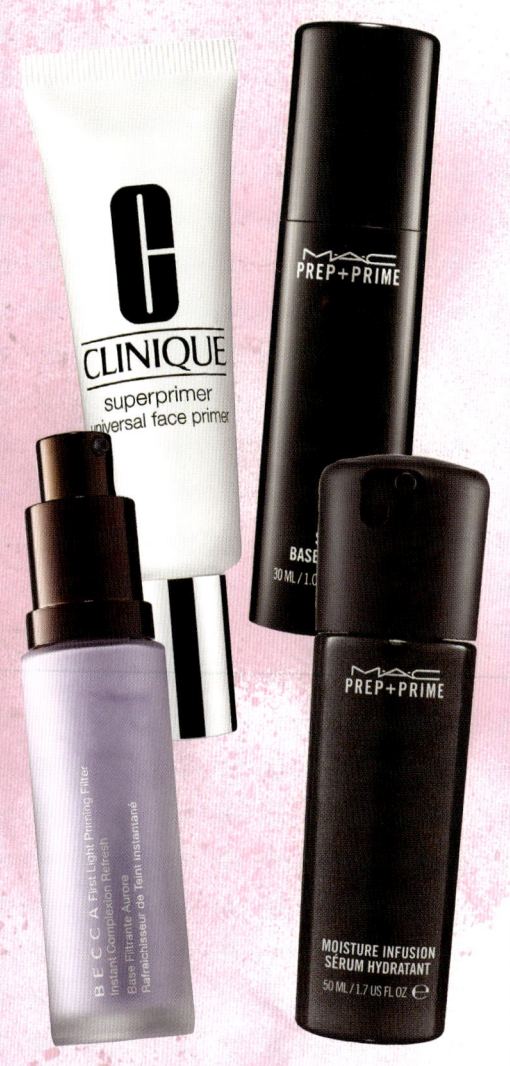

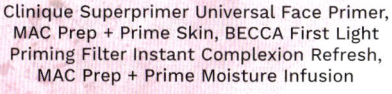

Clinique Superprimer Universal Face Primer, MAC Prep + Prime Skin, BECCA First Light Priming Filter Instant Complexion Refresh, MAC Prep + Prime Moisture Infusion

SKIN IS A THING

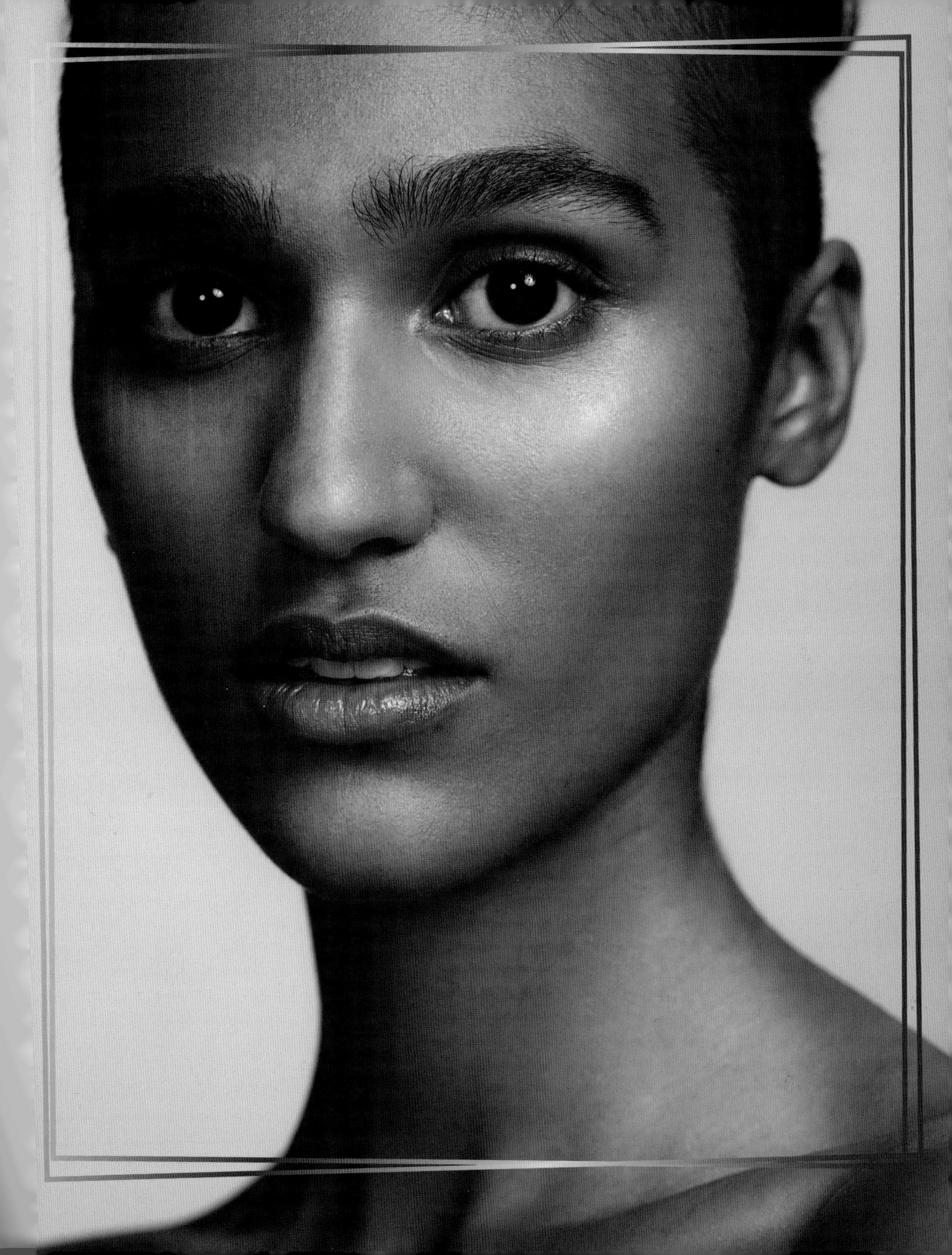

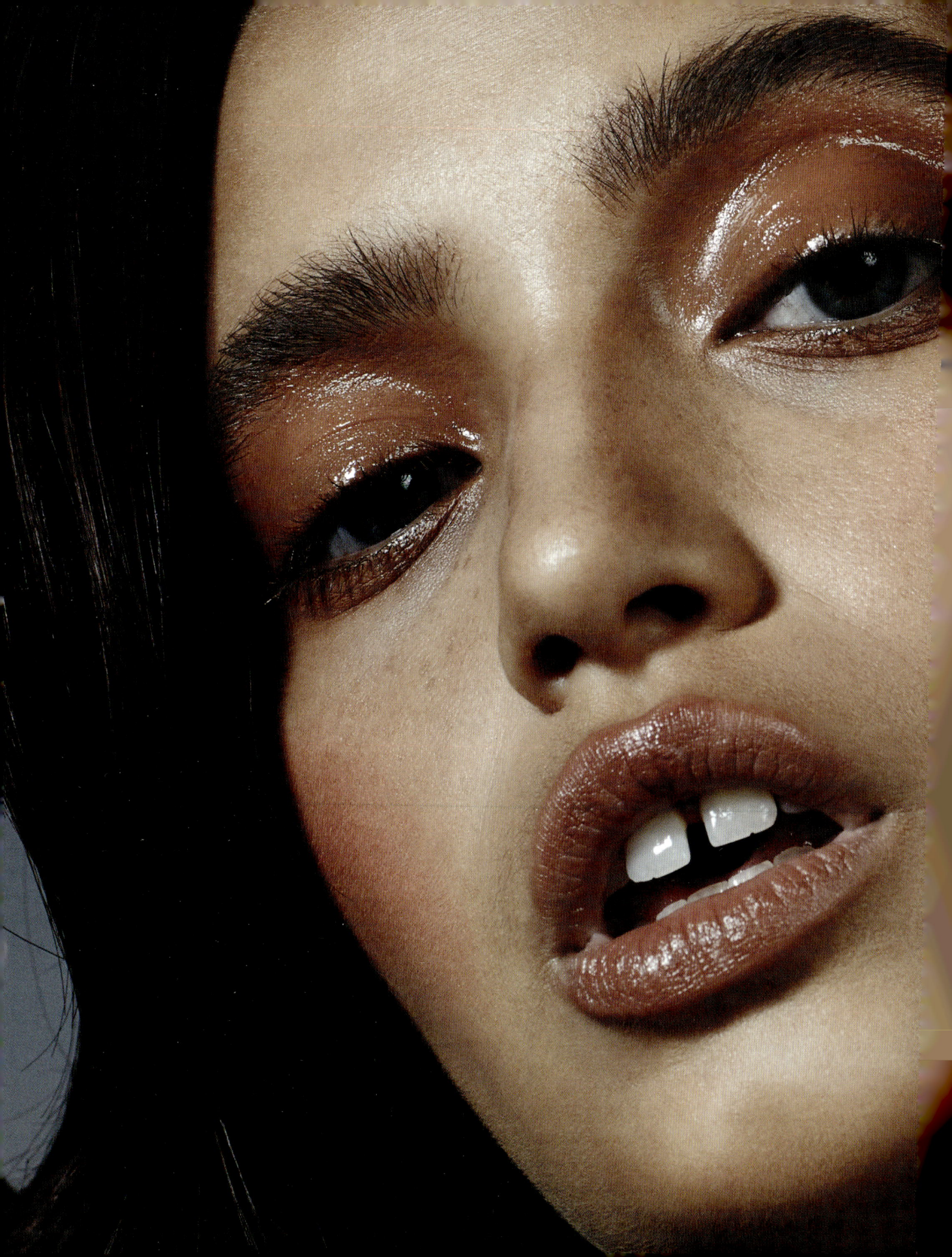

All about that base

If only it was easy to find 'The One'. There would be no need for online dating, or being set up with the nice chap who lives next door to your parents, hell, we wouldn't even need reality dating shows like *Married at First Sight* or *The Bachelor*. The search for true love can be a challenging one, and so to can the search for your perfect foundation.

A makeup artist, YouTube or even the label itself cannot recommend *your* perfect 'foundie' without trying it on your skin. Makeup is like a doctor's prescription, for much of it you don't know whether it is going to work until you try it out. Imagine trying to buy a pair of jeans without trying them on and expecting them to be the perfect fit.

The moral of the story here is test your foundation out first and, if they are available, get someone in-store to help you color match. You can also concentrate the search before you start by asking yourself some key questions.

1. What is my skin type? Oily, dry, normal or combination?
2. How much time to I have? A 30-minute regimented morning beauty routine or just slap it on in the car?
3. How much coverage do I want? Cover it all up or keep it sheer to highlight your freckles or other desirable features?
4. What finish do I want on my skin? Glossed highlights, frosty glow, matte all over, creamy/dewy?
5. What is my dream skin? Who is my skin muse? Even though the makeup consultant unfortunately cannot make you into Bella Hadid, knowing your celebrity muse will give them a good idea of what type of makeup you like! There is a big difference between Giselle and Amrezy, you know!?

Please take your makeup consultant's advice, try some things on, take yourself outside to have a look and see what tickles your fancy. Don't be shy to ask for some samples to take home and have a play with. Find the one for you and never look back.

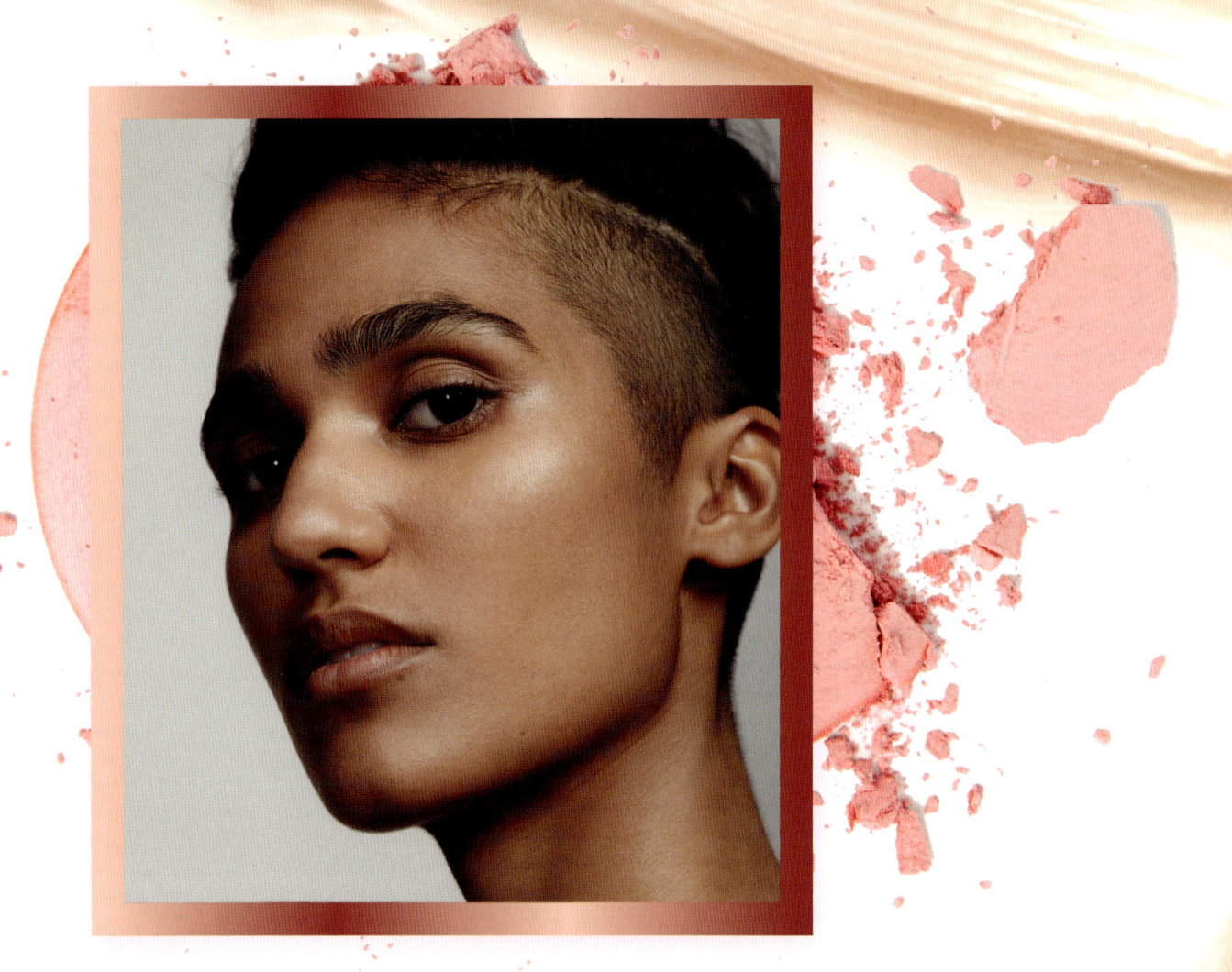

Finding Your Color in the Wall

If you insist in tackling the trickiest foundation job ever, and picking your personal color from a wall of foundie shades, make sure to swatch the testers onto your skin and have a look in good light.

Look at your hand, does it look the same as your face? If you answered yes here I applaud you! This means you have taken impeccable care of your hands over the years for them to look like your delicate facial skin! The majority of you will have answered NO, as our hands don't get cleansed, toned and moisturized like our faces, they get washed a million times more and they spend a whole lot more time in the sun, so why do we try foundation on our hands?

Try the color of your décolletage – this is the color you want to match. This will ensure an even color traveling between both and will mean you don't end up with the whole white face thing! If you can't do décolletage, do lower jawline. But make sure to bring your shoulder up to your jaw while checking the color in the mirror to see that the color match flows.

ALL ABOUT THAT BASE

Where to Contour

Contouring is not new. People have been using the technique of shading and sculpting their face with color for centuries – thank the heavens the products have evolved beyond soot and greasepaint to shape us! Contouring is a retro concept but you can modernize it. By selecting a product with the right color it will create shadows that can slim the shape of the face.

Most people love a powder contour to invisibly deepen the hollows of the face, while others live or die with creams that paint a whole new face shape on! How fun is makeup! Generally the cream or powder works best to create a realistic shadow if the color is a slightly cool toned taupe or brown that is one to two shades darker than your skin tone.

One of the benefits of contouring is that you can utilize products that you may use elsewhere in your overall look. Concealers, contour cream, taupe blushes, eye shadows, face powders or even a matte long-wearing lipstick can all play a role in shaping the face, just be sure they work in with your overall color palette.

Here are the best spots to add color to trim that face!

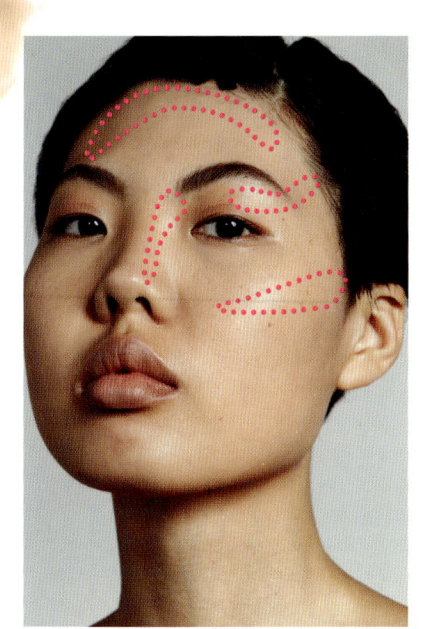

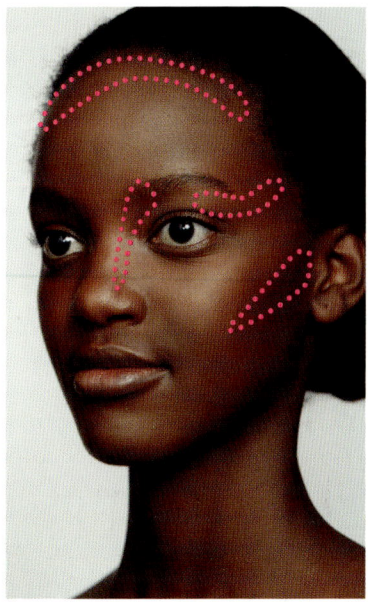

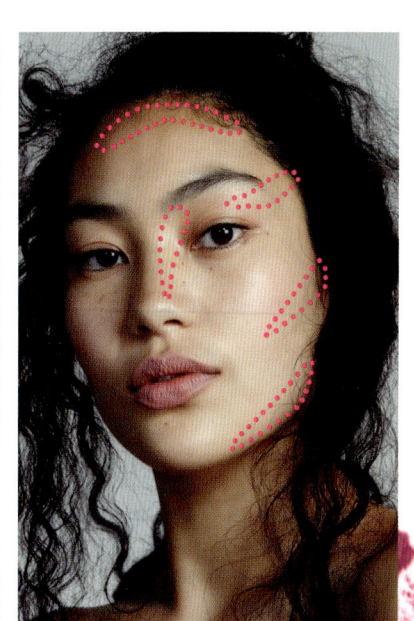

Highlighting

Highlighting is the yin to the contouring yang. Where you pop a contour, throw a light shade next to it, to make that bone structure pop.

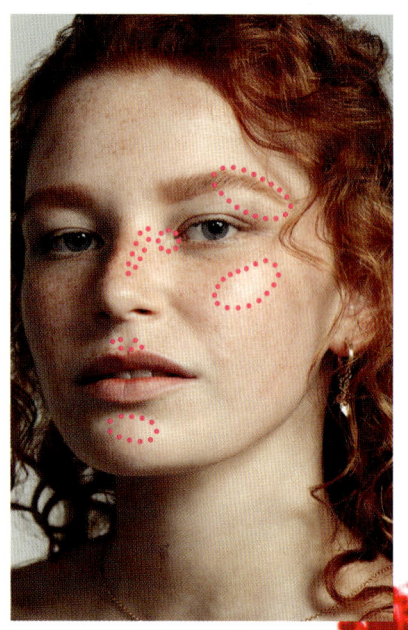

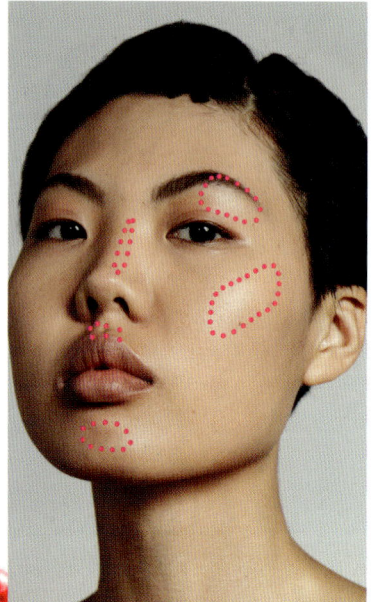

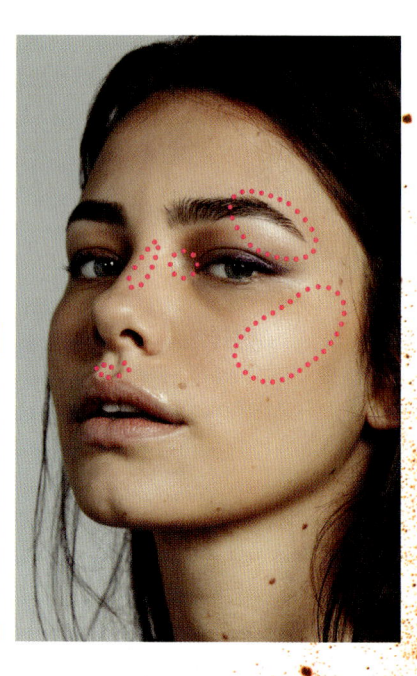

ALL ABOUT THAT BASE

SHEER AND GLOWING

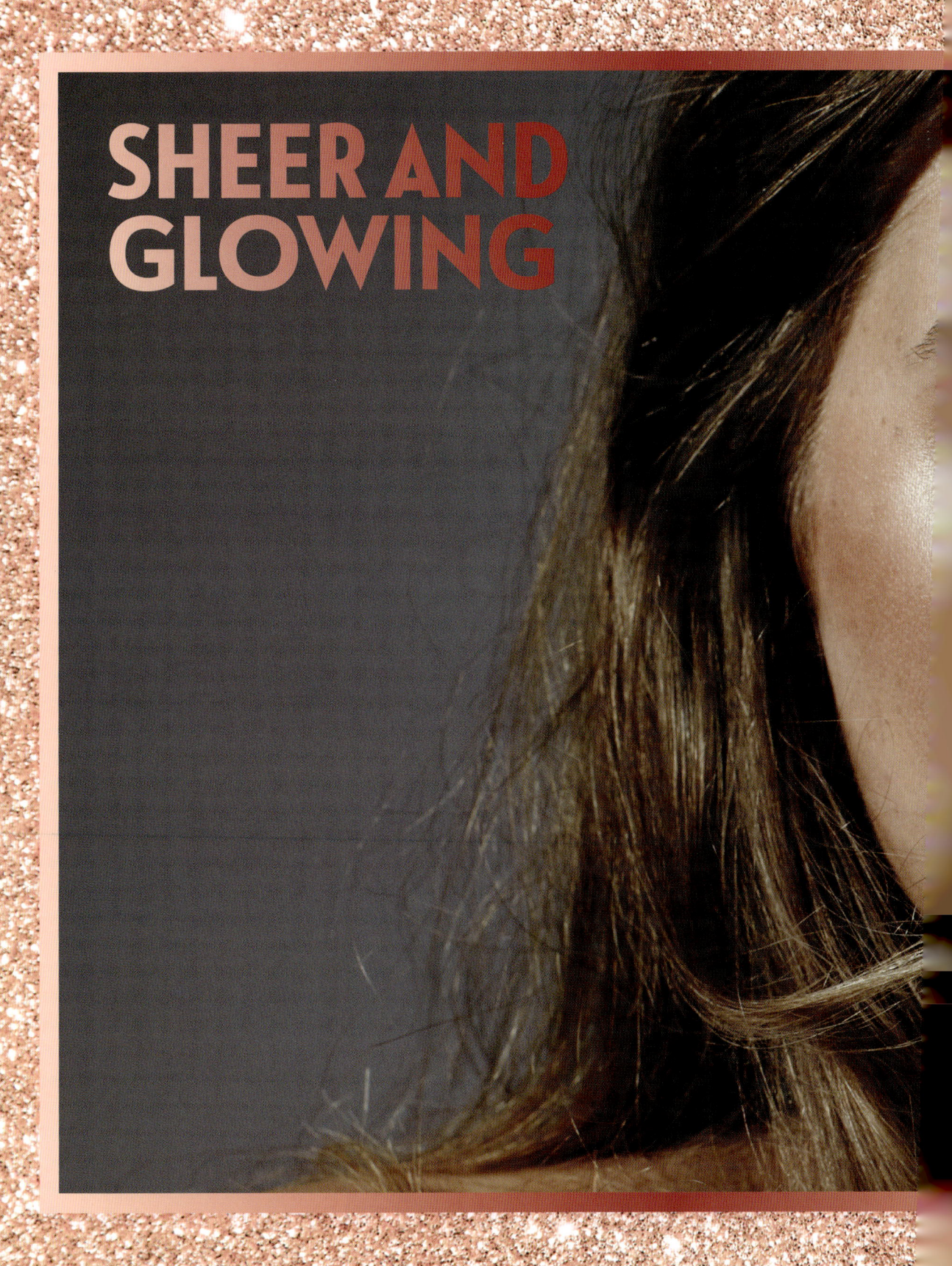

ALL ABOUT THAT BASE

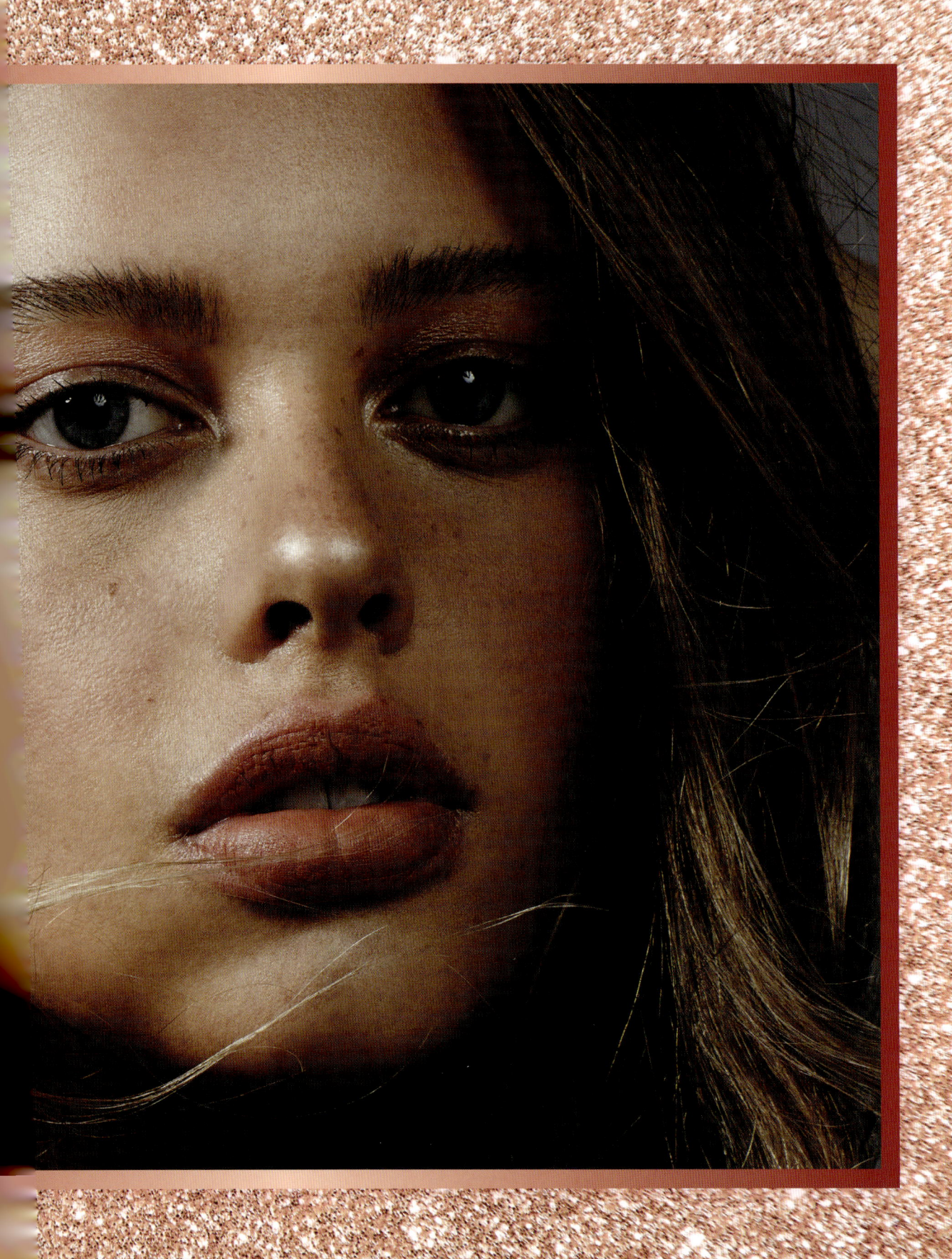

LAY THE FOUNDATION

STEP 1

Hydration station. Start your engines with not one but at least eight sprays of a hydrating face mist and *werk* that bad boy into the skin. Seriously, you should feel soaked. The massage is important here to get that blood circulating, which will help the following product blend easily into your skin.

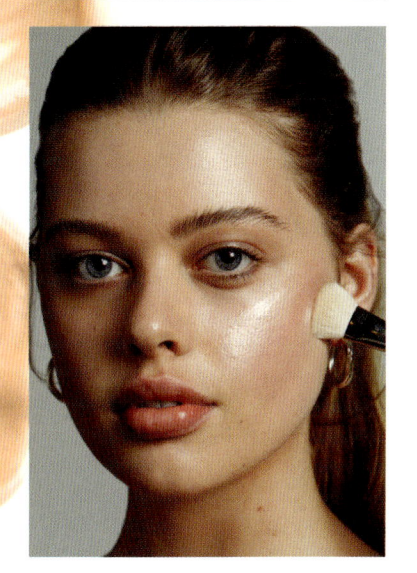

STEP 2

Mix your liquid illuminator into your primer and take over the face, paying special attention to the nose, under eyes and cheekbones. This gives you fast glow and hold in one.

If you get oily skin, separate the primer and the illuminator and pop them on individually. Pat your mattifying primer through the T-zone, chin and jawline, then use your illuminator on all the high points and over the lips. Use a brush to apply the illuminator like you are icing a cake, ensuring a smooth coat. Then, with your fingers, blend the primer into the skin to smooth those pores.

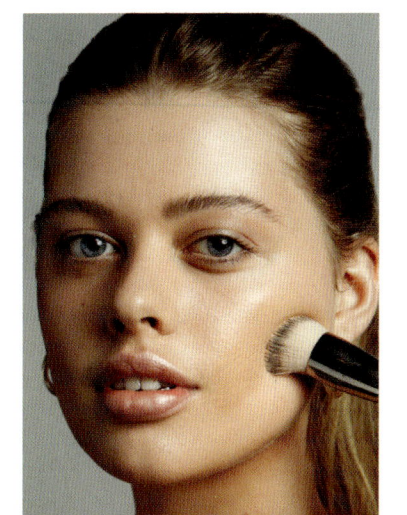

STEP 3

We are using a sheer glowing foundation and I love to blend and stipple foundation on, in this case with a stumpy, soft foundation brush. The round shape stops streaks of color appearing, and the density of this brush will get the most out of a sheer foundation. This enables you to tap and build the coverage in smaller areas where needed.

> **TIP!** Work the foundation around the face beginning at the center and moving outwards. The center of your face is where you need the most coverage so that's where you want to jump in. If you want to get all the glow without feeling bogged down with foundation, do what we do backstage at fashion week – we used a large, fluffy eye shadow brush to take the foundation and concealer ONLY where needed. Healthy skin fake-out!

ALL ABOUT THAT BASE

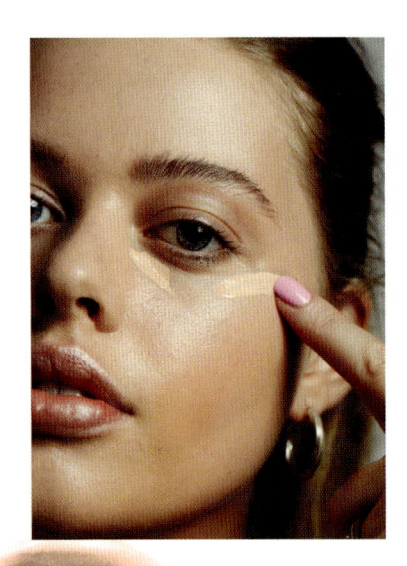

STEP 4

Disguise that fatigued area beneath your eyes and light up dull skin by opting for a brightening concealer pen. Slightly sheerer in texture, these creams are designed to lift and illuminate rather than provide heavy coverage.

When you look into the mirror, you will notice there is a dark diagonal line under our eyes. That's where you swipe the color on then use your finger or fluffy brush to tap away excess product and soften the edges – gently does it!. Work the concealer under the eyes, across the tops of the cheekbones, down the nose and through the center of the lips before tapping away excess with your fingertips. Add and tap, add and tap. Adding is easier than taking away, and this definitely applies to concealer!

> **TIP!** When addressing the area beneath the eye, apply the concealer to the darkest part and blend outwards. Sounds simple enough, yet sometimes we find ourselves falling into the trap of just piling on concealer everywhere and hoping for the best. Now this idea works if you have a makeup light, and softened filter following you around all day (when are they going to invent this?) but for those of us in reality, looking for a reality-worthy skin, please trade in the 'smother and spread' method for this technique immediately!

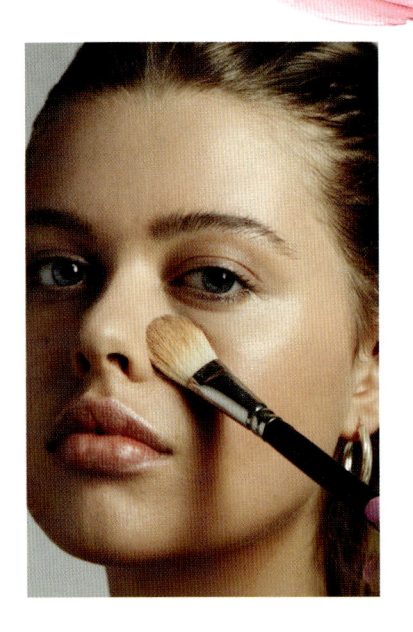

STEP 5

To powder the skin here we need to get specific. Going hell for leather with a giant brush and heaps of powder would ruin all the work we have done so far to get that glow. You want a clean, smooth luxurious finish to the skin so you need some precision.

Using a mineral pressed powder, as they aren't completely matte, use a small powder brush to push the powder into the skin without overloading. Using this powder sparingly, work around the nose, beneath the eyes, in between the brows, over the forehead, jawline and chin and around the mouth.

STEP 6

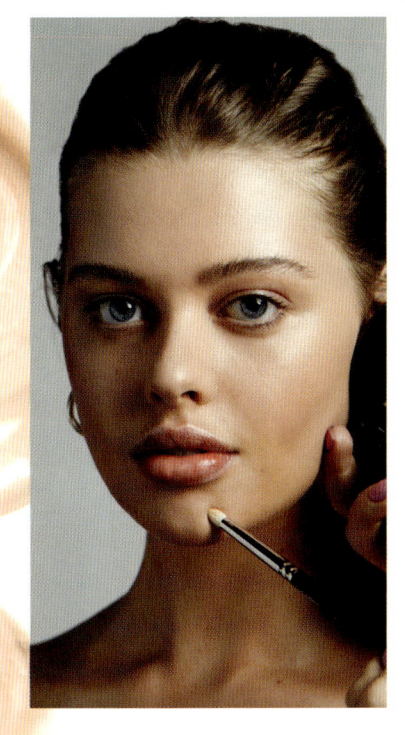

Who has ever had a blemish and you have added so much cream to mask it, it actually ends up either shiny, highlighted or raised to the point where you should just advertise the pimple with a sign. Hands up! This is why I use mineral powder with a pointed brush to conceal. This is especially helpful for raised or slightly dry spots.

Make sure the powder is slightly lighter than your skin color so when it settles in it will blend in perfectly. Using the pointed brush (a soft point or pointed eye liner brush) push the powder onto the blemish. The small brush helps to keep the product directly on the spot, keeping it matte and flat and really disguising the mark brilliantly.

I had to learn this trick for photography and fashion makeup where visible base products are a complete no-no if you want to get booked again! Specific coverage will look more natural and just like *your skin*!

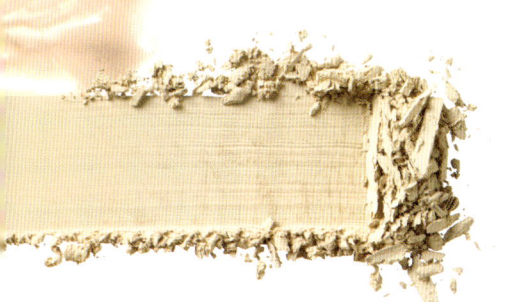

SHAPE IT

STEP 7

'Shaping' the face doesn't always have to be like you are carving brand new features on. Bronzer is the perfect way to continue this effortless look by tinting the skin with warmth and softening the edges of the face.

Use a large splayed brush to sweep the powder bronzer over the parts of the face you want to warm up and enhance. For this look, we are not sitting the color underneath the bone structure to mimic a shadow, we are wrapping the bone structure with warm bronze to fake a healthy tan and soften the framework of the face.

Sweep the color across the forehead, on the cheekbones and on the jawline in the shape of a 3 or an E depending on the side of the face! Under your jaw is usually the lightest part of our body, so hit that area with bronzer and sweep down the neck. Run the brush over the eyelids and over the nose so you aren't

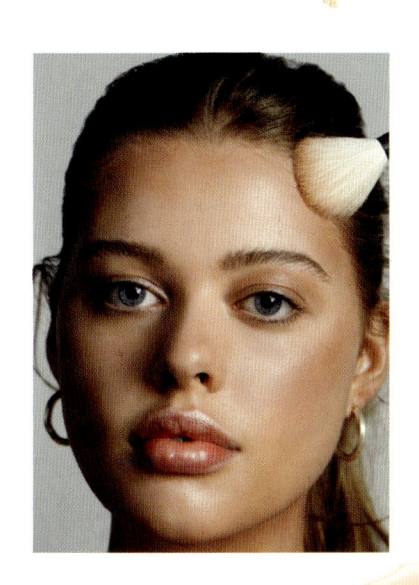

54   ALL ABOUT THAT BASE

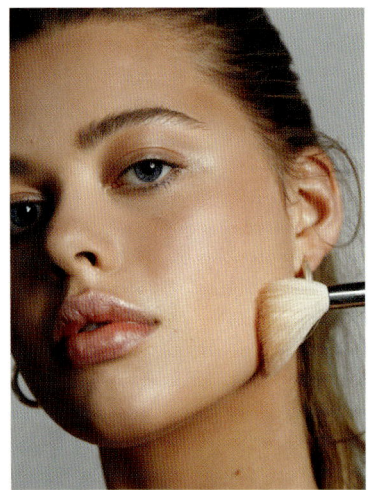

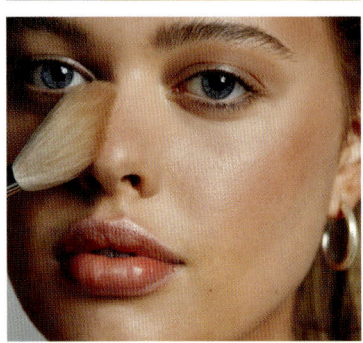

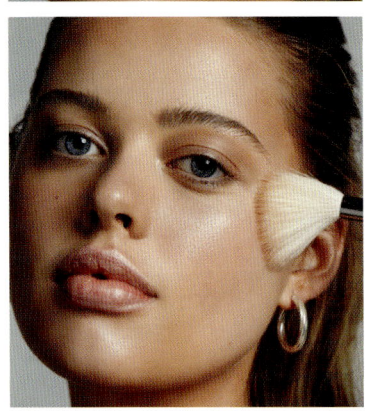

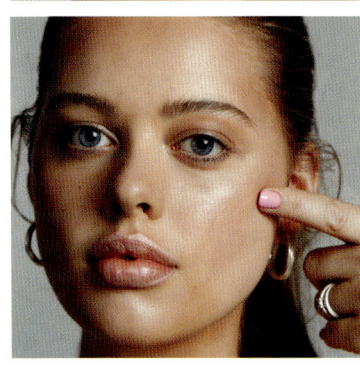

in danger of just creating a bronze circle on the outside of your face. Here I have used a radiant powder bronzer for slight sheen on already pretty creamy skin.

Complete the whole face then repeat. If you add and blend multiple times over one area before moving on, by the time you have hit all areas of the face with color it's going to be crazy dark! Do one layer all around the face first, then step back, and you may notice you only need additional color on the cheekbones not everywhere.

TIP! Powder on top of cream can be seen! But beware of the dangers of wet skin. If the skin is too creamy on the surface the bronzing powder will stick, especially if you are using a small brush or bronzer with strong color pigment. For those two, run the brush lightly through some loose translucent powder first to give that intense bronzer wheels so it glides over the skin evenly.

ENHANCE IT

STEP 8

Ah, if there is one thing in beauty that looks good on almost *everyone,* it is a highlight on the skin. This is my favorite part of the makeup routine, getting that glow on the skin that makes you stop at your reflection in any shiny surface and say 'Oh hey girl'. Highlighting can be done in many different ways, but specifically here we are detailing the easy glow to create a healthy sheen.

I love a cream highlighter in this situation. Now before you go running for the hills at the word cream, there is not just one type and whether you are oily or dry, you can apply it to suit you!

This is the top coat of this skin look so you want to leave it seamless. Just like Step 2, we are going to keep the illuminizer to the outer parts of the face, glazing the cheek bones and shoulder mostly. Use a large soft brush for a sheer and even coat, or your fingertips for a more restrained application of highlight where you need it.

ALL ABOUT THAT BASE

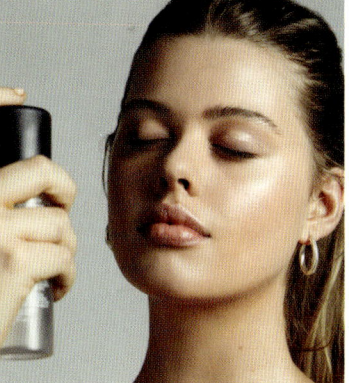

STEP 9

I feel like I should insert this step into every step! Seriously, the hydrating spray has endless uses! Give your skin a good spritz and use the palms of your hands to pat your skin lightly to refresh and set.

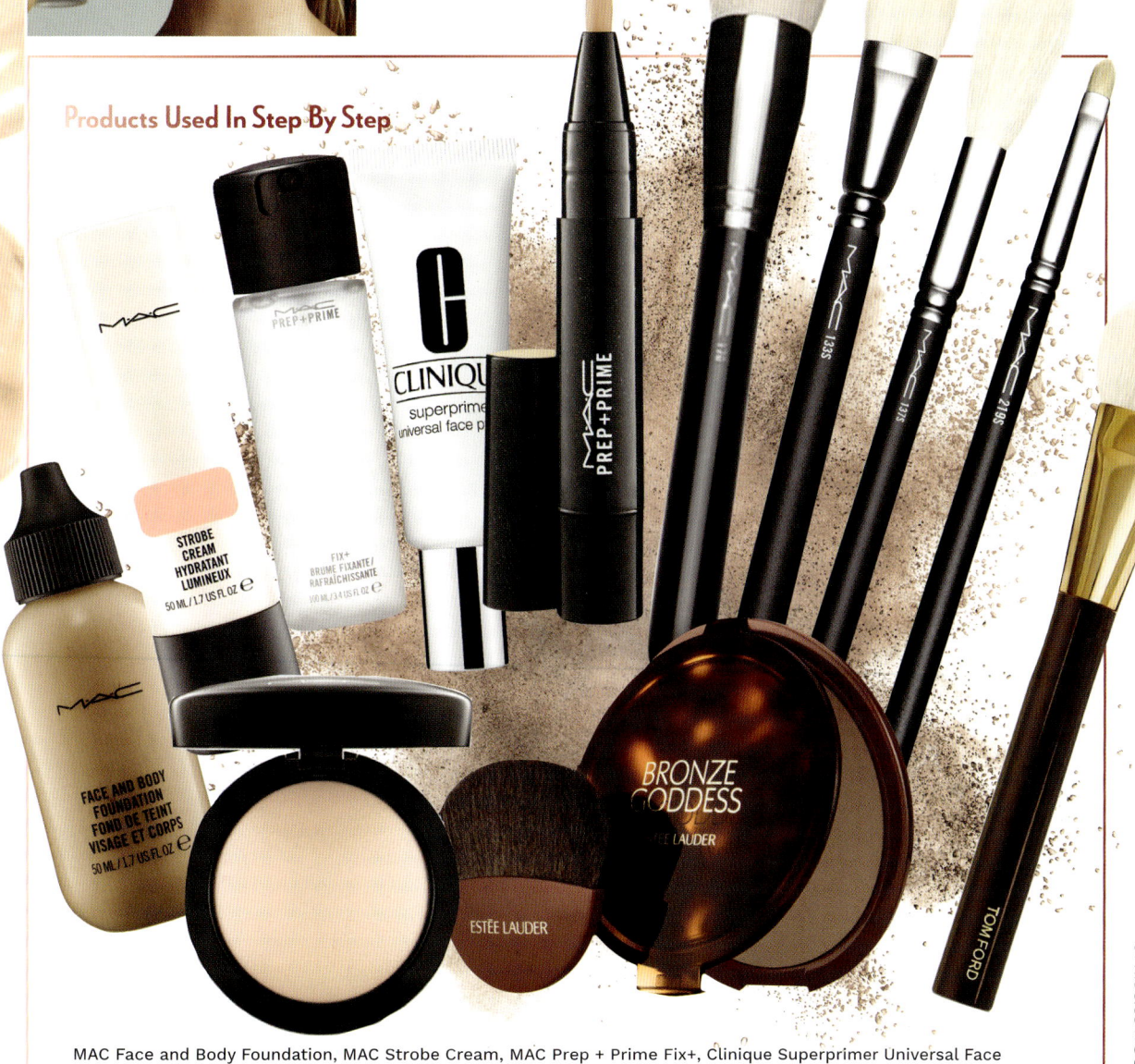

Products Used In Step By Step

MAC Face and Body Foundation, MAC Strobe Cream, MAC Prep + Prime Fix+, Clinique Superprimer Universal Face Primer, MAC Prep + Prime Highlighter pen, MAC 170, 133, 137 and 219 brushes, Tom Ford Cream Foundation Brush, MAC Mineralize Skinfinish Natural Powder to set and conceal, Estée Lauder Bronze Goddess Powder Bronzer

LINNEA FROM PRISCILLAS

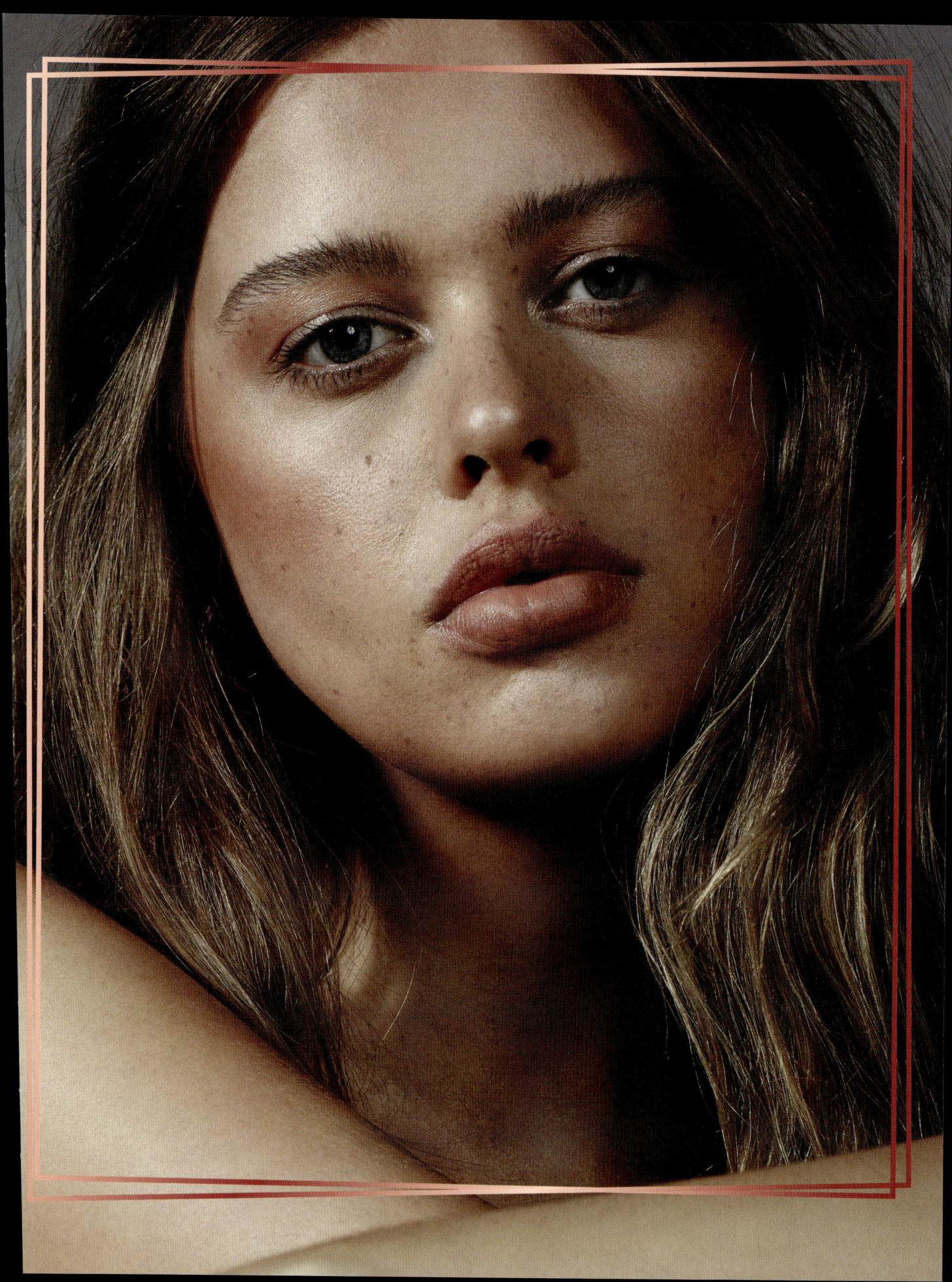

CREAMY COVERAGE

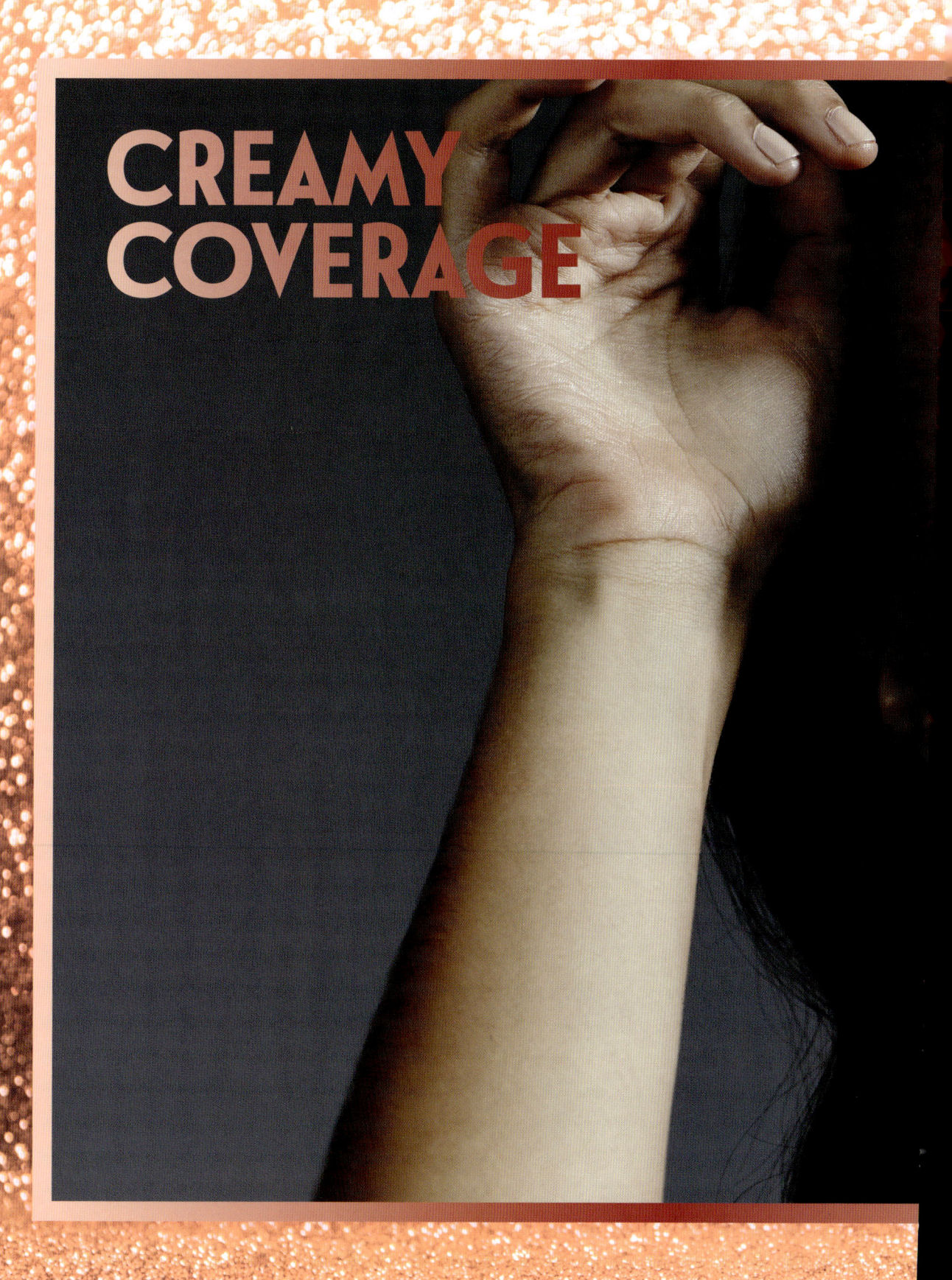

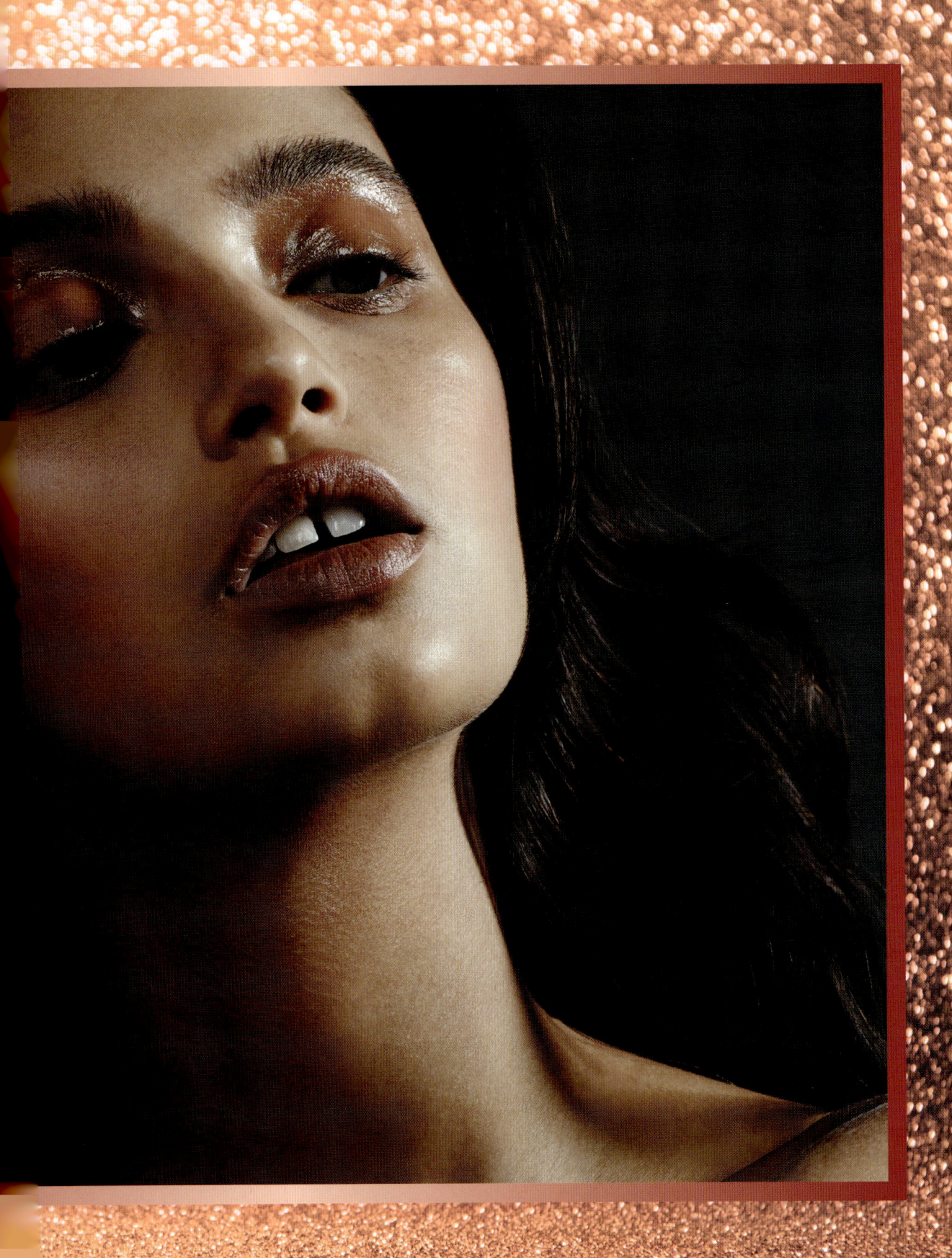

ALL ABOUT THAT BASE

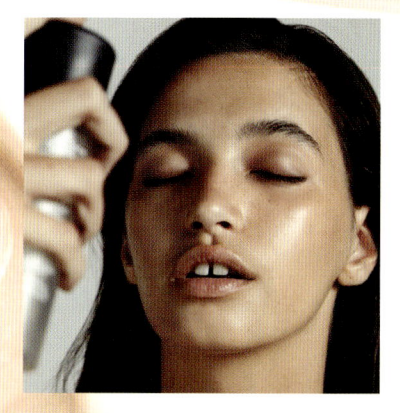

LAY THE FOUNDATION

STEP 1

Do I need to explain this one? Seriously?! Generously spray your face with your hydrating spray across the face and shoulders and massage in. Spray and repeat. This is the start to achieving the 'creamy' part of this makeup look!

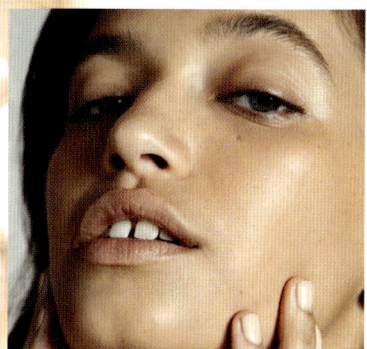

STEP 2

After transforming your face into a hydration station, use your fingertips to apply an oil-controlling primer to the T-zone and jawline of your face. These are two areas you do not want to become shiny during the day.

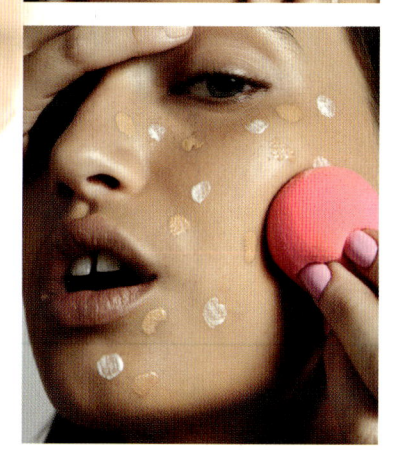

STEP 3

For a fancy look all over your face, do alternate dots all over your face of illuminizer and your liquid fuller coverage foundation with more of the dots being foundation, and blend. For a less festive look, use the back of your hand to mix ⅔ foundation, ⅓ illuminizer and then use your sponge to blend onto the skin.

I love a sponge for this look, as the nature of the sponge is to absorb. You can press and pat all over the face while adding product and it will always ensure you never have too much product sitting on your skin! Add, pat and repeat.

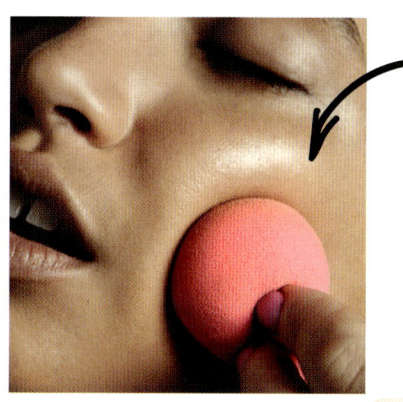

Tip! Wet the sponge and wring out the excess liquid so it remains just damp for a better blend. When the sponge sucks up all the water it is less likely to also suck up all of your foundation. I love to wet the sponge with a hydrating mist so each time you press you are also adding moisture to avoid a heavy, cakey look. Use the smallest part of the sponge to effectively add product, then the larger part to blend in.

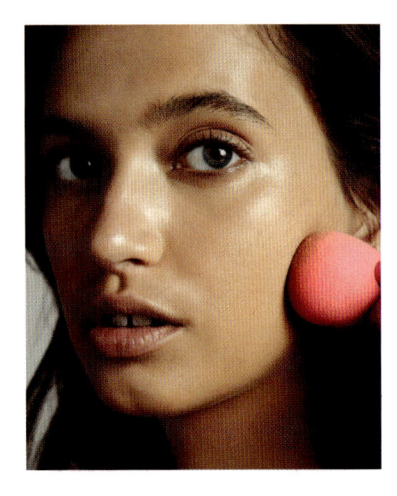

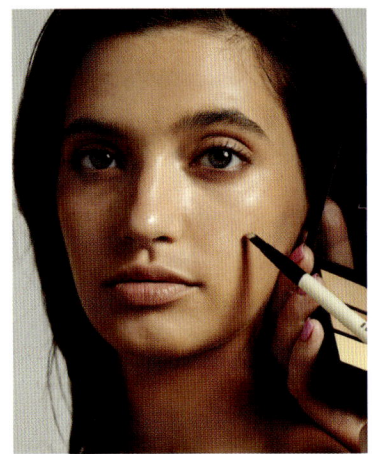

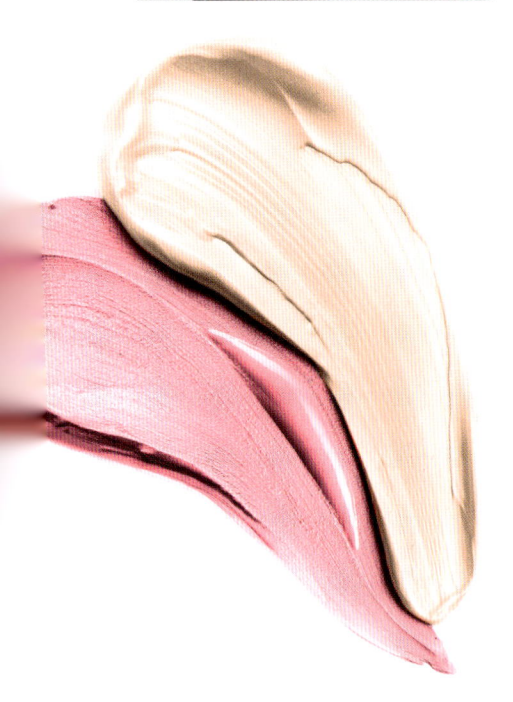

STEP 4

Keep adding and patting. Build that flawless complexion until you get the coverage you desire!

STEP 5

You have now given yourself the most flawless creamy base possible but you still may have some small areas that need a little more coverage. Use a full-coverage cream concealer and a tiny brush to target only the spots you need to hide. This is a backstage trick that works in real life. Most of the time you get all the coverage you need out of your foundation application, using a small eye shadow brush, a pointed eyeliner brush or precise concealer brush just add the concealer onto the blemish or mark and tap the edges away gently.

Gentle is the chosen word!

> *TIP!* Alrighty, if you can't help yourself and you want a dewy coverage that is *flaw*less and *pore*-less use the same damp sponge, take into the cream concealer and blend over your whole complexion. Using the sponge is crucial as it will absorb the excess foundation sitting on top of your skin that you don't need!

STEP 6

Next we are about to set this perfect face with powder. Hold it right there with that powder and brush! Blot your skin first. Wet skin is the enemy of powder, because if it has yet to settle it will be patchy and those patches will be a magnet for powder.

You have two choices with powder here that will make all the difference to how much you need to use on your skin.

1. If you like to powder straight away, make sure you blot your skin first! Use blotting papers or a simple tissue, pat your skin all over to pick up that additional moisture that is sitting there before you go in with powder.

2. The other, and a personal recommendation is to wait as long as you can to powder your skin. When you powder wet skin straight away you will most likely use twice as much as you

ALL ABOUT THAT BASE

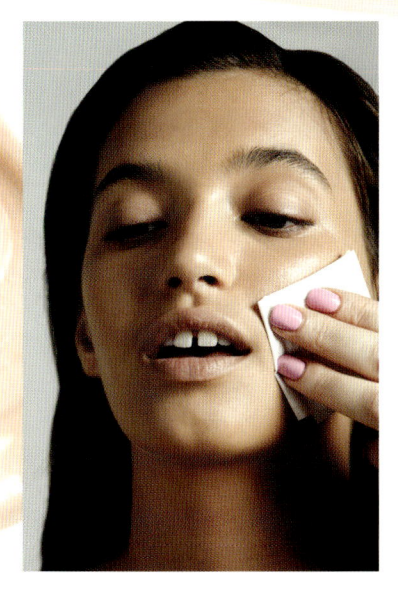

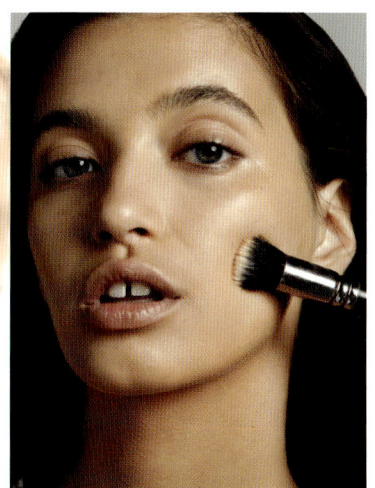

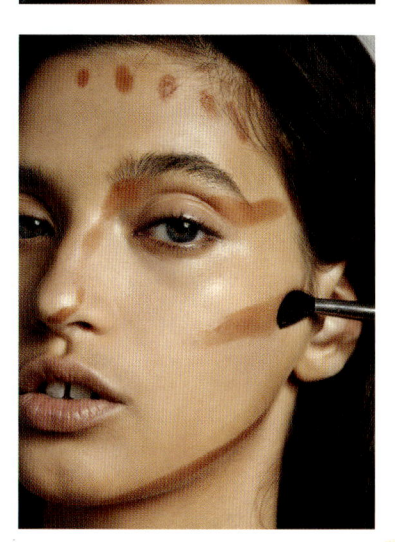

need to as you try to dry your wet skin with powder. By waiting until you have completed your brows and eye makeup, the foundation will have settled into the skin and dried, so you won't need as much product for that desired porcelain effect.

STEP 7

Now we are ready for the powder! You have achieved beautiful mannequin-like coverage, so you don't really need a ton more. To smooth and refine grab a small brush and push in a loose skin-toned powder,

Concentrate the treatment around the nose and mouth, between the brows, center of the forehead and along the lower cheeks. The color can be slightly lighter than the natural skin to give brightening effect in these areas.

> *TIP!* For a double hold in these areas, use the same sponge as before and use this to press a tiny amount of powder over the top to seal the look.

SHAPE IT

STEP 8

Using a cream contour, mark out your contours. Don't worry about exact perfection, you are going to blend it! Choose a cream contour color that is a deeper skin tone, neither too orange nor too pink, as this will stand out too much in a bad way. Choose a specific contouring cream color or a concealer in a much darker color can shape the face well

STEP 9

Blend away edges with a large, soft eye shadow brush. Add more to create a deeper effect where you need it and blend.

Once you have contoured your way to happiness, apply a very light dusting of your loose powder to set. Be sparing.

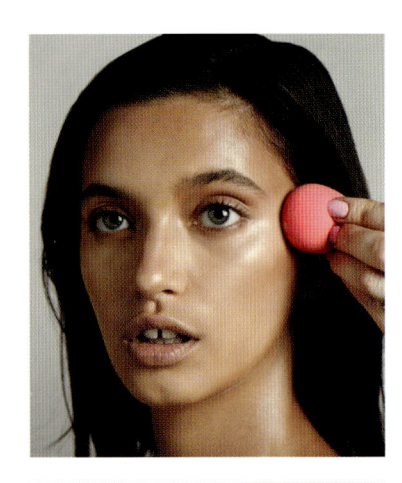

> **TIP!** Beware of the hairline if you have light or blonde hair! This can look terrible if not blended properly. Only use a small amount near the hairline if needed and take the time to blend away the outer edges. My advice is, if you don't really need contouring on your forehead, avoid it with light hair.

ENHANCE IT

STEP 10

You should now be left with a beautiful creamy, flawless coverage that is contoured and matte in the hollows of the face, and the bone structure should be left out with some slight shine. Leave the makeup application here if that is your happy place of skin highlighting.

If you want to continue your journey to mannequin land, grab your trusty beauty blender and finish off the makeup by patting the original illuminizer over the highlights of the face, remembering not to forget the neck and shoulders to complete the look!

If you prefer not to use a liquid to finish this makeup, use a cream highlighter in the same position for a seriously fresh finish.

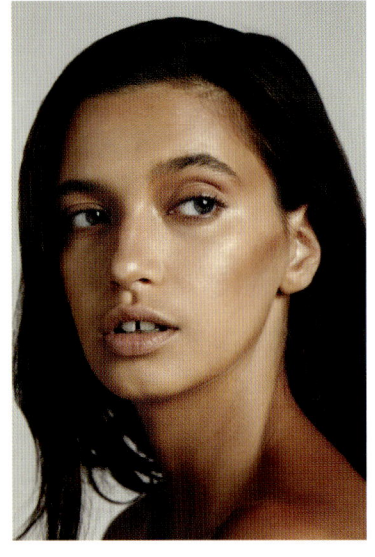

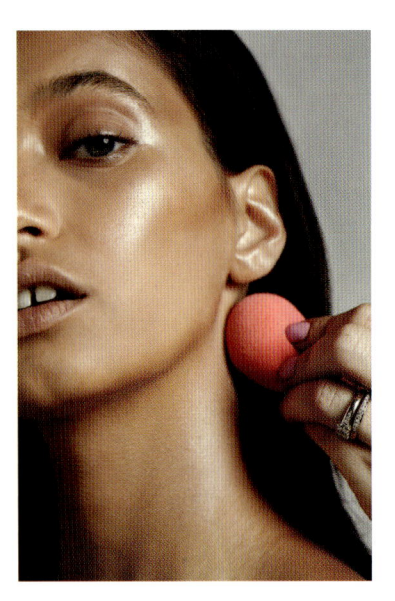

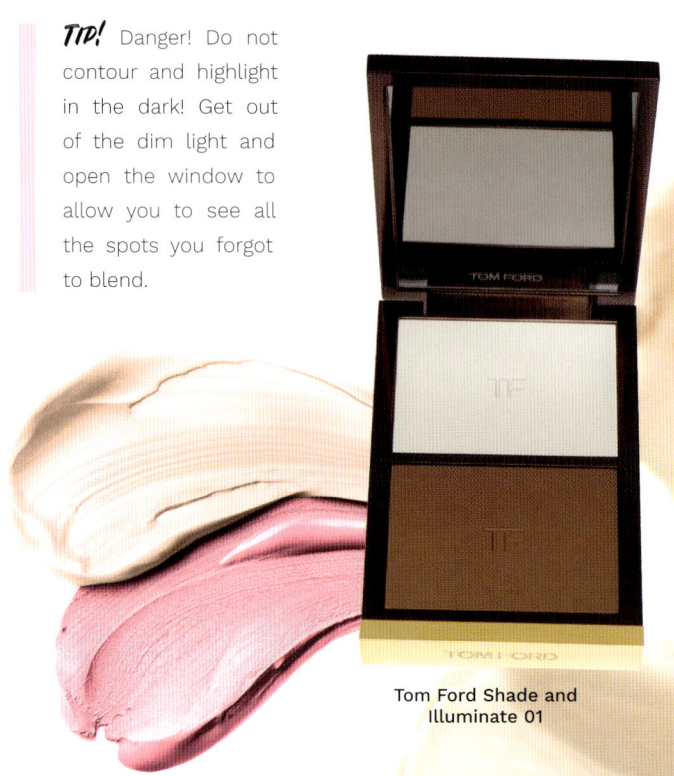

> **TIP!** Danger! Do not contour and highlight in the dark! Get out of the dim light and open the window to allow you to see all the spots you forgot to blend.

Tom Ford Shade and Illuminate 01

ALL ABOUT THAT BASE

Products Used In Step By Step

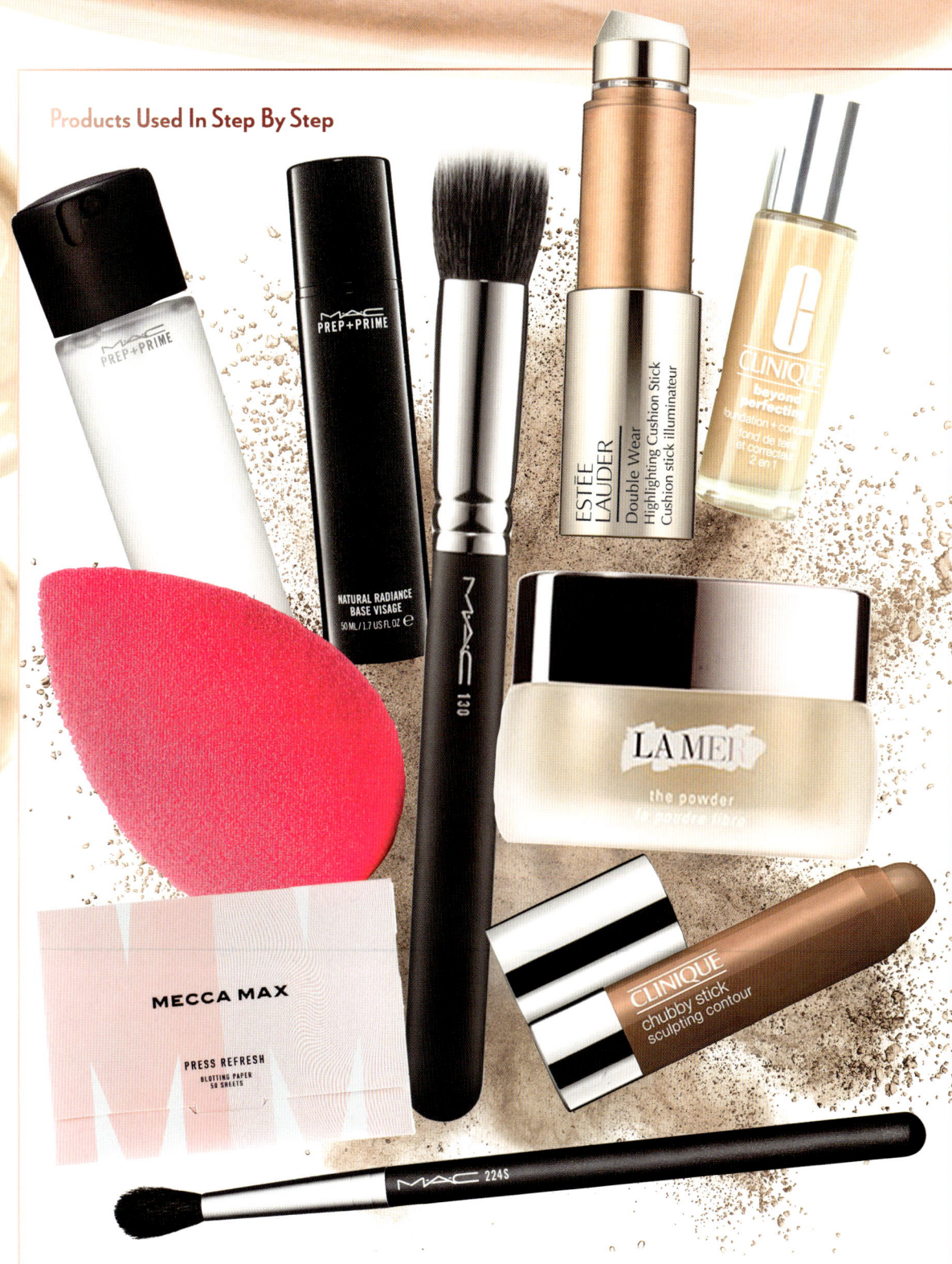

MAC Prep + Prime Fix+, MAC Prep + Prime Natural Radiance, Estée Lauder Double Wear Highlighting Cushion Stick in Champagne Glow, Clinique Beyond Perfecting Foundation And Concealer, Beautyblender sponge, MECCA MAX Press Refresh Blotting Paper, MAC 130 Brush, La Mer The Powder, loose, Clinique Chubby Stick Sculpting Contour, MAC 224 Brush

ALL ABOUT THAT BASE

AZLIN FROM CHADWICK MODELS

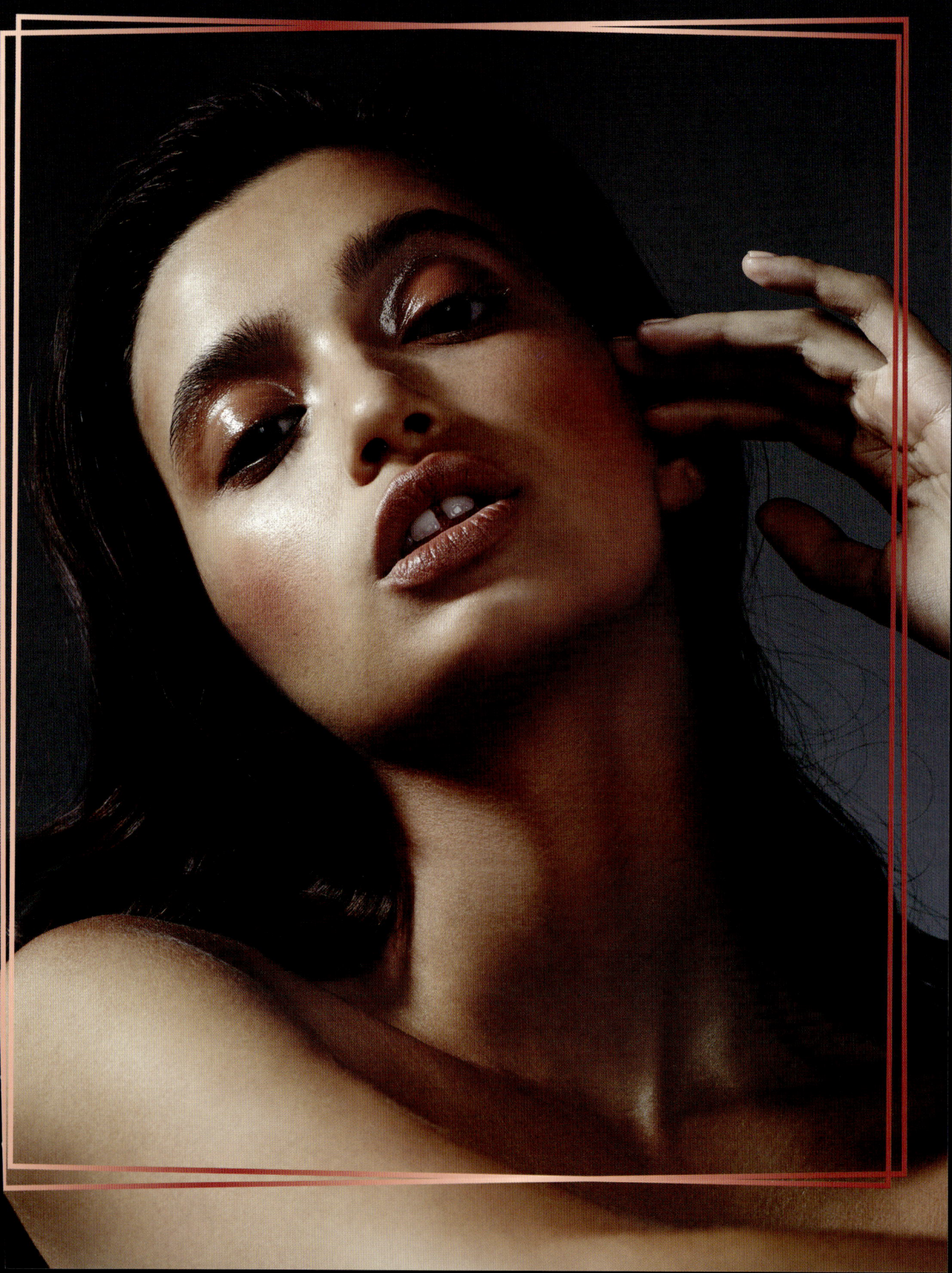

VELVET MATTE WITH HIGHLIGHTS

ALL ABOUT THAT BASE   67

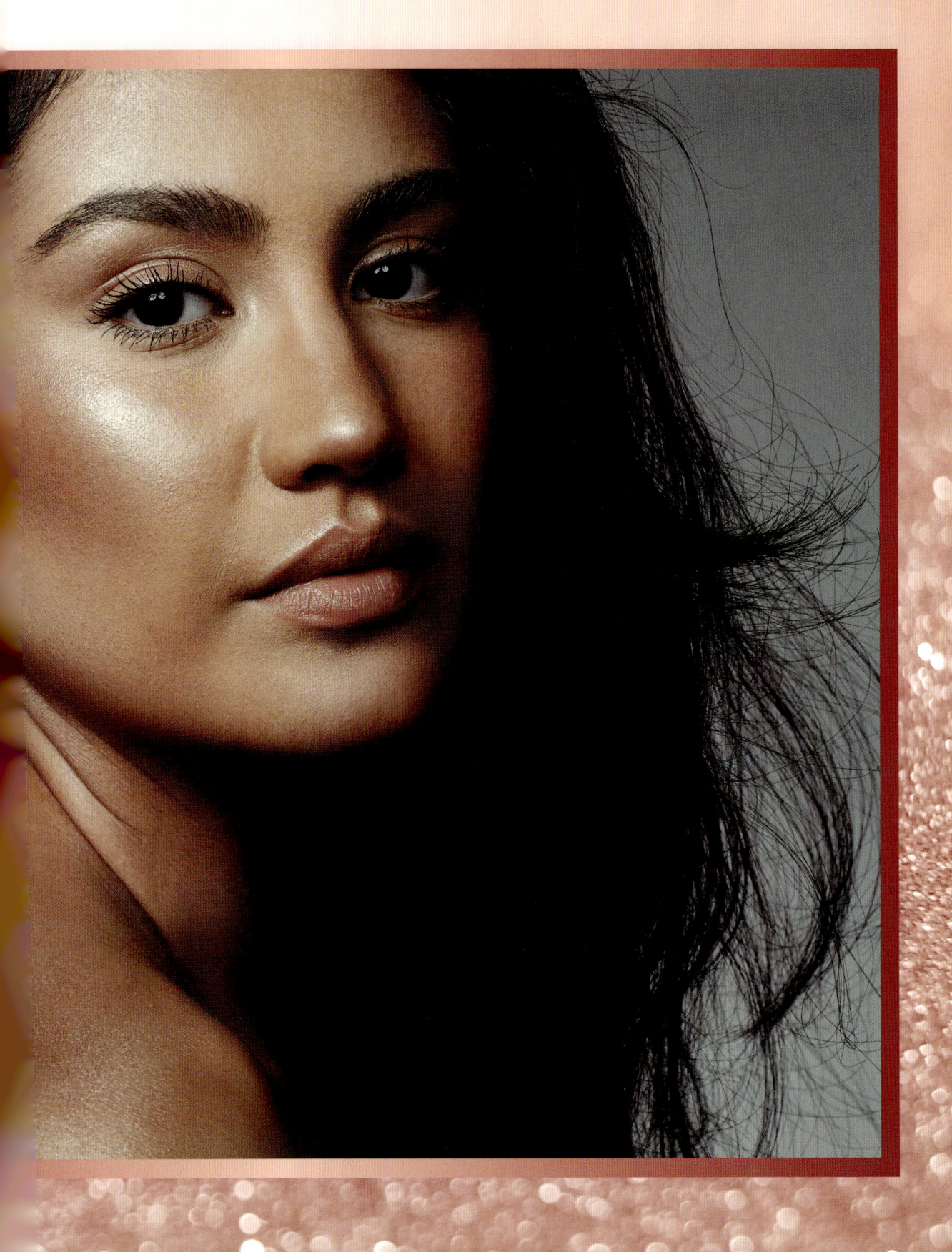

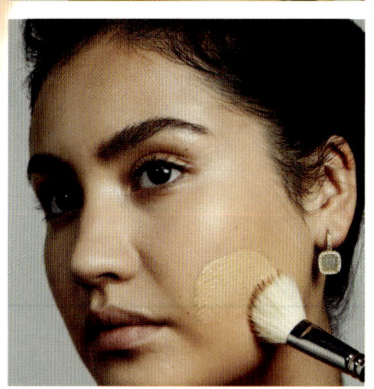

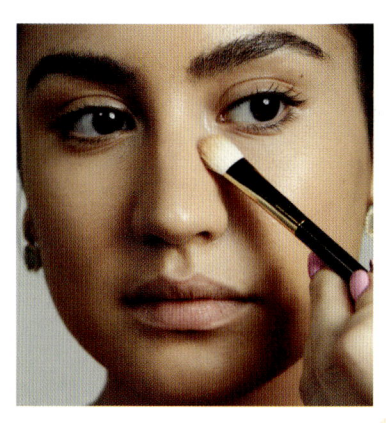

LAY THE FOUNDATION

STEP 1

Moisture is the key to all looks no matter the finish. So by now you are most likely sick of this whole hydration spray thing. Sorry, not sorry, honestly, it is my not-so-secret skin secret! This absorbs fast into the skin leaving it supple and smooth to the touch, it helps so much to get a smooth, matte makeup application, which without moisture will just be a patchy desert face. No good!

STEP 2

Pop on a matte oil controlling primer through the centre of the face with a large, soft eye shadow brush or the fingertips. Make sure to rub into under eyes, nostrils, around the mouth and between the brows for the smoothest possible base.

STEP 3

Next up matte full-coverage foundation! Exciting words to some, frightening for others. How do you build up a smooth, matte, full-coverage look without ending up with a finished look that a clown would be jealous of? LAYERS.

Buff in sheer layers of a foundation with a large soft brush over your entire face and décolletage. If you have dry skin spritz your face in between each layer of foundation to help it glide on and not dry with a flat and dull finish.

> ***TIP!*** Think of this like a great manicure. A good one lasts weeks because of the right base coat and three sheer layers built up to an opaque color rather than just chucking it on in one gluggy thick layer. Who wants gluggy foundation? Not me! So I encourage you to do the same with your foundie.

STEP 4

Smear on your concealer, in one shade lighter than the skin color, to the areas of the face you need to lighten and brighten. Use a

soft flat brush to stipple and lightly blend. Patting and stippling the product pushes it into the shine while retaining the coverage.

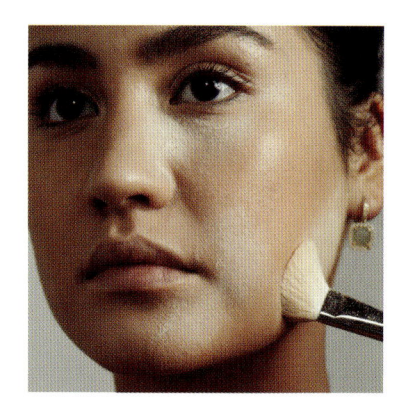

STEP 5

Give the skin another spritz with your hydrating spray and pat to make sure the products are not sitting on top of the skin, then go in with your powder. To get an immaculate matte base I love to double powder. Now this does not mean heavy, this means complete. Take a sheer loose powder all over the face with a fluffy brush. Tap it on blending away the excess and polishing it into the skin.

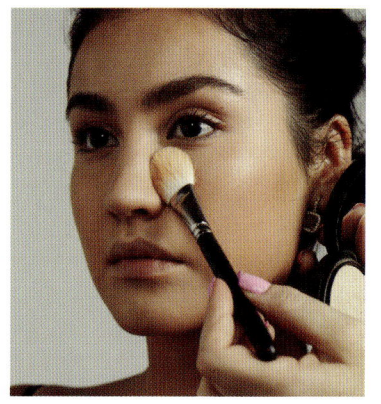

STEP 6

Now with a small brush apply a sheer, skin-colored powder through the center of the face where makeup tends to move during the day, to give you that extra coverage security blanket.

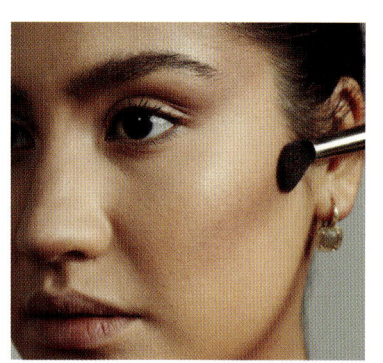

SHAPE IT

STEP 7

With a small powder brush or large eye shadow brush sweep the contour powder under the cheekbones, through the crease of the eye, up into the temples, down the sides of the nose, the corners of the forehead and just under the jawline.

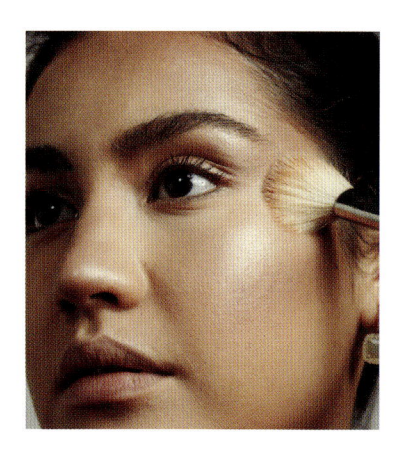

ENHANCE IT

STEP 8

With a damp brush, glide the powder highlighter over the skin hitting those cheekbones, brow bone (both under and above the brow), down the nose, over the lips and across the collarbones.

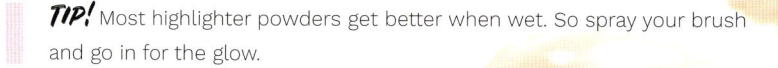

> *TIP!* Most highlighter powders get better when wet. So spray your brush and go in for the glow.

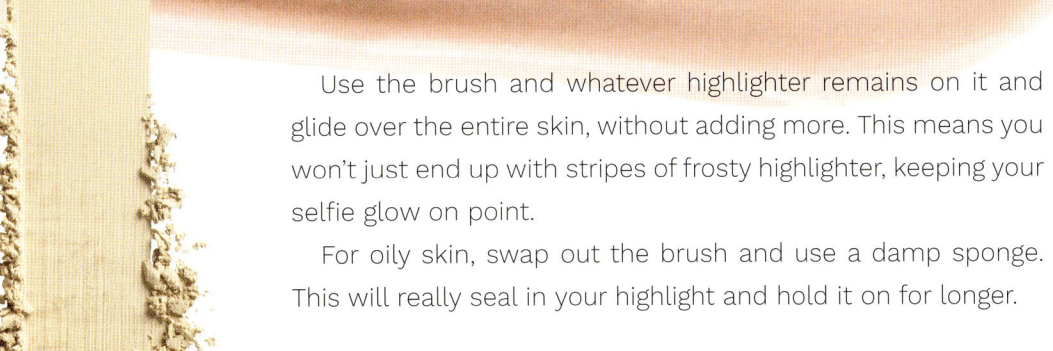

Use the brush and whatever highlighter remains on it and glide over the entire skin, without adding more. This means you won't just end up with stripes of frosty highlighter, keeping your selfie glow on point.

For oily skin, swap out the brush and use a damp sponge. This will really seal in your highlight and hold it on for longer.

TIP! When you want to get more shine, often you don't actually need to dig into your shiny powder for more product, you just need to wake up what you have applied! Simply dampen your brush and polish over the spots you have hit already – watch that shine double!

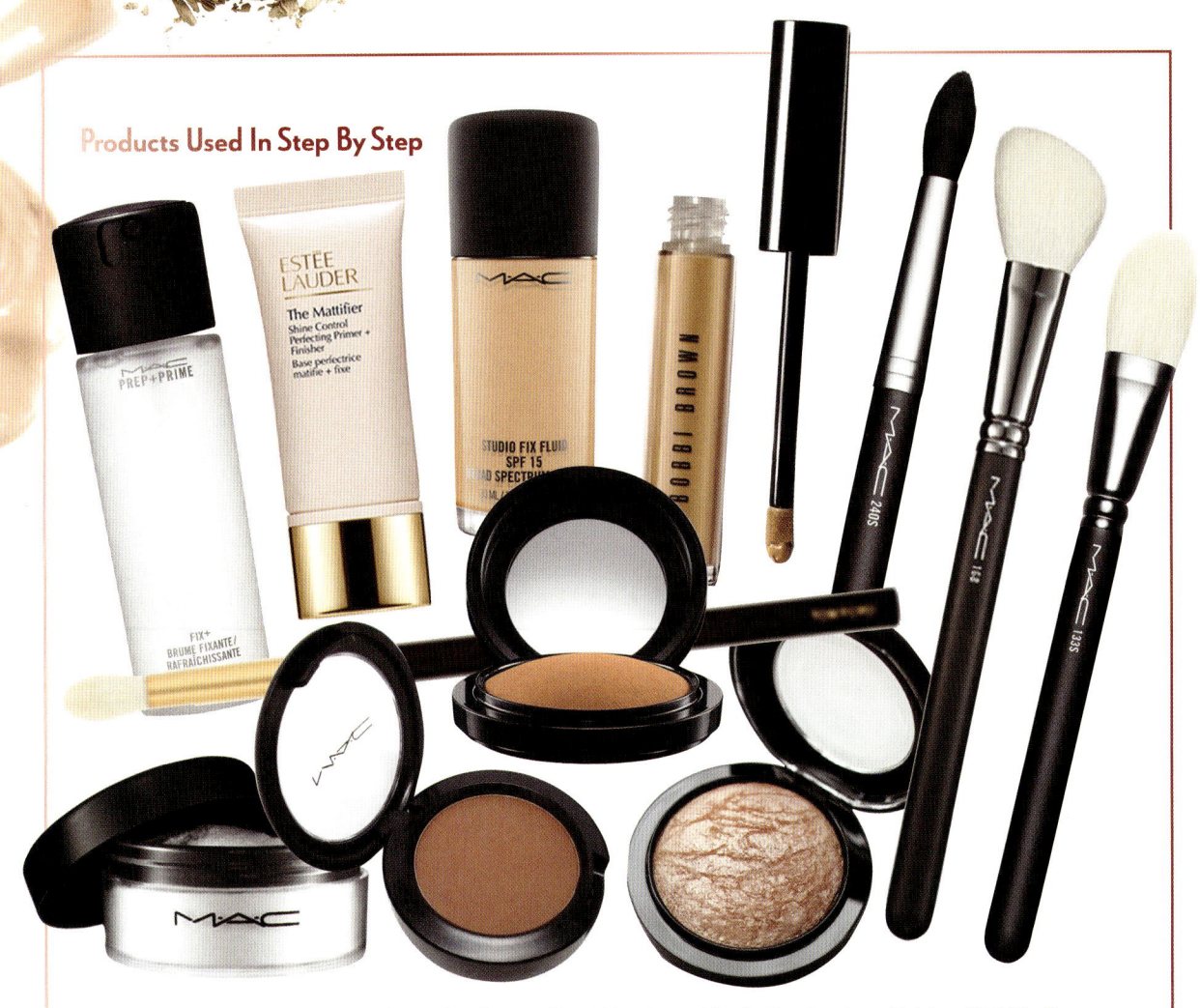

Products Used In Step By Step

MAC Prep + Prime Fix+, Estée Lauder The Mattifier, Shine Control Perfecting Powder + Finisher, MAC Studio Fix Fluid Foundation, Bobbi Brown Instant Full Cover Concealer, MAC 240, 168, 133 brushes, Tom Ford Eye Shadow Blend Brush, MAC Prep + Prime Transparent Finishing Powder, MAC Mineralize Skinfinish Powder in Natural, MAC Poweder Blush in Blunt, MAC Mineralize Skinfinish Powder in Soft and Gentle

TIARE FROM BELLA MANAGEMENT

ALL ABOUT THAT BASE

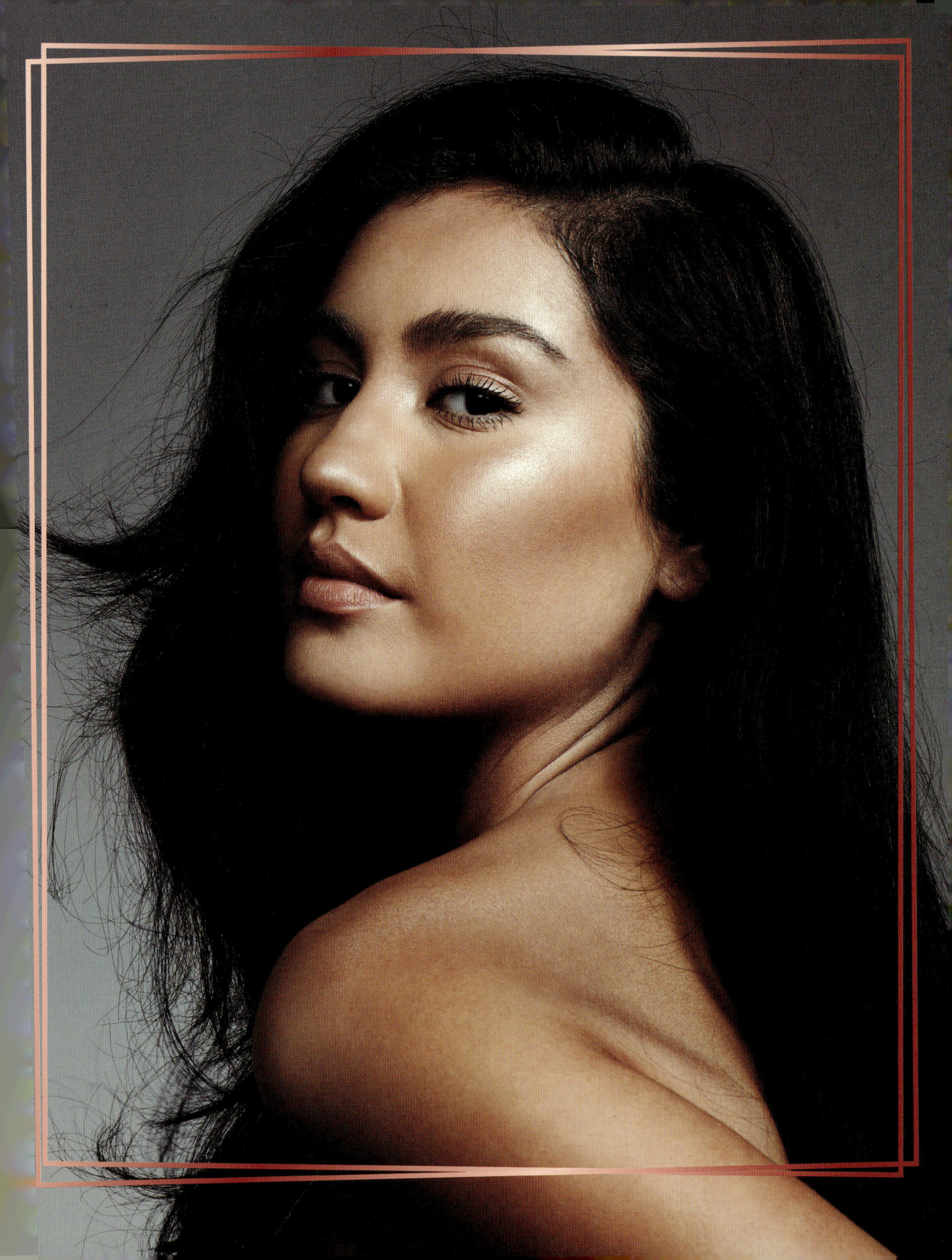

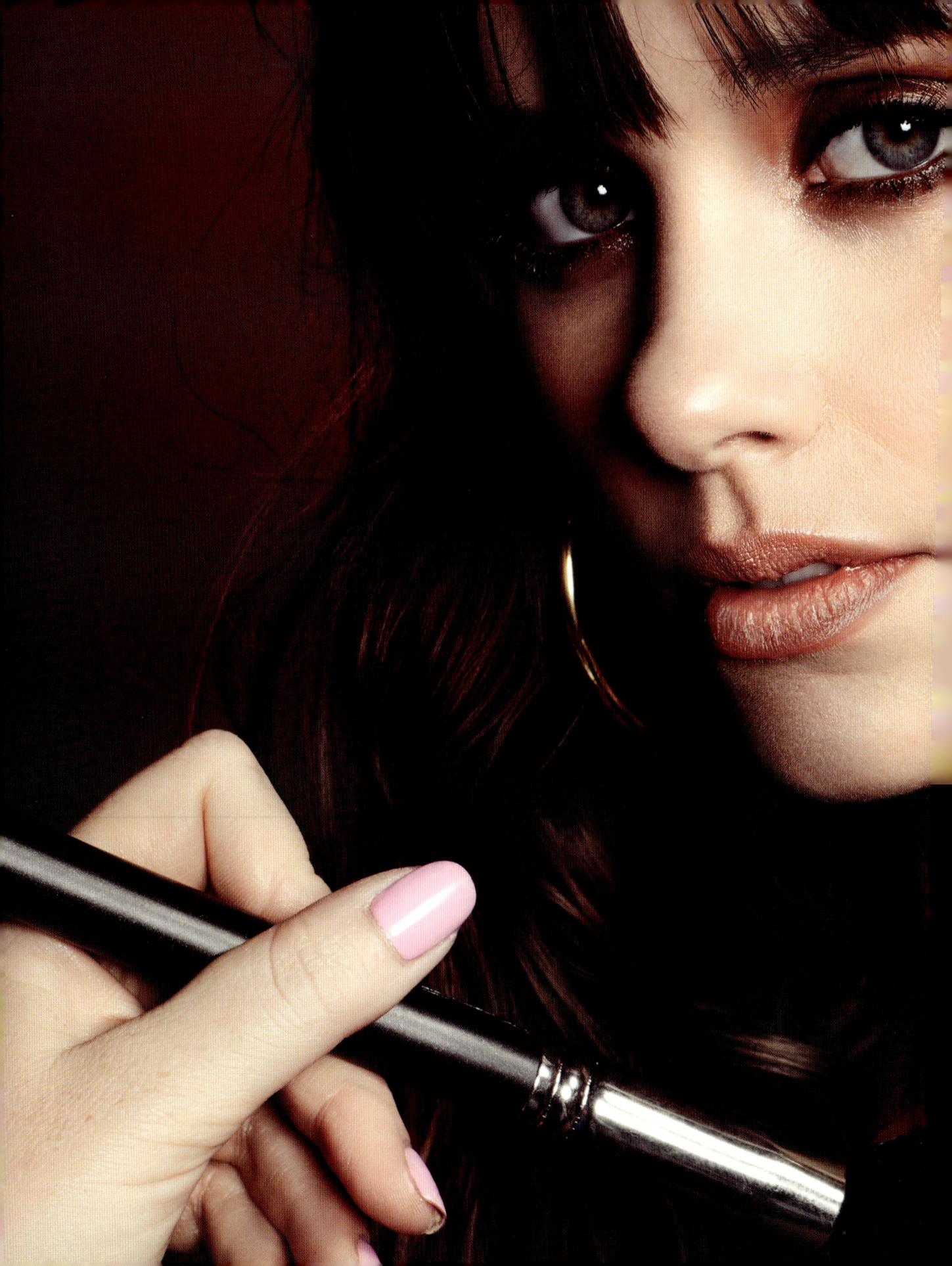

A body of work

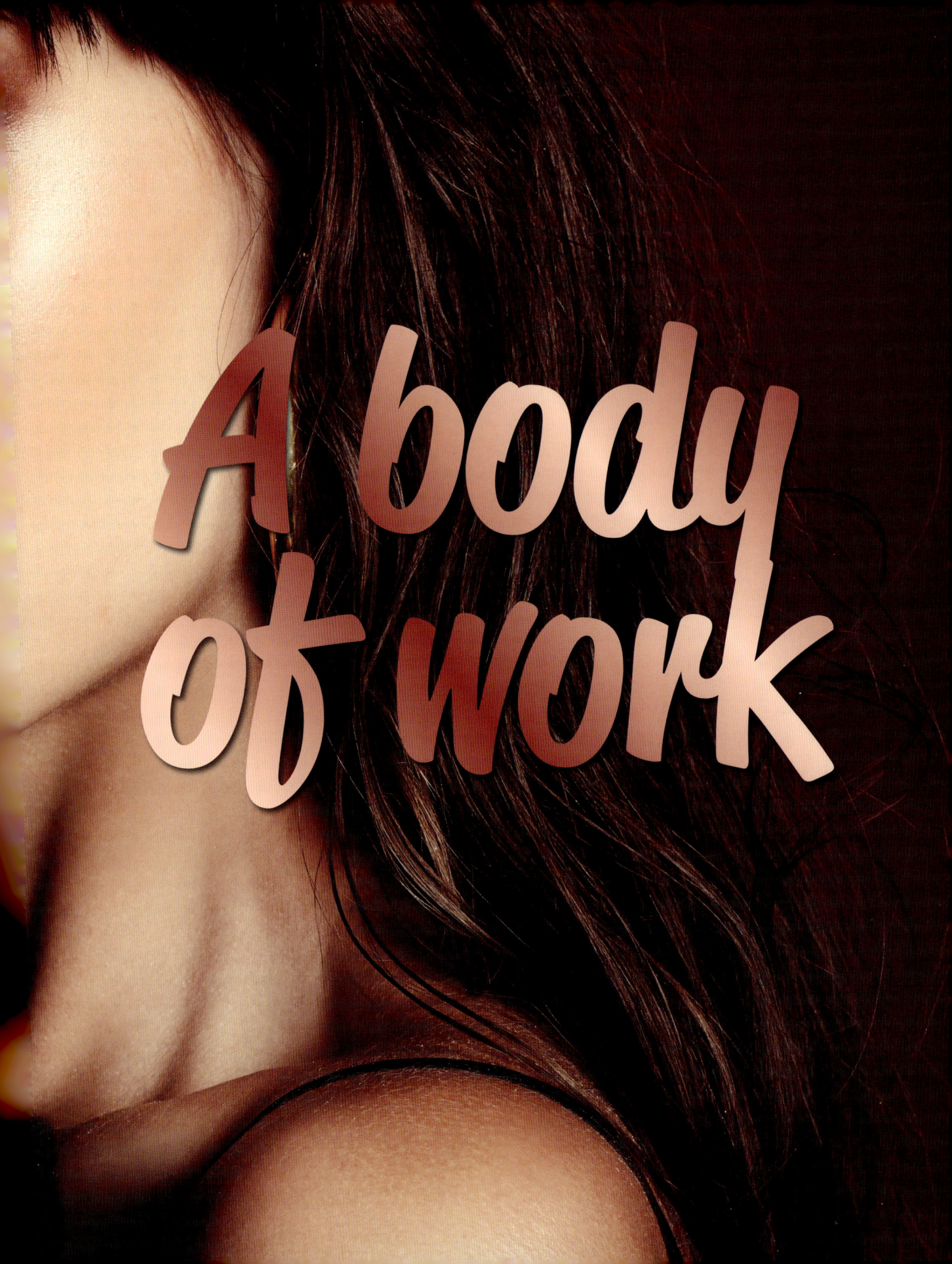

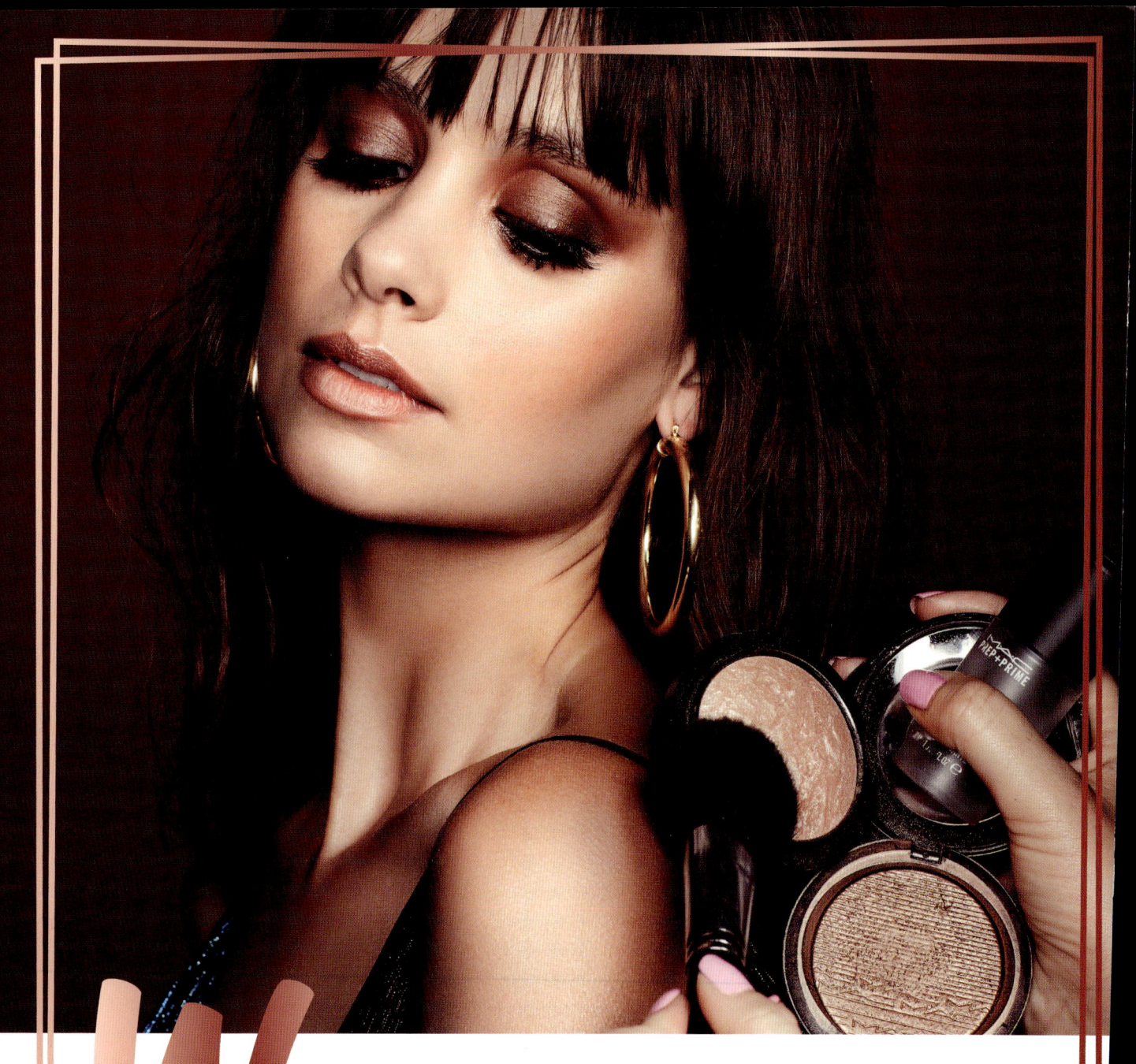

When you hear the words 'body makeup' you could be forgiven for instantly conjuring up thoughts of glitter painted-on abs. While I would hate to rain on your imaginary parade, it really is more about giving you a complete and flawless appearance from head to toe.

We spend so much money and time on skincare, masks, injections and treatments for our faces, why don't we apply the same attention to other exposed areas of our body? I'm certainly not suggesting that you should create a new makeup kit specifically for your body but you should definitely make it a part of your preparation rituals each day.

EMILIE FROM CHADWICK MODELS

A BODY OF WORK

Exfoliation

Continue that buffing and smoothing down onto the body! Just like the face, the results are instant and you will really notice your skin looking smoother with a tone more even for when you dare to bare. Grab yourself a body scrub and take a moment to do it once a week, or make your own scrub! I love to mix sugar with some olive, almond or coconut oil, creating a deliciously effective body scrub. Scrubbing with purpose, I concentrate on the knees, elbows, shoulders and legs.

You don't always have to have a separate body scrub or wash, you can simply use your favorite soap with one of my personal favorites, exfoliating gloves. These gloves work so well to gently exfoliate and work just as well on the body as they do on small areas of the face like the lips.

Exfoliating doesn't always need to be a wet experience either. Grab yourself a face and body dry brush to really polish your skin all the way to sparkling!

TIP!
Now that you are exfoliating every inch of your body that you can reach, don't neglect the body part doing all the scrubbing – your hands! Whether you are shaking hands, holding hands or posing with a peace sign for Instagram, dry and flaky is something you will want to avoid.

Aveda Beautifying Radiance Polish, Clinique Sparkle Skin Body Exfoliating Cream, Aveda Tulasara Radiant Facial Dry Brush, Exfoliating gloves, Oil and sugar exfoliator mix

A BODY OF WORK 75

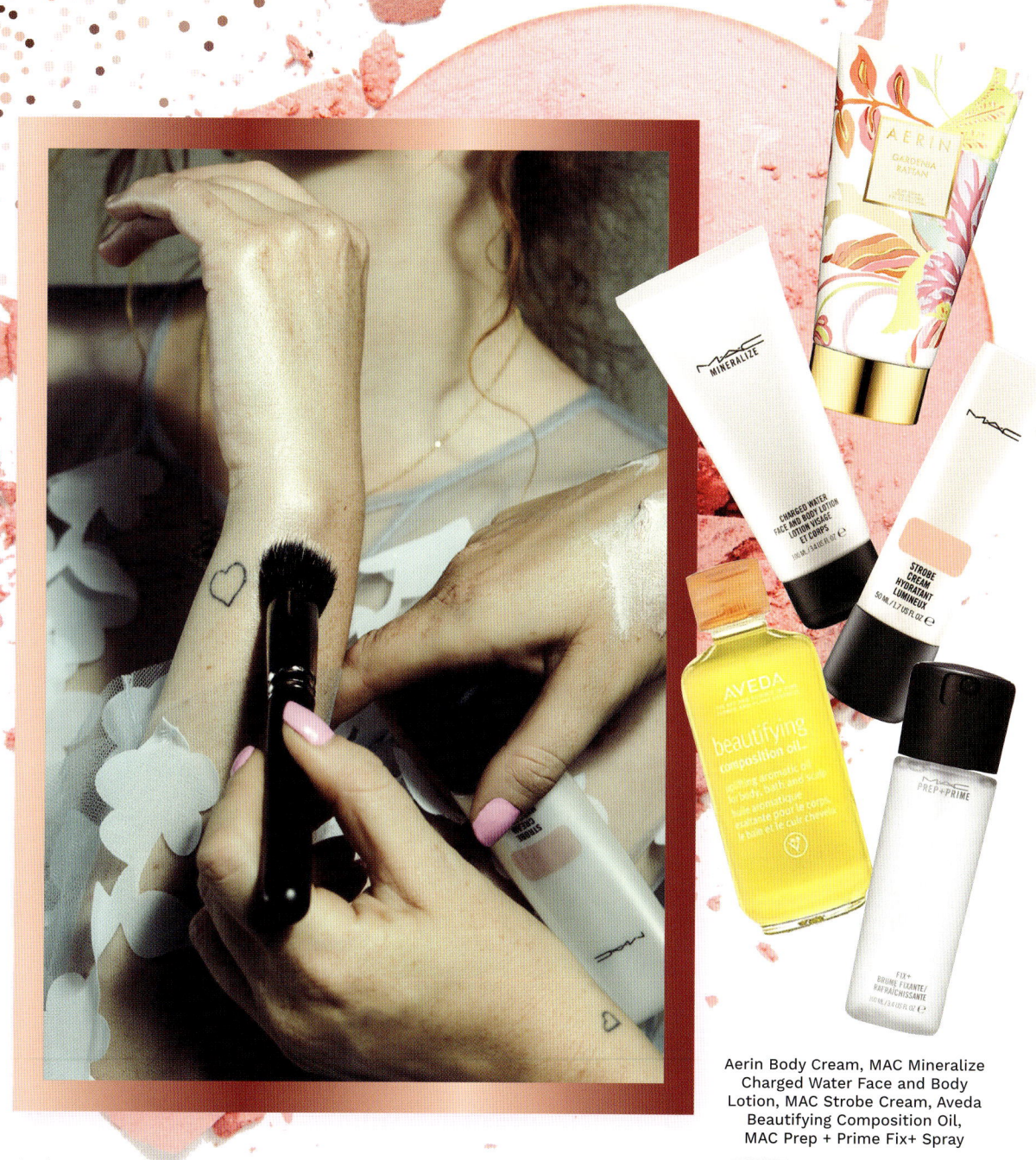

Aerin Body Cream, MAC Mineralize Charged Water Face and Body Lotion, MAC Strobe Cream, Aveda Beautifying Composition Oil, MAC Prep + Prime Fix+ Spray

Moisturizing

Hydration is the not so secret secret to young skin, so why do we forget?! We all have 30 seconds to slap some moisturizer onto our bodies when we get out of the shower. Try to do it every day if you can, every week at the very least. You will definitely notice the difference.

TIP!
I love to add a few drops of my face oil into my body cream. I'm a once a week kind of gal so I need all the help I can get!

A BODY OF WORK

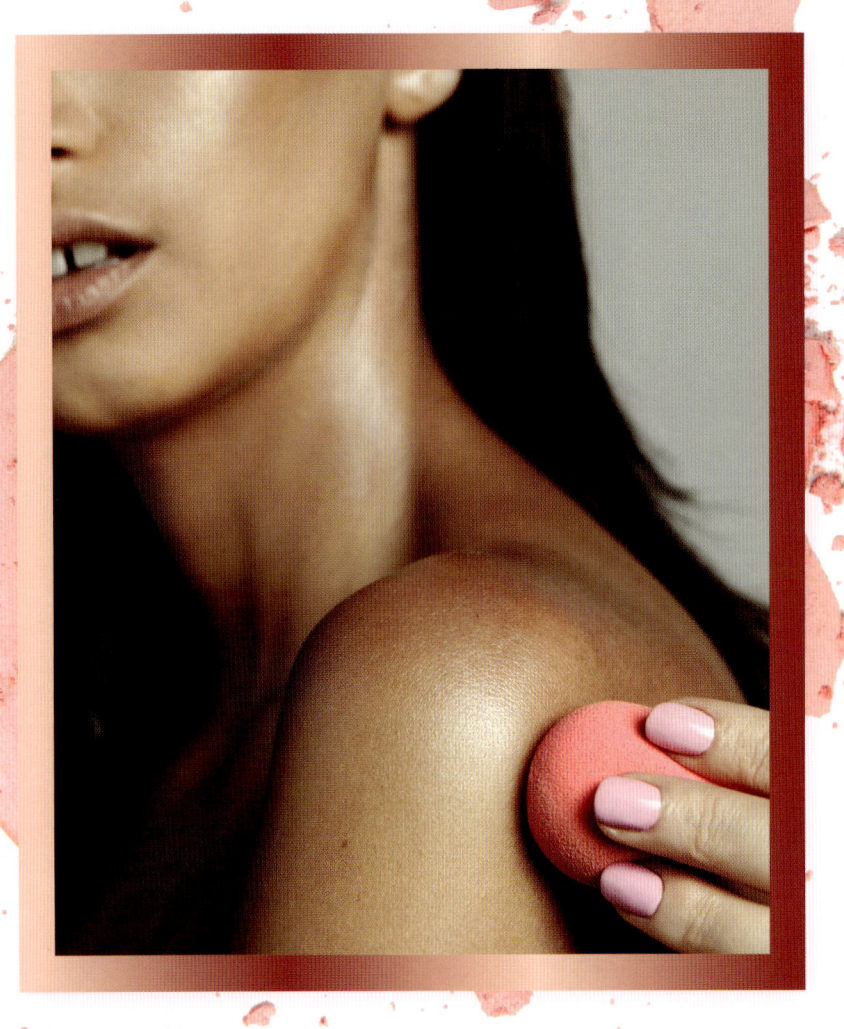

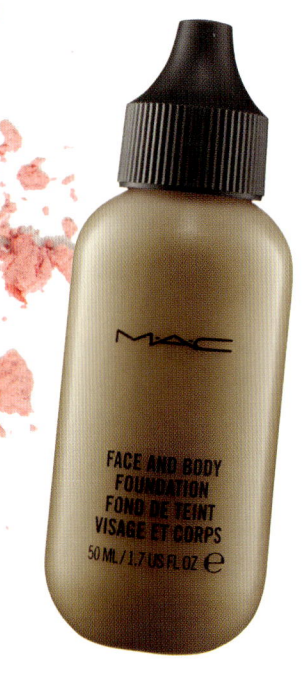

MAC Studio Face and
Body Foundation

Foundation

Let me introduce you to an iconic, long-time backstage product for *perfect* bodies on the catwalk, red carpet and on set – the waterproof MAC face and body foundation. It is undoubtedly the unsung hero of my makeup kit.

Being sheer in texture it will not look like you have taken a bath in a tub of foundation. Nobody has time for that. If you have matched it to your skin you will look like you are wearing a body stocking! Go one to two shades darker to give you a healthy boost of color.

TIP!
I have been caught out before a media appearance and realized I had forgotten to pack my body makeup. Just mix some of your foundation and moisturizer (hotel cream if you are like me!) to even out body skin tone.

A BODY OF WORK

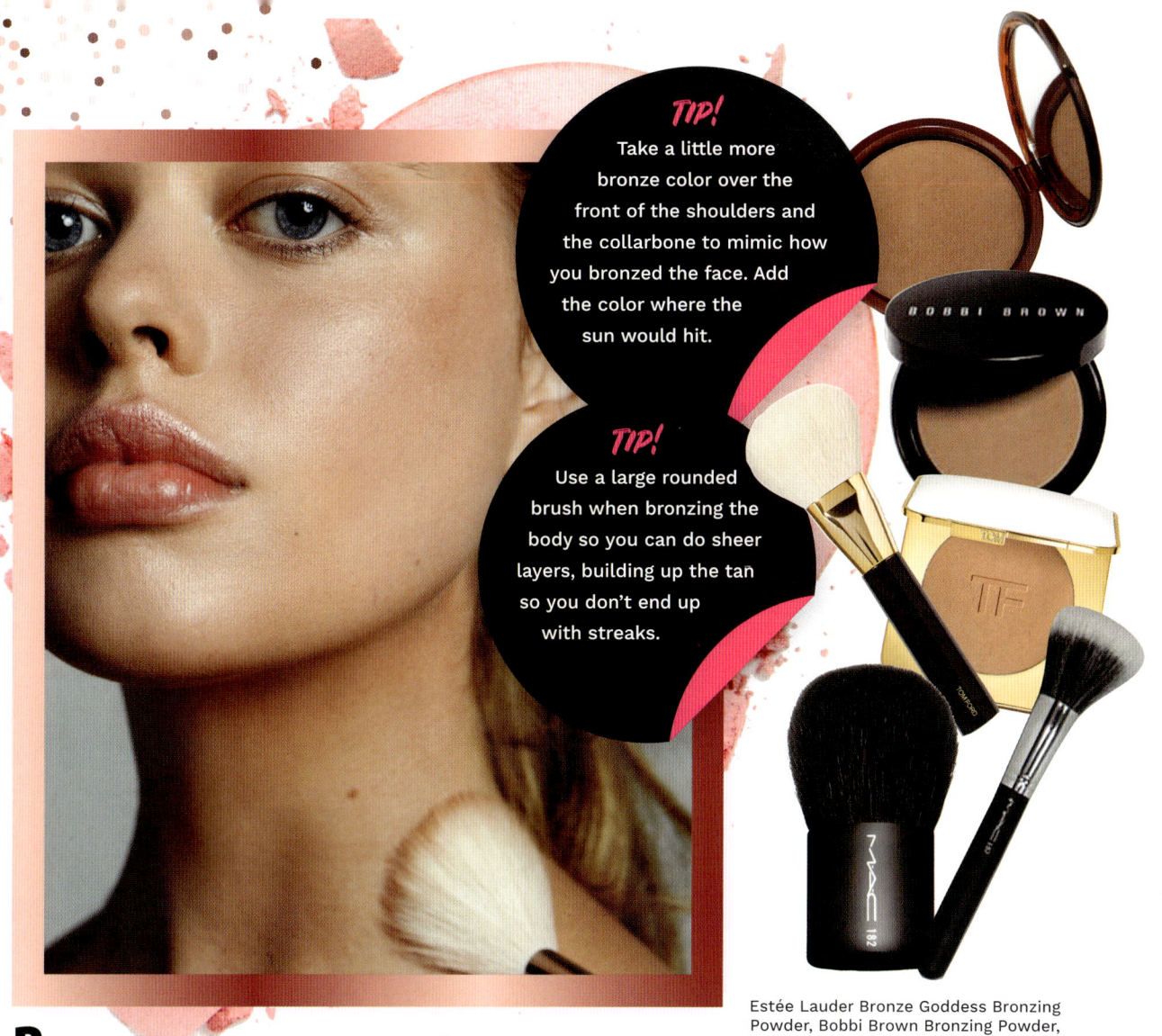

TIP!
Take a little more bronze color over the front of the shoulders and the collarbone to mimic how you bronzed the face. Add the color where the sun would hit.

TIP!
Use a large rounded brush when bronzing the body so you can do sheer layers, building up the tan so you don't end up with streaks.

Bronzing

Estée Lauder Bronze Goddess Bronzing Powder, Bobbi Brown Bronzing Powder, Tom Ford Large Bronzing Powder, Tom Ford Bronzer Brush 05, MAC 187 and 182 brushes

Your bronzer is the marriage between your body and your face. If you have tanned your body, spreading your bronzer over your face before makeup will stop white floating-head syndrome! It's the same the other way around – if you have bronzed and contoured your face, you *must* take it down the neck on onto the décolletage.

Under our jawline and the top of the neck are usually the most pale. Blend your powder or cream color down the neck and across your shoulders, concentrating the color onto the bone structure before blending outwards with a fluffy brush to avoid streaks or edges.

TIP!
When you are tanning your body, run a small amount of the tanner over moisturized facial skin to lightly tint the face the same color as the body. This will give you a head start in matching the color with your bronzer and make the whole thing a lot easier!

A BODY OF WORK

Highlighting

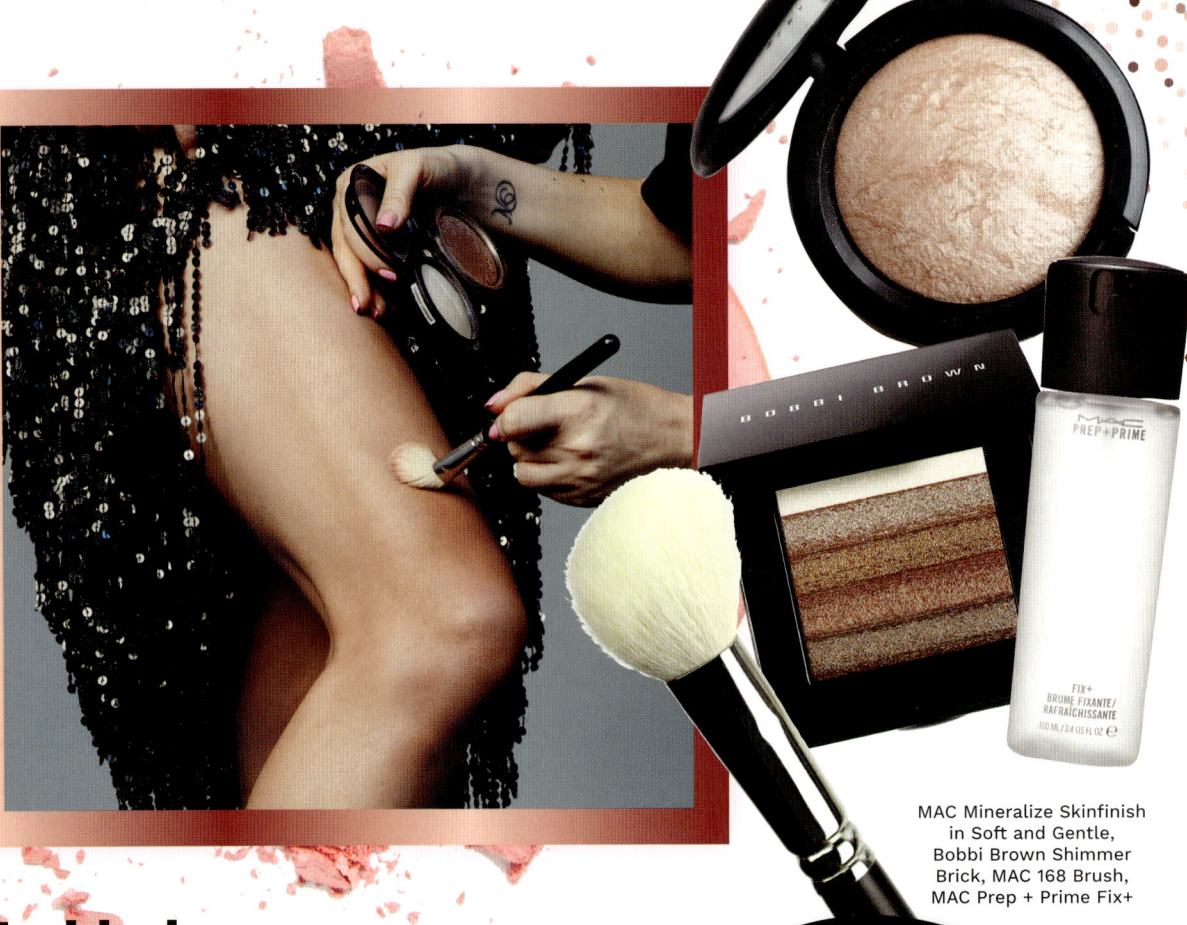

Highlighting on the body has become just as important as the makeup to my clients. Just like with the face, we highlight the parts of the body we want to bring forward, on top of the bone structure. Before I leave any wedding, I make sure that the bride's shoulders are gleaming and her hands are smooth and shiny ready to show off that new ring! I check that the legs look the same color as the face and they have the same sheen.

Backstage at fashion week, we take it up another notch. Before I let any of the models set foot on that catwalk, I make sure that we have highlighted every muscle they have exposed, particularly arms and legs. Brush the highlighter onto clenched muscles – flex your arm and highlight what shows, clench your leg and do the same! In photos you will look slimmer and more toned – winner!

MAC Mineralize Skinfinish in Soft and Gentle, Bobbi Brown Shimmer Brick, MAC 168 Brush, MAC Prep + Prime Fix+

TIP!
Applying cream illuminator with a fluffy brush will give a glossy shine to the skin. Mix it with a little body moisturizer to sheer it out if it is too frosted for you. Choose a powder highlighter with a damp brush for that impressive mannequin shine we have created in the opening image!

Bigger is not always better

If you want something to stand out that little bit more, like your collarbones or shoulders, use your finger or a smaller brush to run the highlighter along that feature – it will apply a more intense amount of shine to that specific spot!

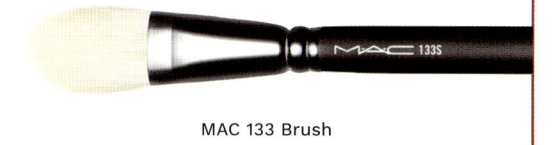

MAC 133 Brush

Oily goodness

Like to be a little more natural with your highlight? Body oil as a finishing touch over the bone structure works a treat. The excess absorbs and you are just left with subtly glossed skin. For added gleam, use a body oil with a shimmer within it.

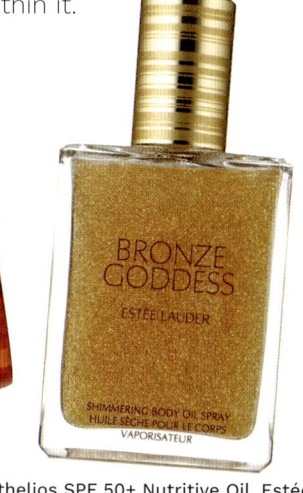

La Roche-Posay Anthelios SPF 50+ Nutritive Oil, Estée Lauder Bronze Goddess Shimmering Body Oil Spray

Fake it till you make it!

Beach ready! While I would love to be on the beach au natural looking fabulous, my pasty white skin needs a little help! I like to mix some illuminizer in with my sunscreen to make me feel a lot better up against all these tanned beach bodies.

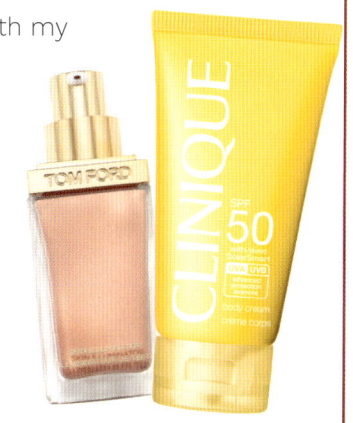

Tom Ford Skin Illuminator, Clinique Body Cream SPF 50

Get creative!

Don't be afraid to mix and get crafty! Do you have a face mist? Yes! Do you have a shimmer eye shadow or loose pigment? Yes. Shake some of the shimmer up in that bottle and go bananas spritzing your body!

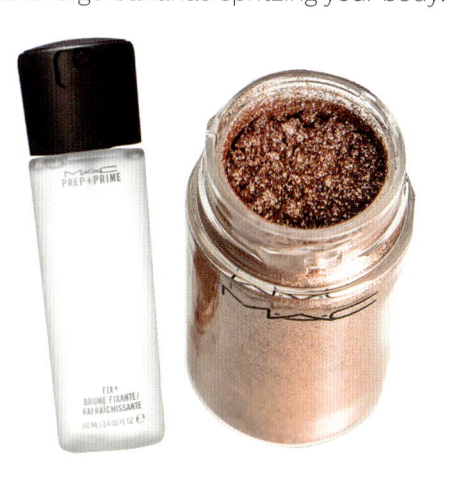

MAC Prep + Prime Fix+, MAC Pigment in Tan

A BODY OF WORK

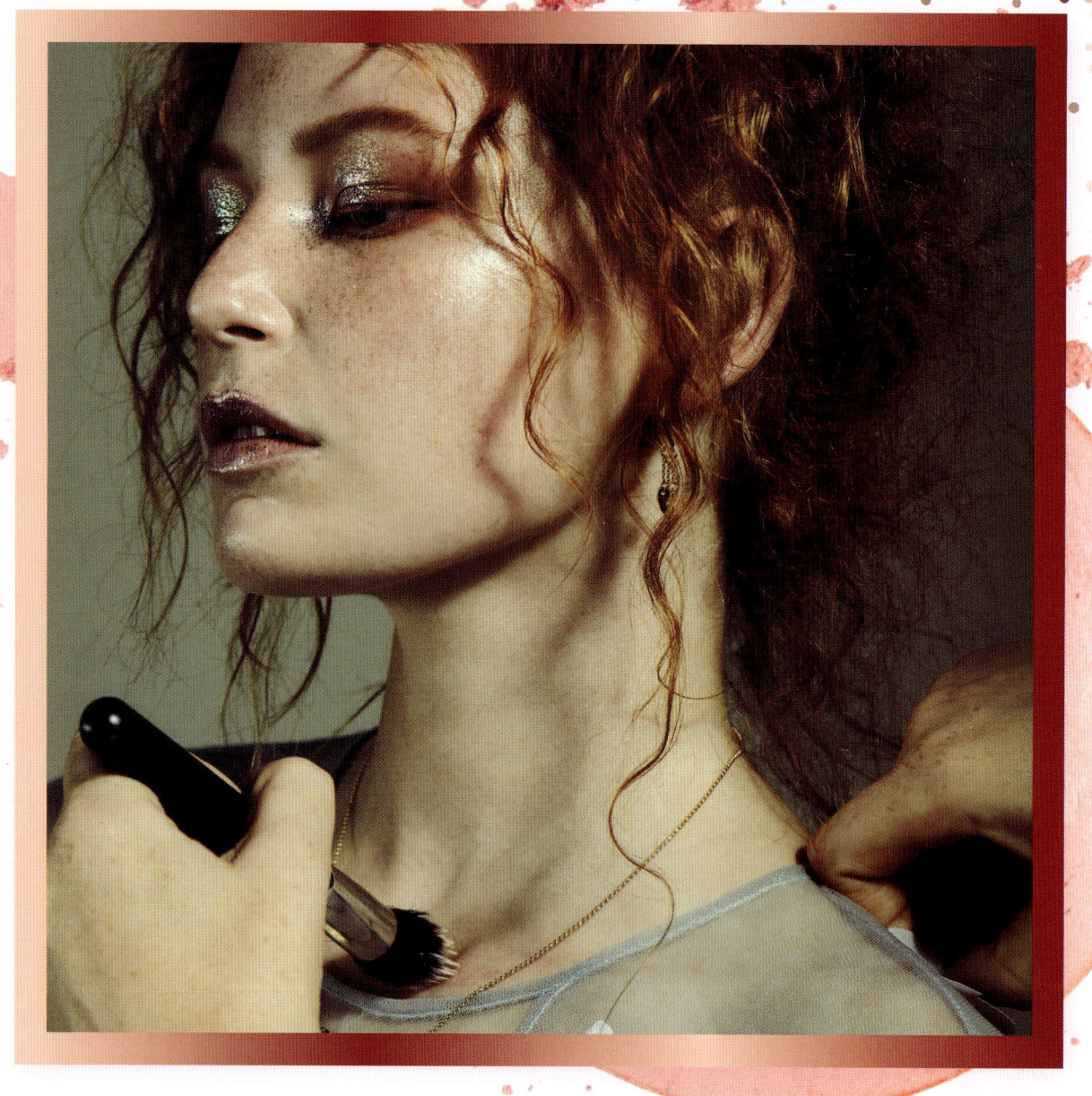

Keep It Consistent

Whatever finish you have on the face, continue it onto the body! For me in makeup, there is nothing weirder in a photo than a perfect matte face with a shiny body. When I am doing makeup on a client, I literally follow them on to set with all the same skin products (face powder, highlighter, moisturizer etc.), I wait to see what skin is showing, and then I take those same products to hit every bit of exposed skin!

Keep in mind I am talking about the challenge of close up high definition photography – real life is much simpler!

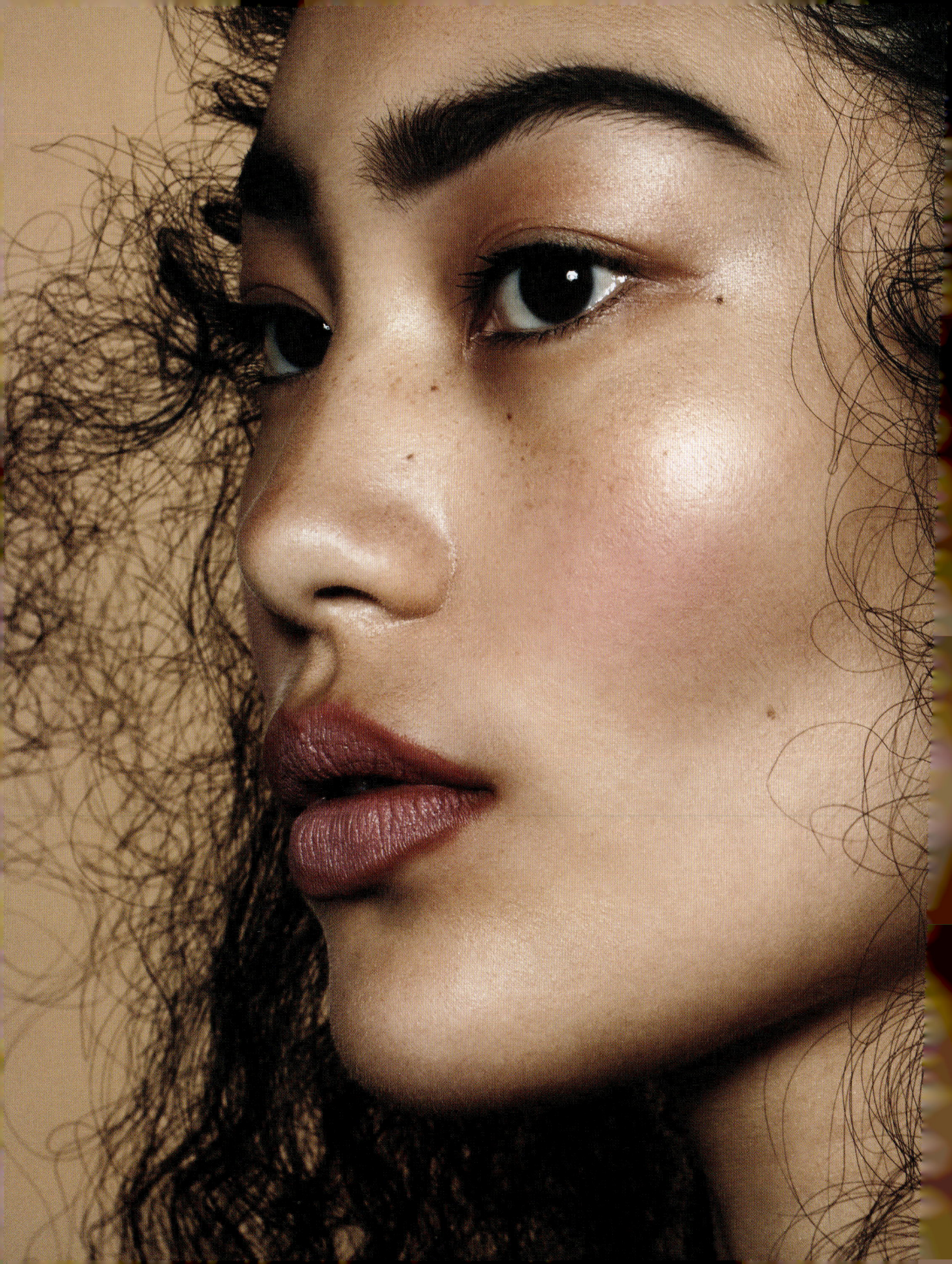

Brows like a boss

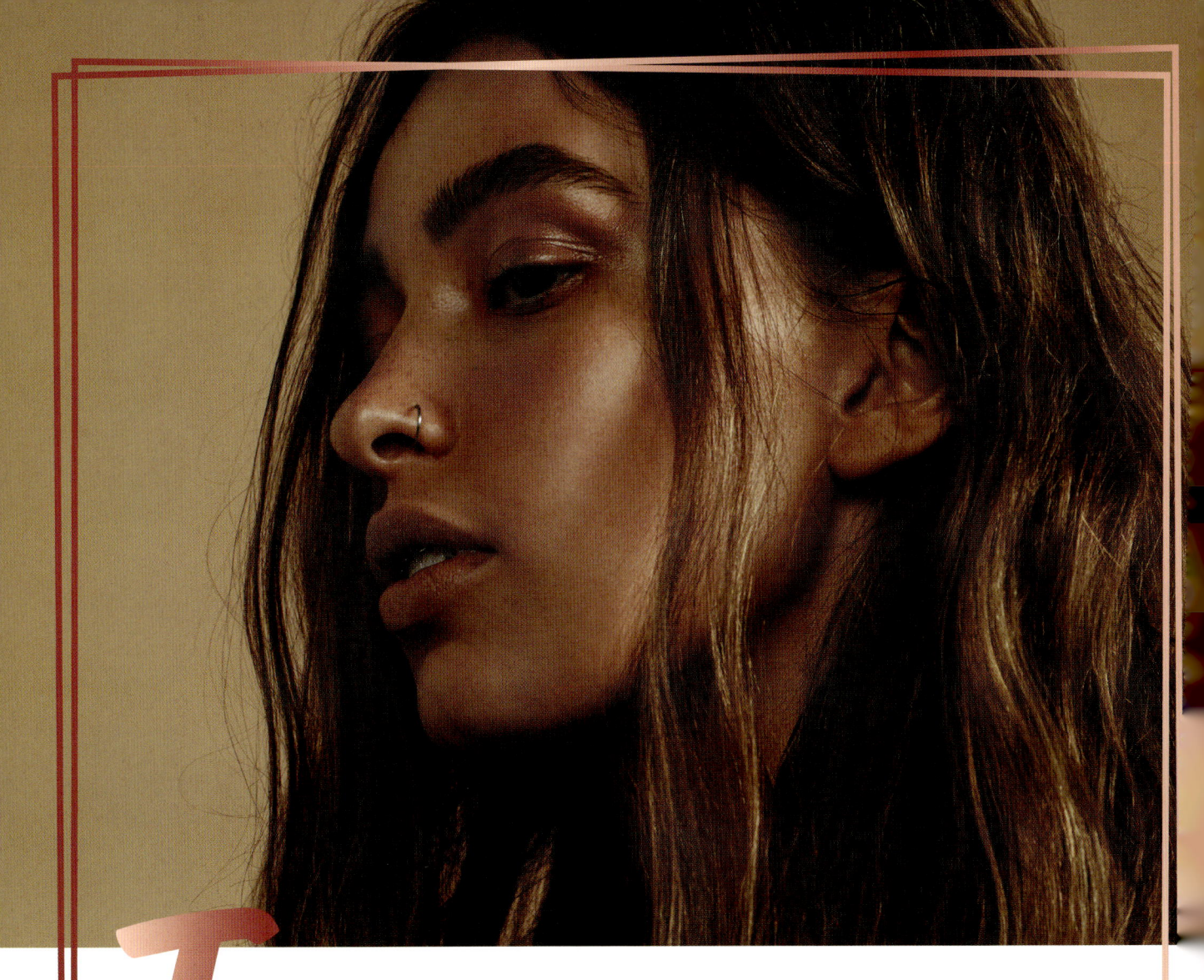

If eyes are the windows to your soul then brows are the frames or window to your personality for that day! You can alter said personality with the flick of a brush. Changing up the technique of your brow game can take you from softly defining your features to bold defined power brows to give you that 'I'm ready to ask for that pay rise' kind of look.

I woke up one morning to the latest makeup 'trend', it was called the halo brow. This brow consisted of a brow, where the line continued to form a semicircle on one's forehead. This is not on trend people, this is outrageous! Some other faves include the 'squiggle brow', where brows are replaced by a squiggly pencil thin-line and then there are the ever-complex 'plaited brows', which while incredibly skillful to execute, look as though some braided weaves have fallen down your forehead.

Now please don't let my 'judgy face' stifle your creativity. Remember, the only rule is there are no rules, but for me *shape and color choice* are the two most important things to consider when it comes to creating great brows.

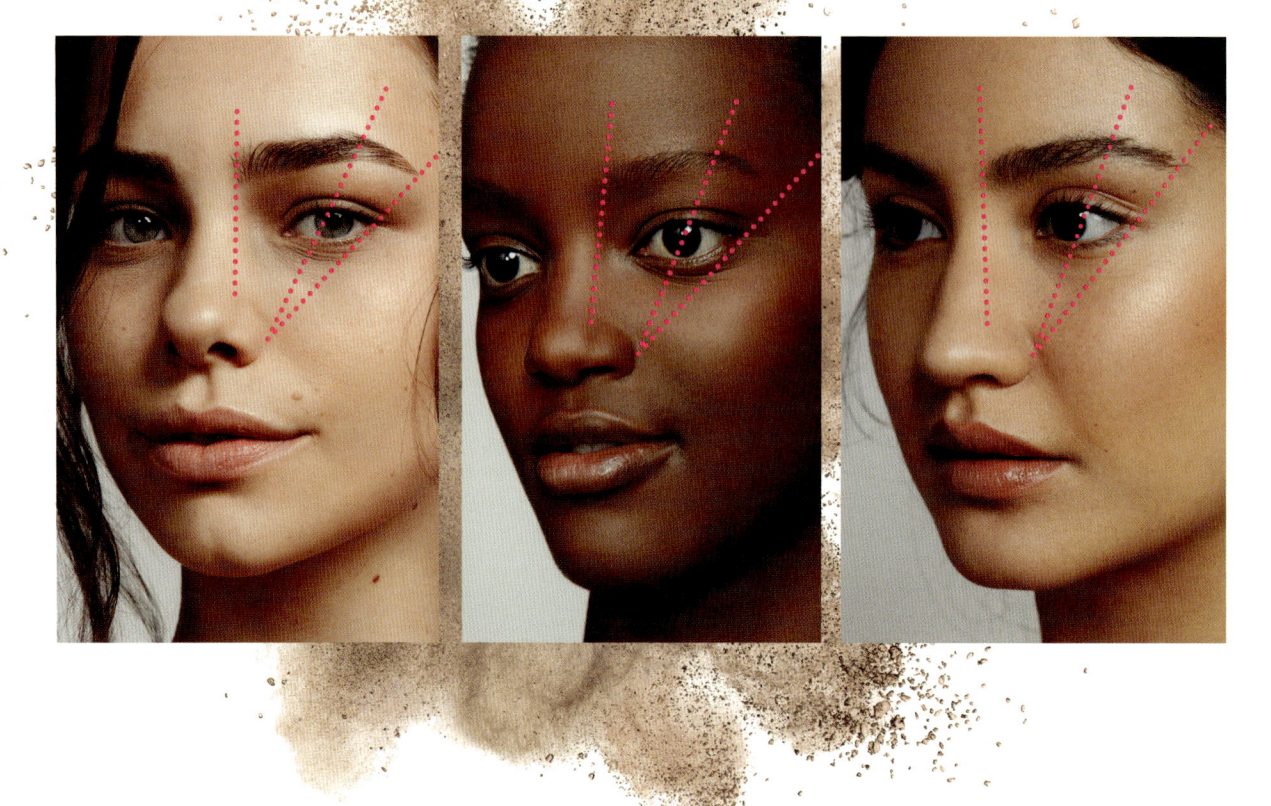

Shape

I have seen many a brow shape in my time (many of them were different shapes on my own face over the years – eek!) and what I have noticed is that this tried and true shaping technique has worked on them all as it uses YOUR face as the guide!

See the lines on the faces above to see how the diagram works with each face. To apply the three main points on your own face, use a pencil or makeup brush as your guide.

1. Imagine a vertical line that goes from the side of your nostril straight up – this is where your brow should begin.
2. Now imagine another line going from your nostril straight up through the pupils of your eyes and this will give you the point of the brow arch.
3. Another line starting at the nostril and this time running diagonally outward skimming the outer corner of your eyes will show you where your brow should end.

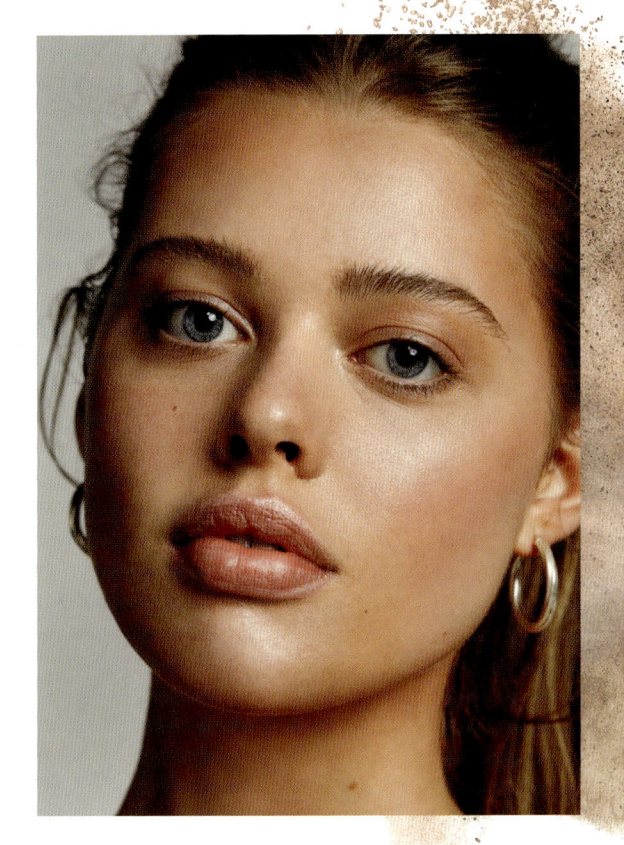

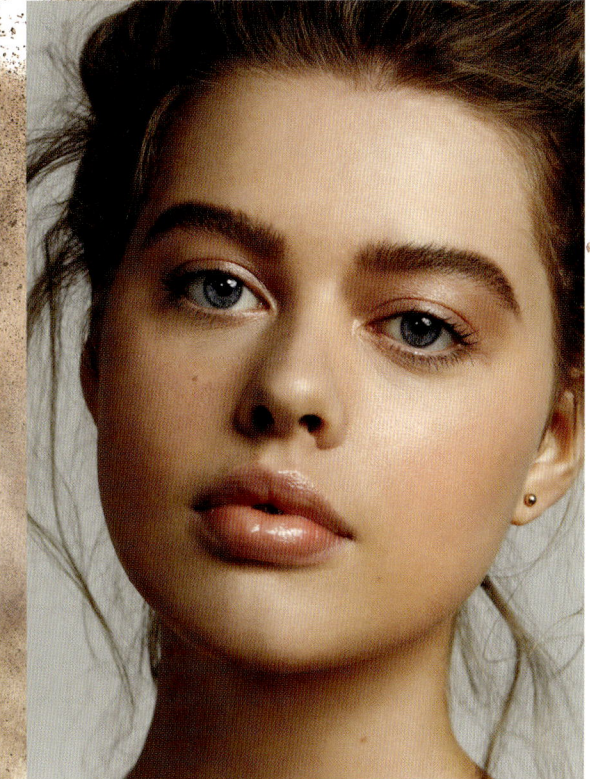

Do a tiny dot of brow product at each position point, and there you have your guideline! BAM!

Now time to add your brow product. Whether using a pencil, shadow or crème product, the basis of your brow shape should remain the same. It is super difficult to take the brows back to natural after you have applied so much product in them that you could be an extra in *The Muppet Show*. Build color as you go. Beware of long dark lines, instead start with soft strokes of color that mimic the hair growth, following that guide line while slowly making the shape wider and longer as you go.

Step back from your mirror and check – and then stop when you are happy!

I love to do the brows *first*, when it comes to color on the face. Adding them first will give you the framework for your eye makeup, and really the rest of your face as well, so you don't look and feel color-heavy at the end.

Remember: The more you practice the better you get! (This applies to most things in life! No-one is just born knowing how to ski, am I right?)

Color Choice

There are more than just light, medium and dark hair colors in this world! Thank god we now have so much choice when it comes to products and the colors they offer. Use this as a guide for color tone, but remember always try before you buy any makeup!

Just like the hair on our head, there are many colors running through the hairs in our brows. I find that using at least two colors works well to accurately impersonate your natural brow. One shade that is lighter than the brow hairs to build up shape, and the other the same color as your brow hairs to add depth for a more realistic brow.

If you do the whole thing with a light color, it won't give you the defined shape you are after, and if you attack with only a dark color, your look will be heavy and may give you an angry look that many may mistake for a 'resting bitch face'.

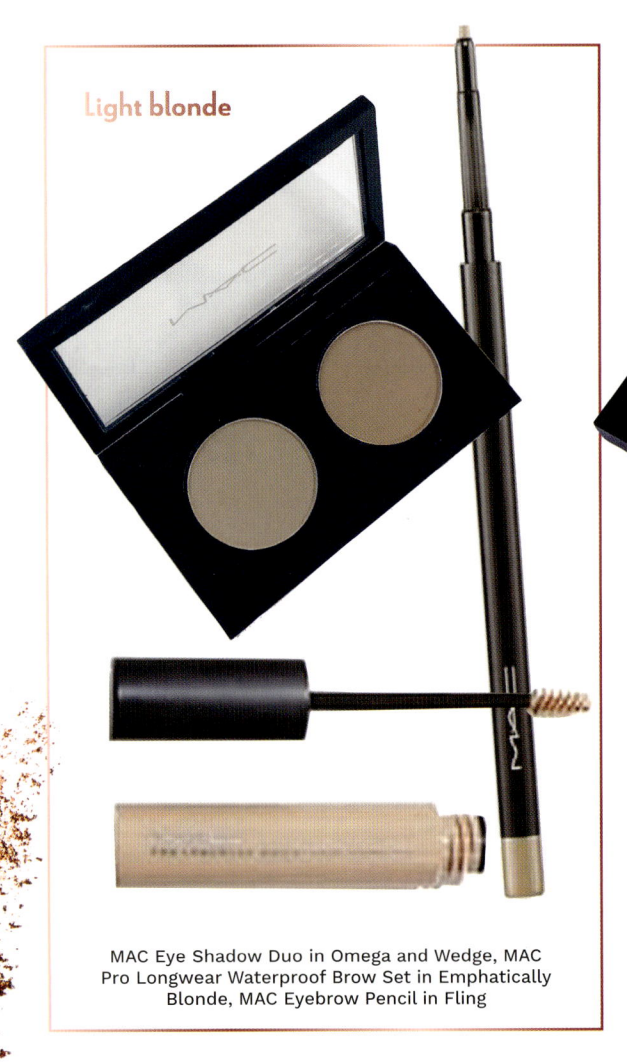

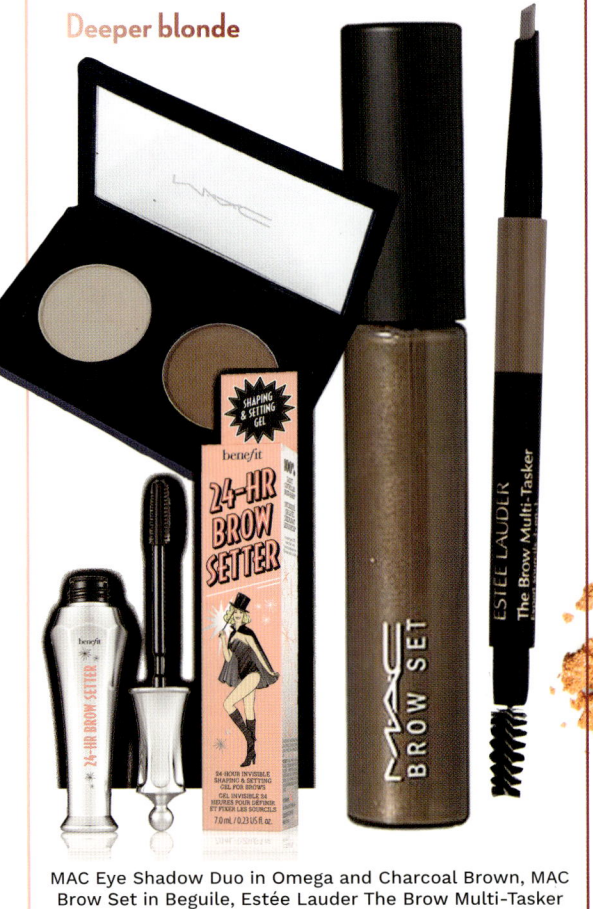

Light blonde

MAC Eye Shadow Duo in Omega and Wedge, MAC Pro Longwear Waterproof Brow Set in Emphatically Blonde, MAC Eyebrow Pencil in Fling

Deeper blonde

MAC Eye Shadow Duo in Omega and Charcoal Brown, MAC Brow Set in Beguile, Estée Lauder The Brow Multi-Tasker in Blonde, Benefit 24-Hr Brow Setter Clear Brow Gel

BROWS LIKE A BOSS

Red head

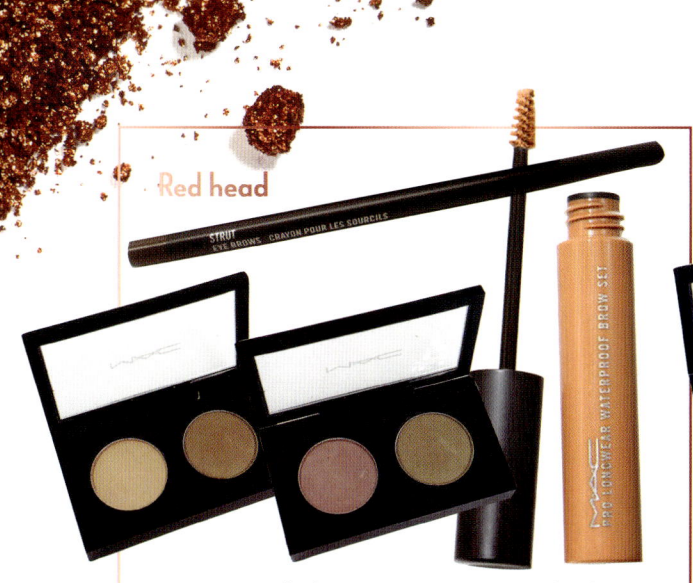

MAC Eye Shadow Duo: WARM REDHEAD (Cork and Soft Brown) DEEPER REDHEAD (Haux and Cork), MAC Pro Longwear Waterproof Brow Set in Toasted Blonde, MAC Brow Pencil in Strut

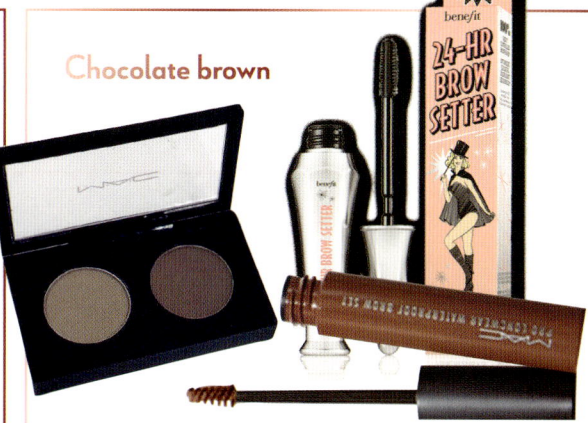

Chocolate brown

MAC Eye Shadow Duo in Coquette and Espresso, Benefit 24-Hr Brow Setter Clear Brow Gel, MAC Pro Longwear Waterproof Brow Set in Quiet Brunette

Sandy brown

MAC Eye Shadow Duo in Charcoal Brown and Wedge, Estée Lauder The Brow Multi-Tasker in Light Brunette, MAC Brow Set in Beguile

Ashy brown

MAC Eye Shadow Duo in Coquette and Brun, Estée Lauder Brow Now Volumizing Brow Tint in Brunette, MAC Brow Pencil in Spiked

Black

MAC Eye Shadow Duo in Brun and Print, Benefit 24-Hr Brow Setter Clear Brow Gel, MAC Pro Longwear Waterproof Brow Set in Bold Brunette, Estée Lauder The Brow Multi-Tasker in Black

TIP!

Add a scribble of pink pencil, turquoise pencil, royal blue pencil and red pencil. If you are like me and have had a rainbow of hair colors over the years, think outside the box when it comes to what you use in your brows! Sometimes the perfect color match will come in the form of a lipliner, eyeliner and eye shadows!

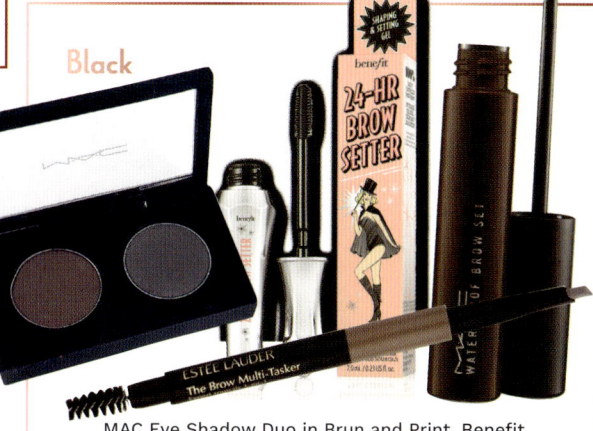

My Favorite Brow Tools!

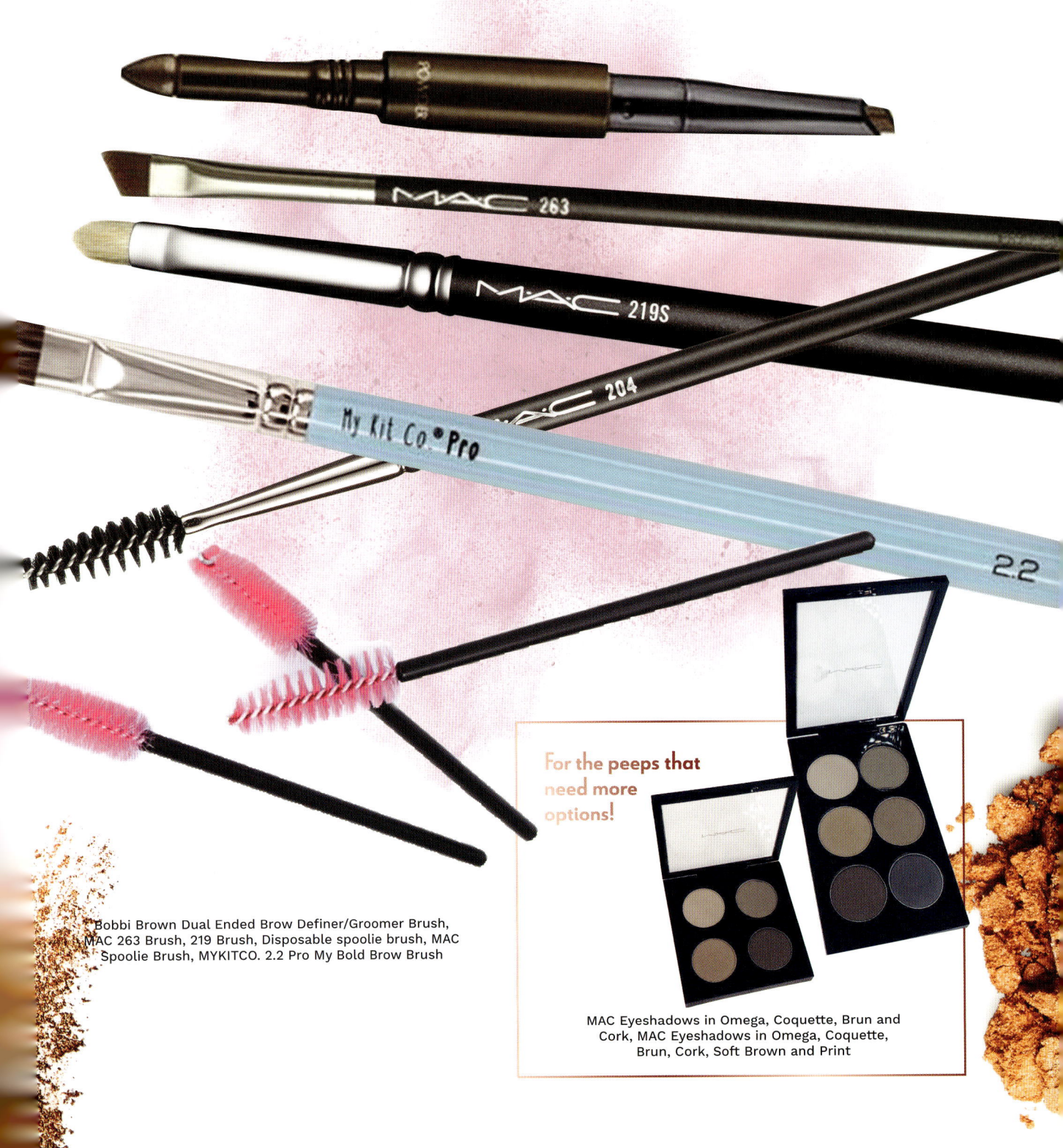

Bobbi Brown Dual Ended Brow Definer/Groomer Brush, MAC 263 Brush, 219 Brush, Disposable spoolie brush, MAC Spoolie Brush, MYKITCO. 2.2 Pro My Bold Brow Brush

For the peeps that need more options!

MAC Eyeshadows in Omega, Coquette, Brun and Cork, MAC Eyeshadows in Omega, Coquette, Brun, Cork, Soft Brown and Print

BROWS LIKE A BOSS

BROWS FROM NOTHING

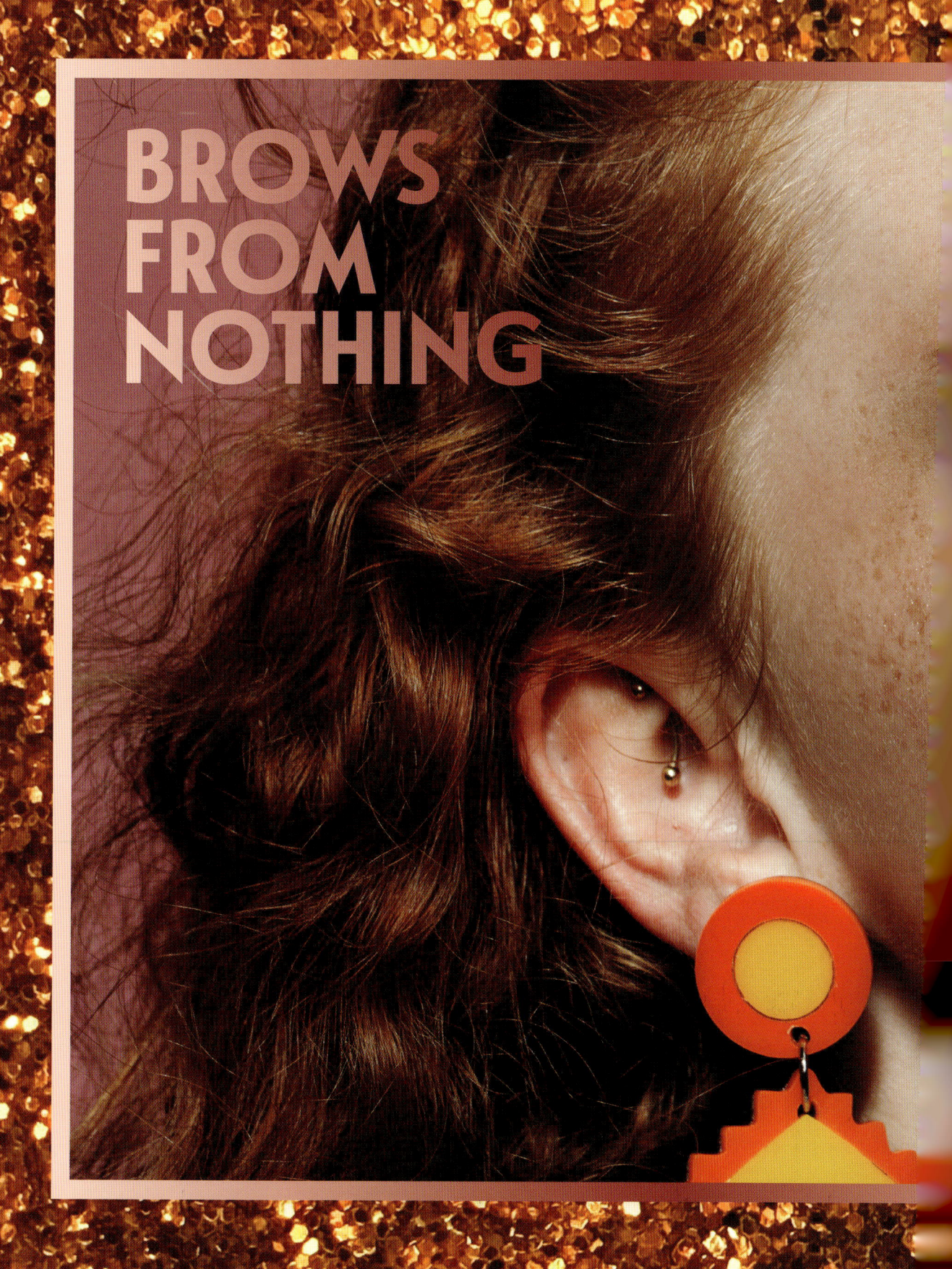

BROWS LIKE A BOSS

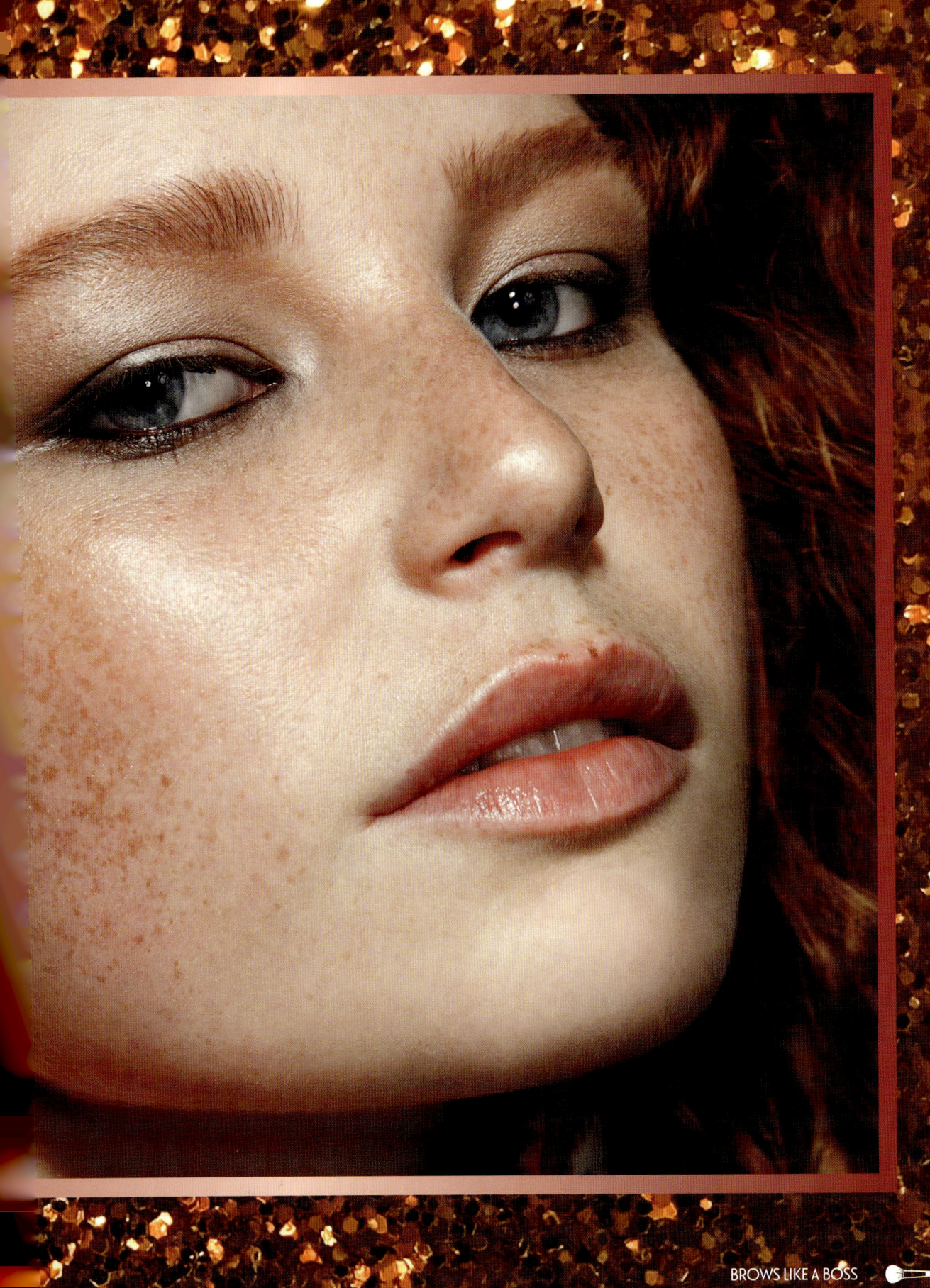

BEFORE

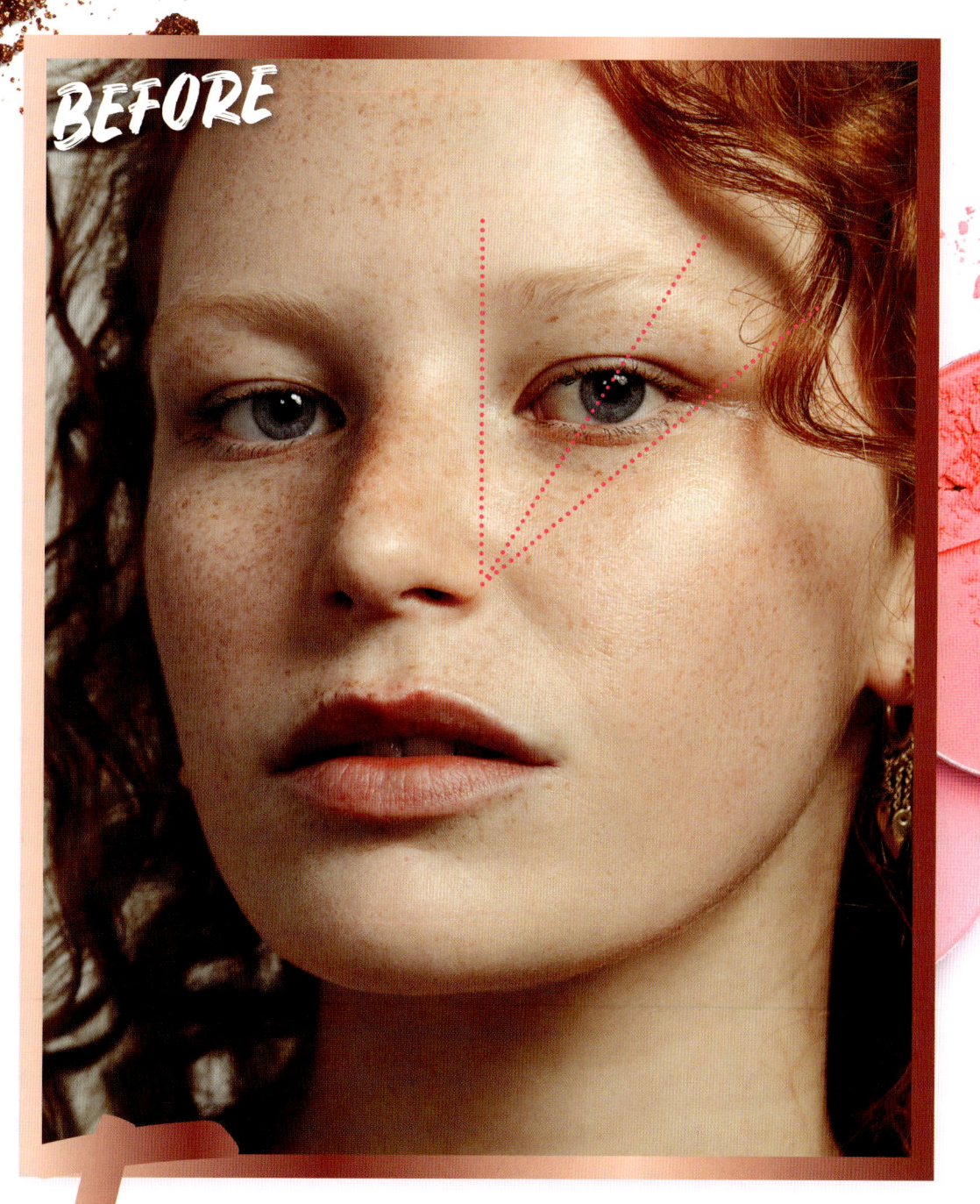

For those of you out there who wake up like me in the morning, devoid of a single brow hair (okay, well I have four brow hairs, but they are super tricky to manipulate into the full luscious brows of my dreams!), have no fear! The next few pages are dedicated to you.

After years of playing around with all different techniques, I have used the below steps on myself and my clients with much success.

STEP 1

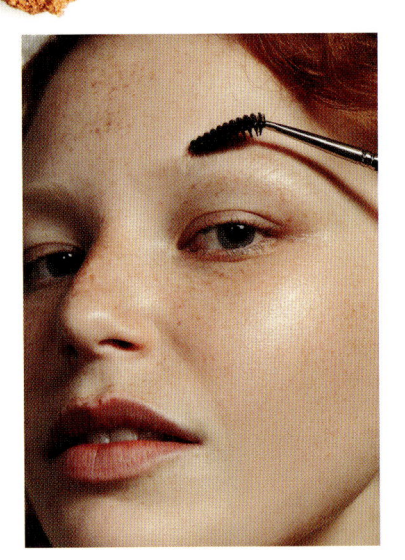

Well, you've already got the ultimate clean canvas – no brows! Give your brow hair a quick brush through to have them all going in the same direction to start. Now, we need to lay down something on the skin for our products to stick too. No-one wants a moving brow! MAC 24-Hour Extended Eye Base is perfect. No color and smoothing finish, it will eliminate uneven pores and texture. Use your finger or a fluffy brush to go over your eyelids and up over your brows – buff that guy in! You should not be able to see it on the skin.

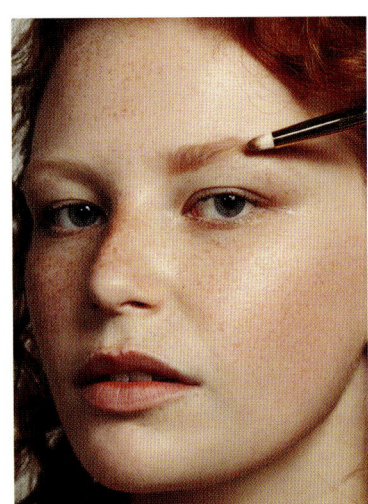

STEP 2

Okay…starting from *no* color is tricky, so adding color softly and slowly to build up the shape is the most flattering way to apply your brows. If you go straight in with strong color, any mistakes, or lopsided application will be obvious and tougher to correct. Get out your trusty soft-pointed eyeshadow brush (the one we used for powder as concealer previously!) and gently stroke the shadow color into your brows. At the front of your brow, start from the base and move upwards and outwards following the shape on the brow guideline.

As always I love to have at least two colors for each brow – and with a redhead the color choices are important! You want to mix the ginger shade with a color that will neutralize it, so the whole brow does not end up too orange. Mix warm tones with cool ones, using my color guide at the start of this chapter as a reference.

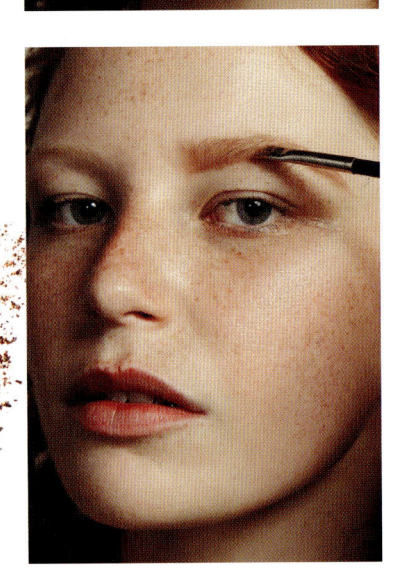

STEP 3

Use a different brush for a different effect, this time a small angle brush for intense color application. Use the shadow colors alternately and stroke the shadow through in a hair-like motion.

BROWS LIKE A BOSS

STEP 4

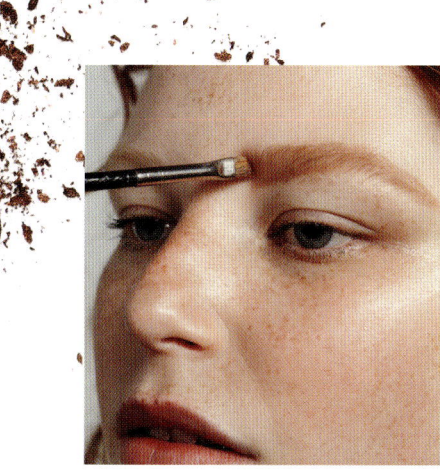

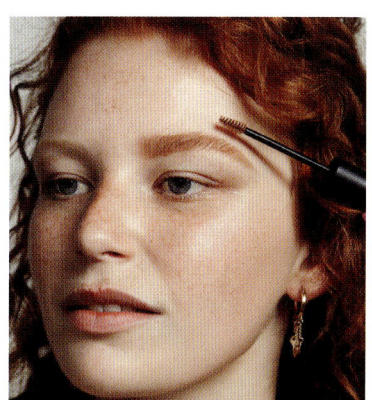

Switch up the angle of your brush and now add the same product in soft, hair-like strokes flicking the brush upwards at the beginning of the brow and moving outwards.

STEP 5

Brush a colored brow mascara through the brows to coat the light hairs and bring the whole brow look together to form one complete, natural look.

Make sure to wipe the brow mascara wand. This is the one time you do *not* want a completely coated mascara wand – it will be goop city! Gah! Give the brush a quick wipe through with a tissue before you start so the color on the wand tints the hairs naturally.

> *TIP!* Your brow shadow can also double as the perfect eye shadow. As they generally match your hair color, it will create the ultimate natural shade.

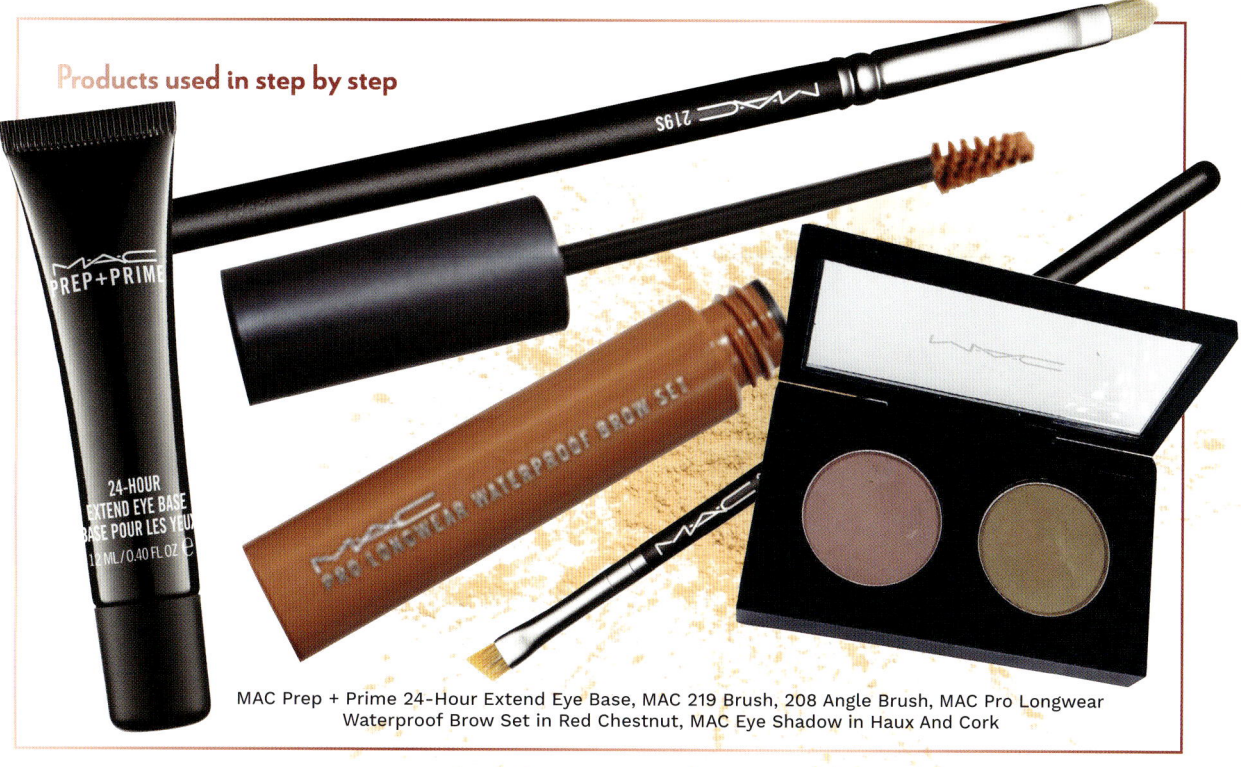

Products used in step by step

MAC Prep + Prime 24-Hour Extend Eye Base, MAC 219 Brush, 208 Angle Brush, MAC Pro Longwear Waterproof Brow Set in Red Chestnut, MAC Eye Shadow in Haux And Cork

BROWS LIKE A BOSS

GEE GEE FROM KULT MODELS, EARRING, DOODAD AND FANDANGO

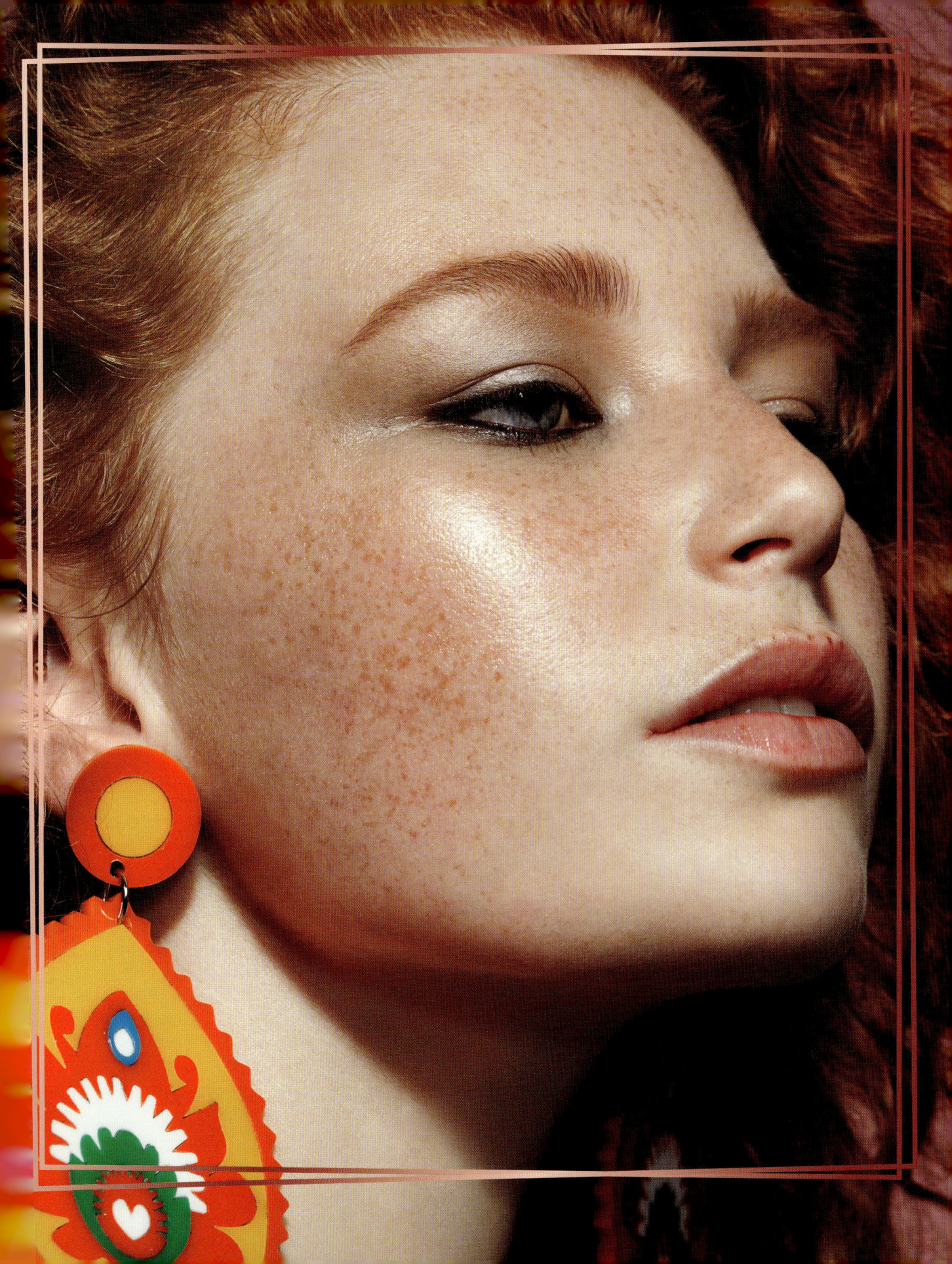

FLUFFY FARSHUN BROW

BROWS LIKE A BOSS

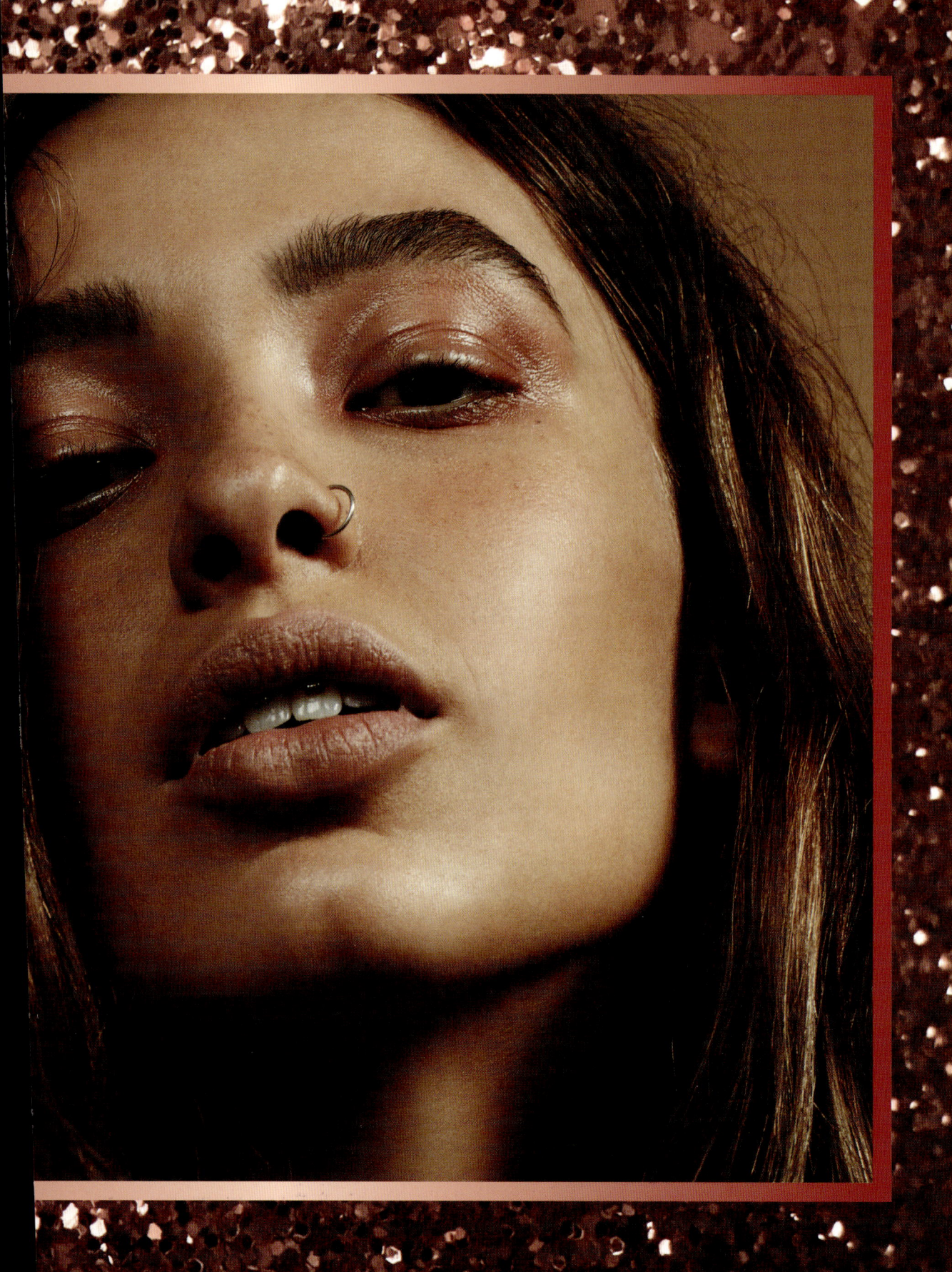

BEFORE

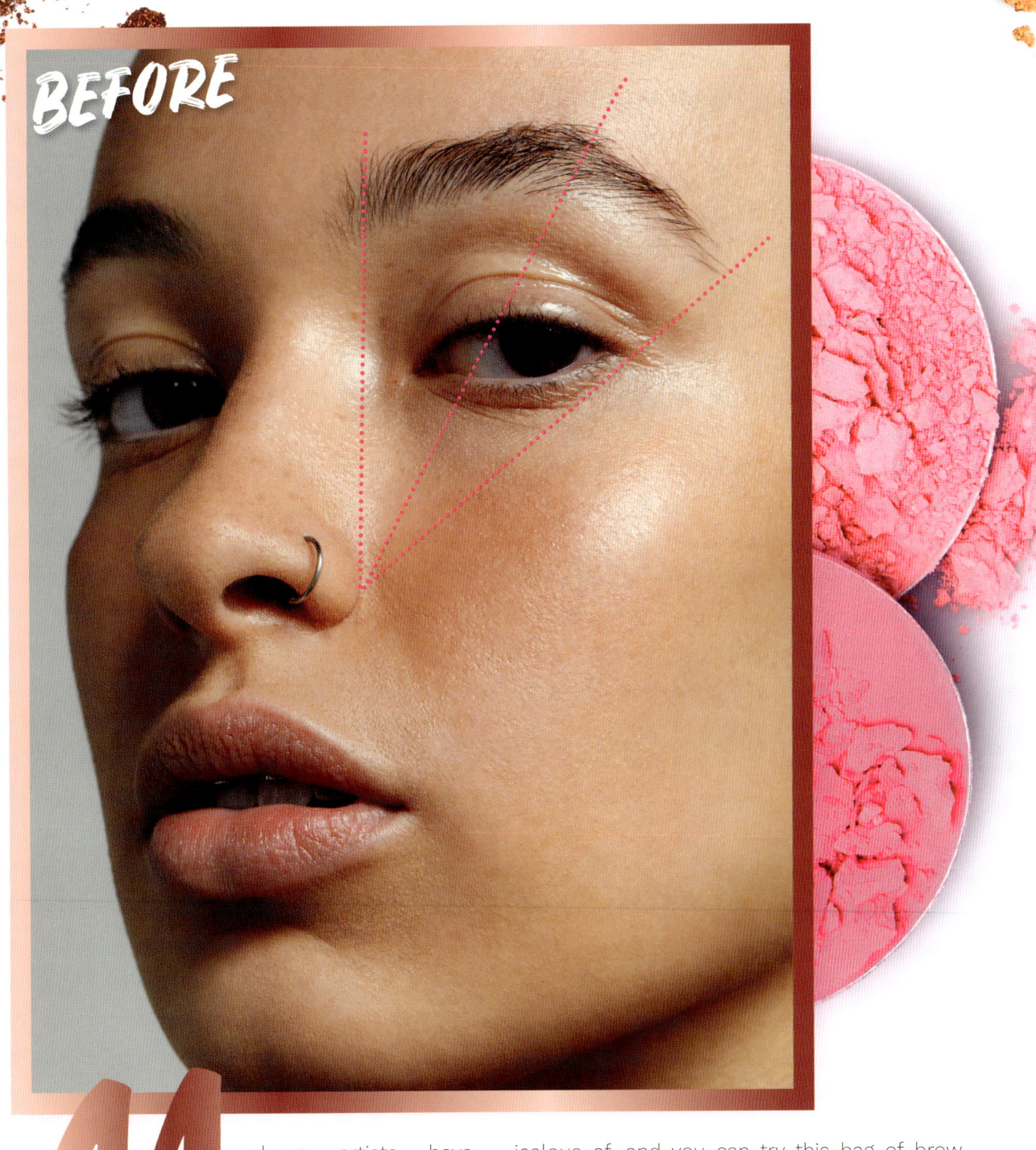

Makeup artists have been wielding brushes and products to fake a bushy, full brow Cara Delevigne would be jealous of, and you can try this bag of brow tricks yourself. It's all about creating a strong shape with soft edges, which will look youthful, yet is surprisingly easy to apply.

BROWS LIKE A BOSS

STEP 1

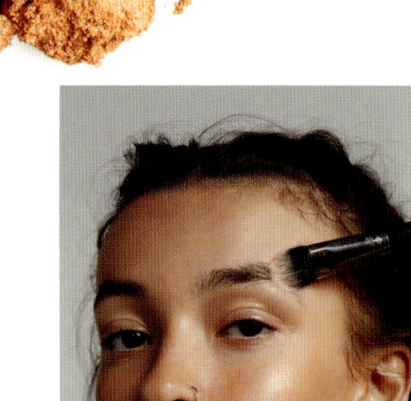

Powder the brows first. If there is too much moisture on the skin before you apply it will cause the products to slide around. Apply with a light hand otherwise the products you add on top will feel super heavy. Use a loose invisible powder or your usual face powder.

> **TIP!** If you have uber oily skin, try a waterproof eye primer instead. Give the MAC Prep + Prime 24-hour Extend Eye Base a go and use your fingers to take a small amount over the brow area. It is equal parts perfect and lightweight while also being colorless to work on any skintone or hair color.

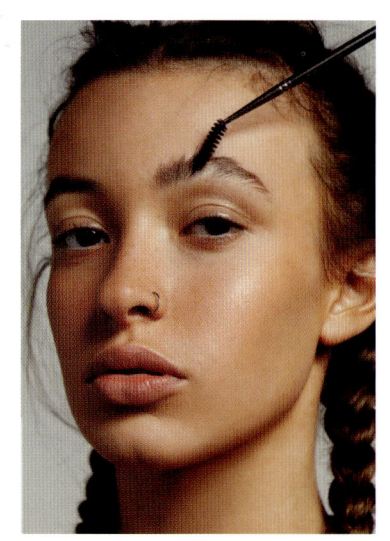

STEP 2

Brush through the brows to see what they can do. Guide the hairs into the shape you want to create first.

STEP 3

Using your soft-pointed eye shadow brush, add a sheer layer of brow shadow, starting with the lightest shadow color first. What you are doing is creating a sheer, full shape first that you can add the detail into afterwards and keep the whole thing looking natural. I cannot believe I am saying this, but there is no place for shimmer here. Gasp! Shimmer shadows will not give you definition or a natural look with your brows. Matte shadows work best.

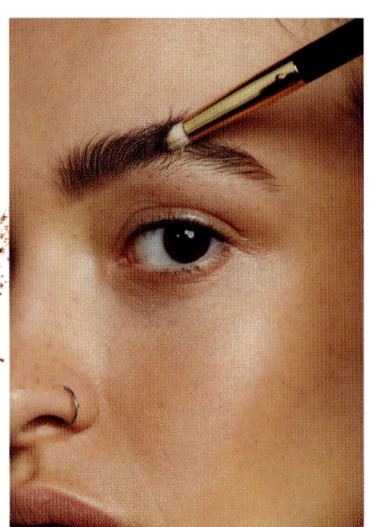

> **TIP!** As soon as brow color products hit the brow hairs, they appear darker on the face so start lighter than you would think. You can always make it darker or stronger – but it is hard to take it away once you have gone full Bert from *Sesame Street*!

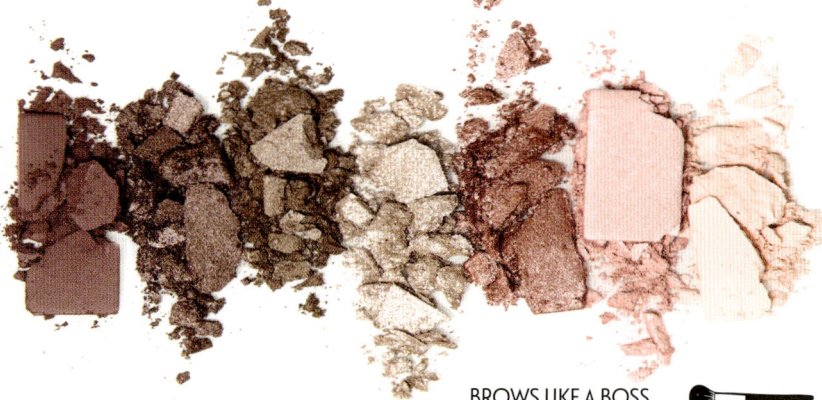

BROWS LIKE A BOSS

STEP 4

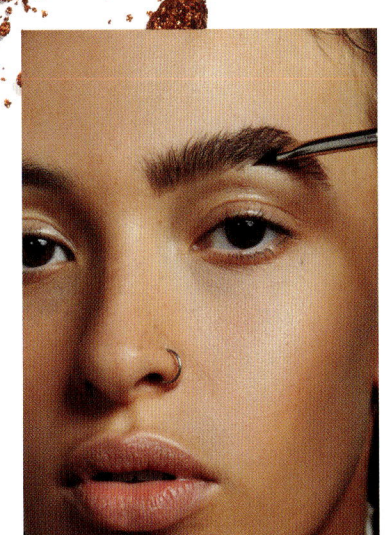

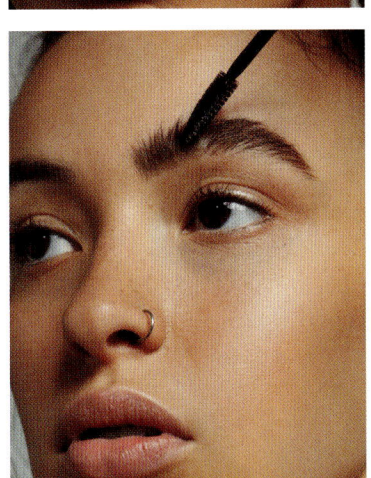

Using the thinnest angle brush in your kit (mine is a #263 angle brush from MAC) you can create imitation brow hairs that look as real as it gets. Lightly spritz your brush with a little setting mist – do not drown the brush as it will sheer out the color, and ruin your eye shadow – and dip into the shadows. Then take the color in feathery strokes through the brows at the same angle as your natural hair growth, starting light, then adding in the darker color in between to create the illusion of fuller brows.

STEP 5

Brush false lash maximizer through the brows to give a fuller texture to each hair and also to give a strong hold, like you've taken to them with a can of hairspray. This product is actually a lash primer. It thickens and doubles the lash size, so why not try it in the brows! Multipurpose magic!

> *TIP!* The spoolie is a great tool! Amazing to comb through the darker shadow color and cover the grey hairs, or fill in color between hairs and even out the hair line. If you have been a little aggressive with your color application and want to soften the look, put down your remover and cotton tip and pick up your brow spoolie! Be sure to brush through the entire brow as this will soften the lines, pick up excess product and have the whole thing looking really natural.

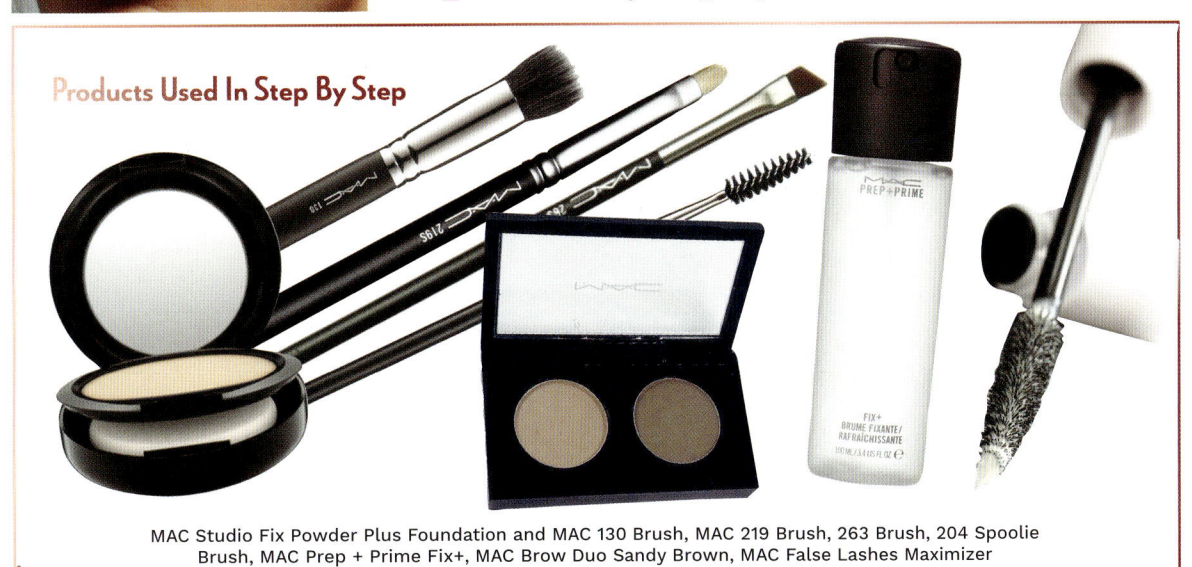

Products Used In Step By Step

MAC Studio Fix Powder Plus Foundation and MAC 130 Brush, MAC 219 Brush, 263 Brush, 204 Spoolie Brush, MAC Prep + Prime Fix+, MAC Brow Duo Sandy Brown, MAC False Lashes Maximizer

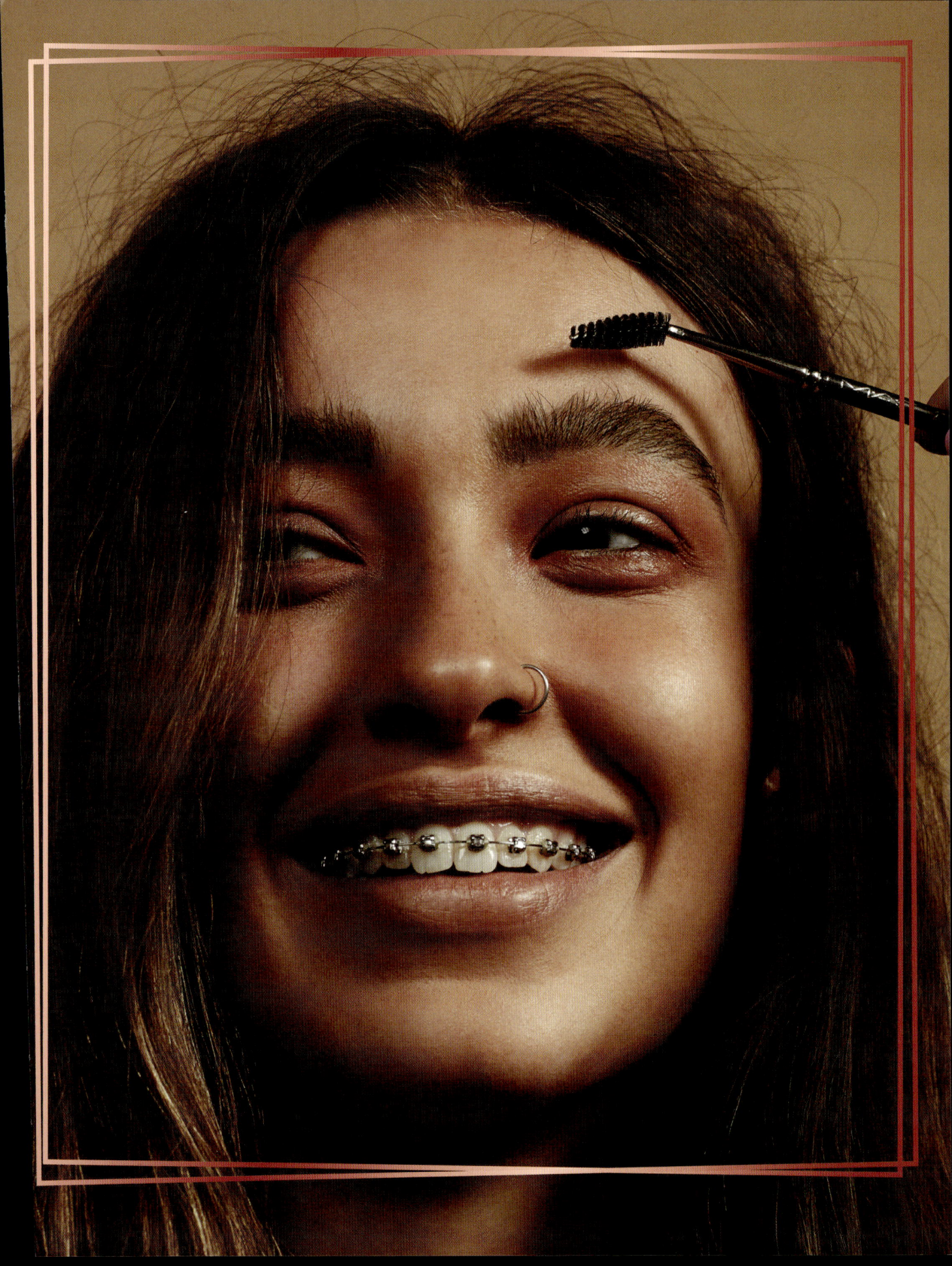

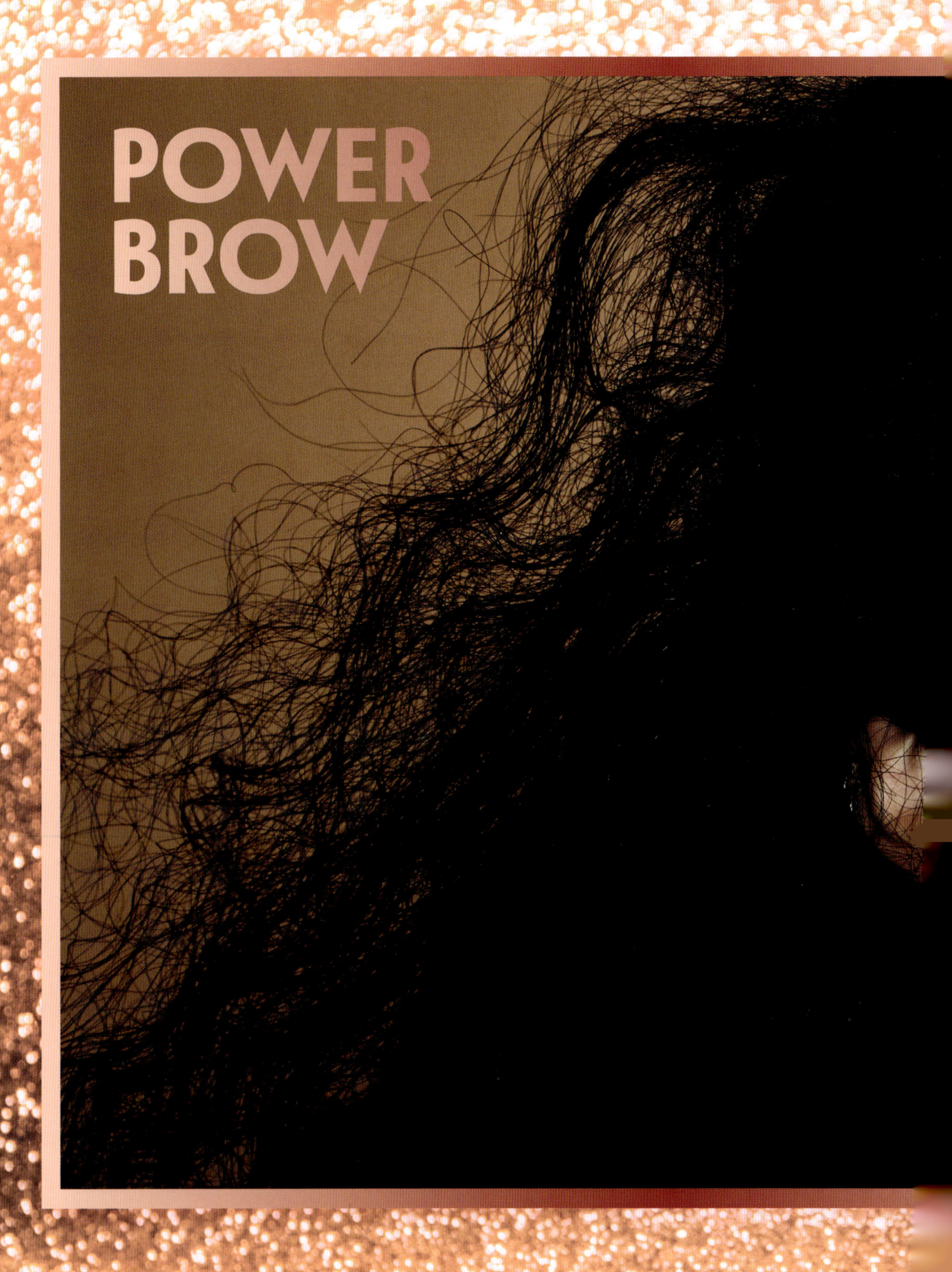

POWER BROW

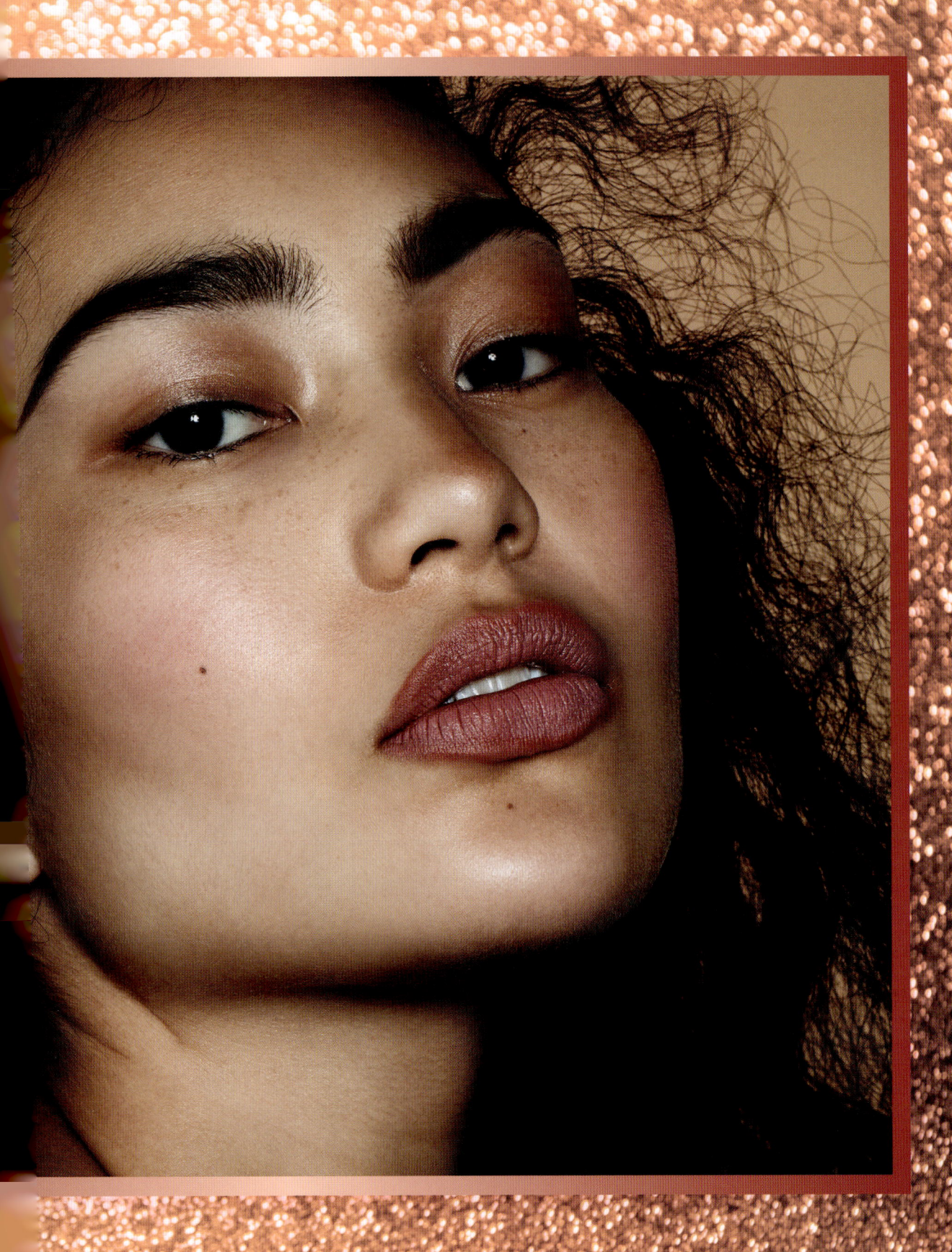

BROWS LIKE A BOSS   103

BEFORE

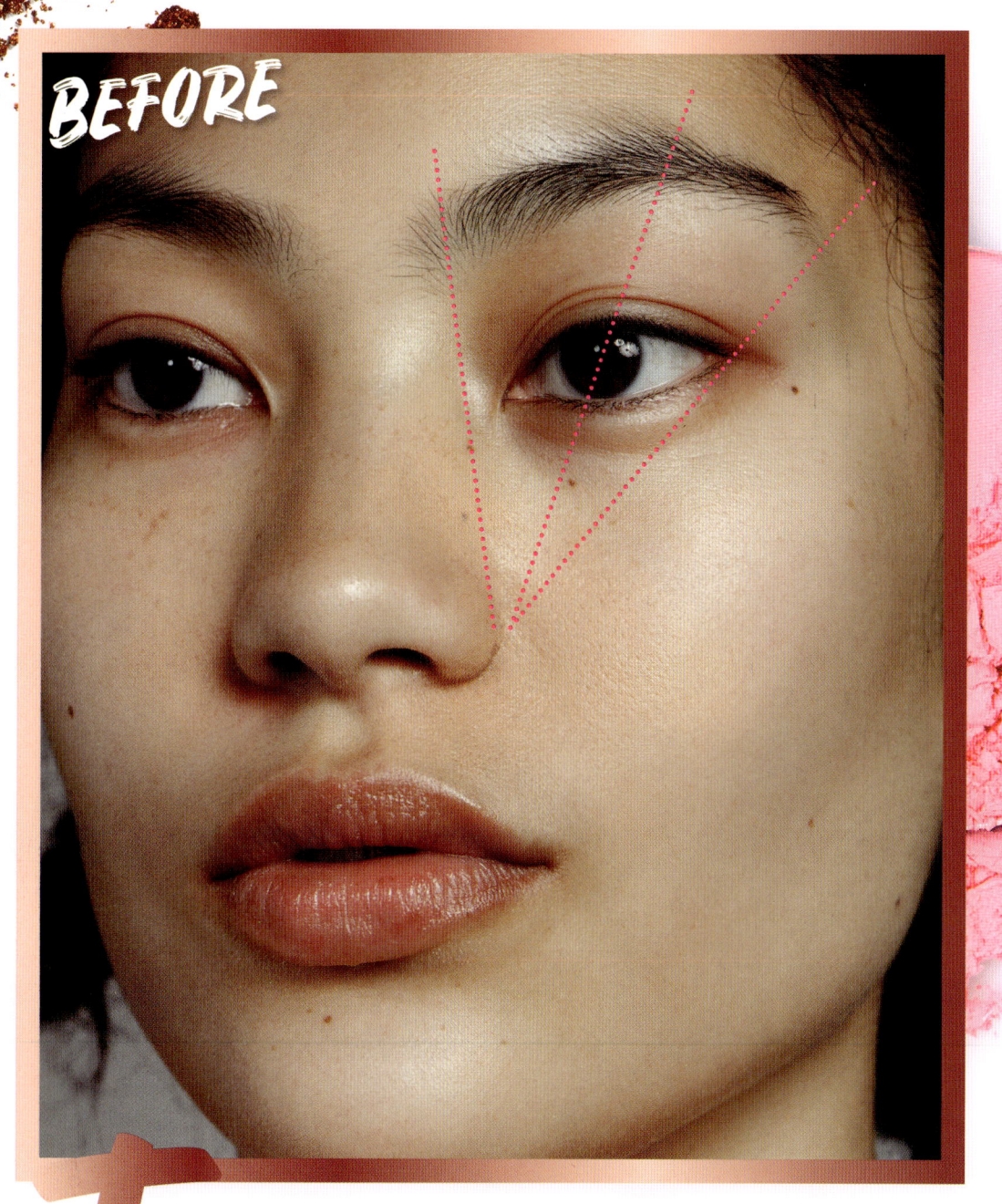

1

he brow that is everything we want it to be: defined, strong and in perfect shape. Oh the dream! Fortunately for you, achieving this won't take seven days a week at the gym and some guy with 2% body fat yelling at you.

You see, the defined brow works as effectively in the boardroom as it does on a Friday night, and in both instances, it is a look that means business. But as bold as this brow may appear, it is equally effective as the feature of your look or sharing the stage with a lip or eyeliner moment.

STEP 1

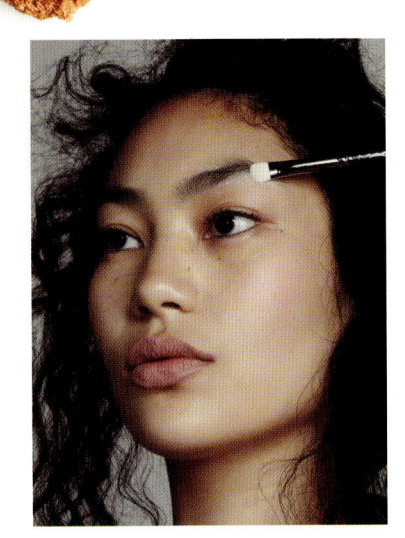

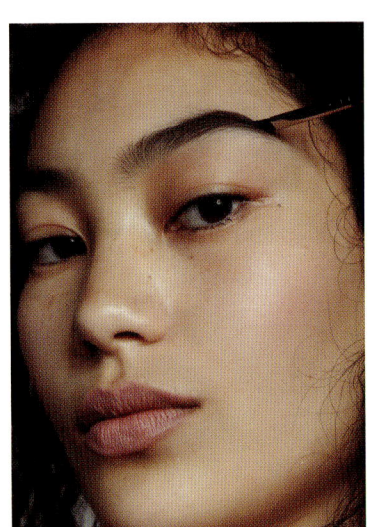

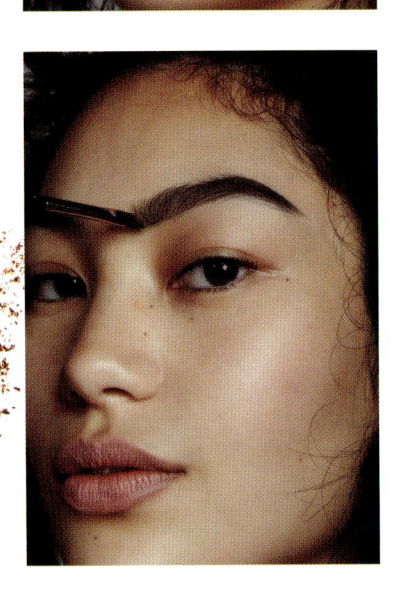

Clean canvas! Yes this old thing again! I'm telling you, this is my consistent brow secret. Start with that clean, smooth color and the brow you put on top will be 100% better! You can use a concealer or your face powder – whatever you like! I would suggest powder if you get oily skin, or concealer if you get dry skin.

STEP 2

With a thin angle brush, dip into the brow cream and follow the guideline of where to apply color, this time starting at the underside of the brow in the center and working outwards from there.

Brow creams are designed to be rich in color so be careful not to pick up too much product straight away. Wherever your first swipe of the brush hits the skin, that is where the bulk of the color will be, so make sure to start at the underside. If you start from the inside of the brow you may finish looking like you are in phase one of building a veranda above your eyelids!

> **TIP!** If the idea of brow cream freaks you out, use the same technique and use a brow pencil.

STEP 3

Move the angle brow brush around to follow the natural direction the hair grows in.

MAC 239 Brush

STEP 4

Using the same brush and powder or cream product as Step 1, apply the color lightly around your brows to polish up the edges and create a subtle contrast to the brow color for maximum power brow action!

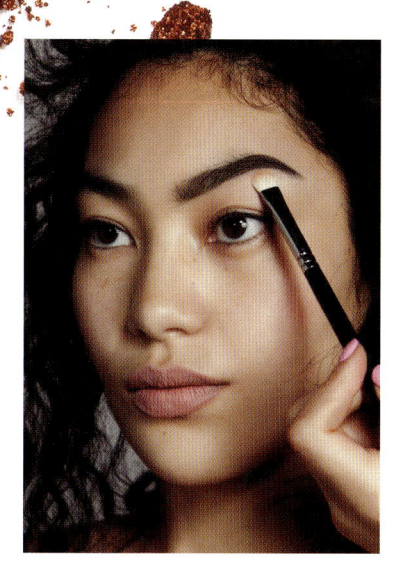

You only need to choose a color one or possibly two shades lighter than your skin tone when highlighting around the brows! We want to create a subtle contrast to the brow so it looks clean and tidy.

If the edge of the brow ends up *too* defined, and it looks a little hard on your face, especially if you have paler skin, use a small, soft eye shadow brush to rub over the edges slightly to soften the look – makes a huge difference!

TIP! Had one to many coffees before painting on your brow? Fix any dodgy edges with a little MAC Prep + Prime Fix+ on your flat brush. This, rather than a remover, will help you soften the edge and clean up the color without removing everything around it.

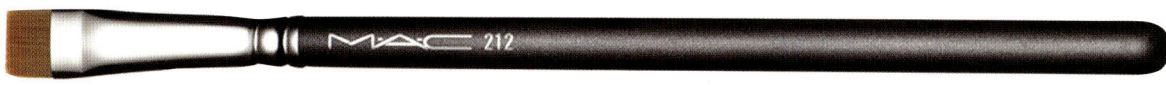

MAC 212 Flat Brush

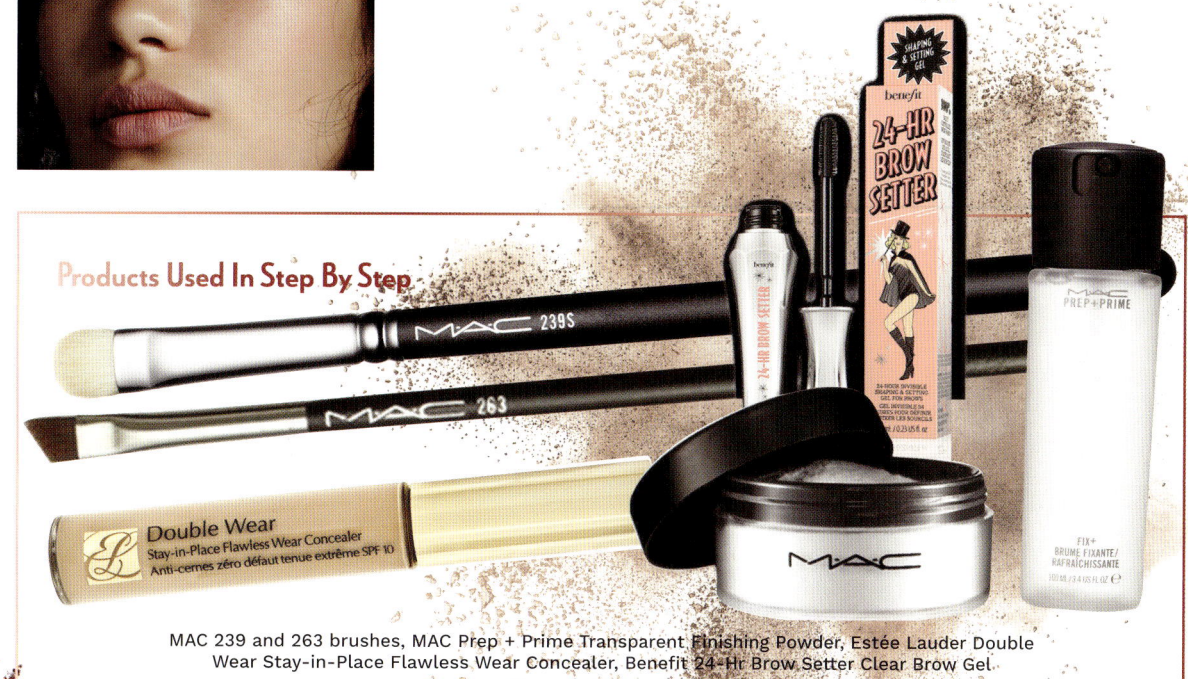

TIP! We love to get close to the mirror when doing our brows to see all that detail. Make sure while you are busy applying, that you pause and take one step back from the mirror to see the whole brow and what you are creating. Remember it's much easier to add more color, than it is to take it away when you look start looking like a villain from a James Bond movie.

Products Used In Step By Step

MAC 239 and 263 brushes, MAC Prep + Prime Transparent Finishing Powder, Estée Lauder Double Wear Stay-in-Place Flawless Wear Concealer, Benefit 24-Hr Brow Setter Clear Brow Gel

BROWS LIKE A BOSS

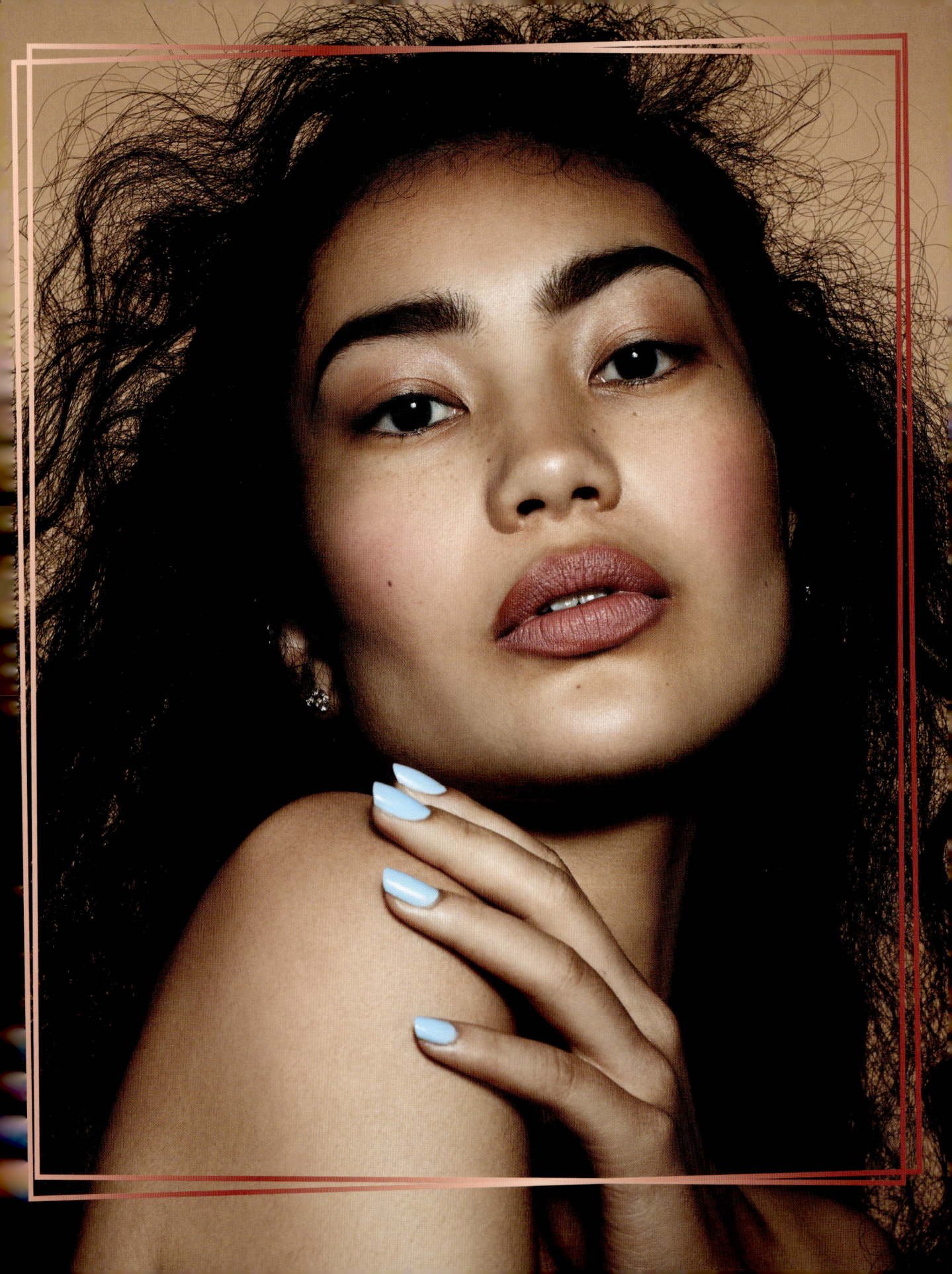

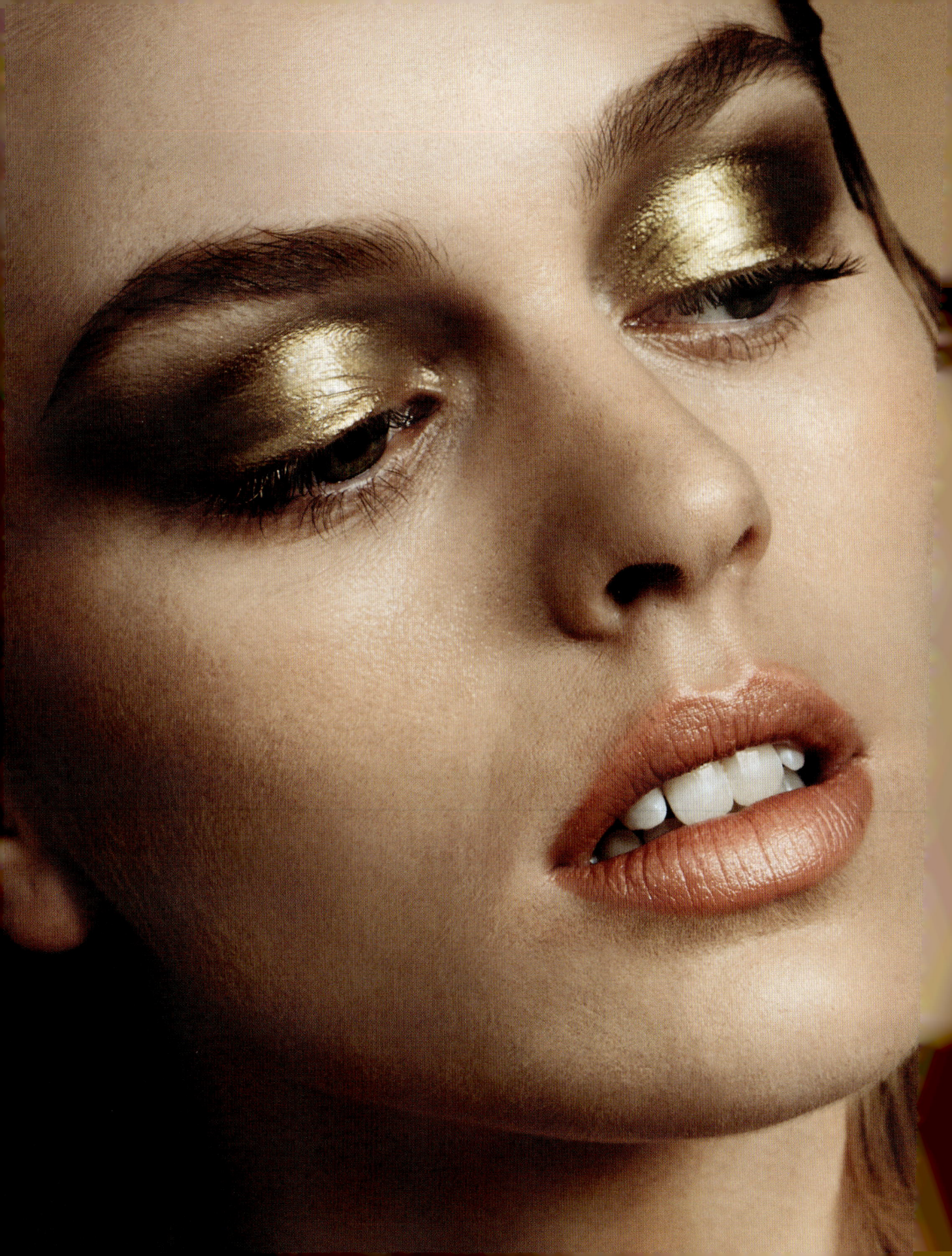

Eye spy with my smoky eye

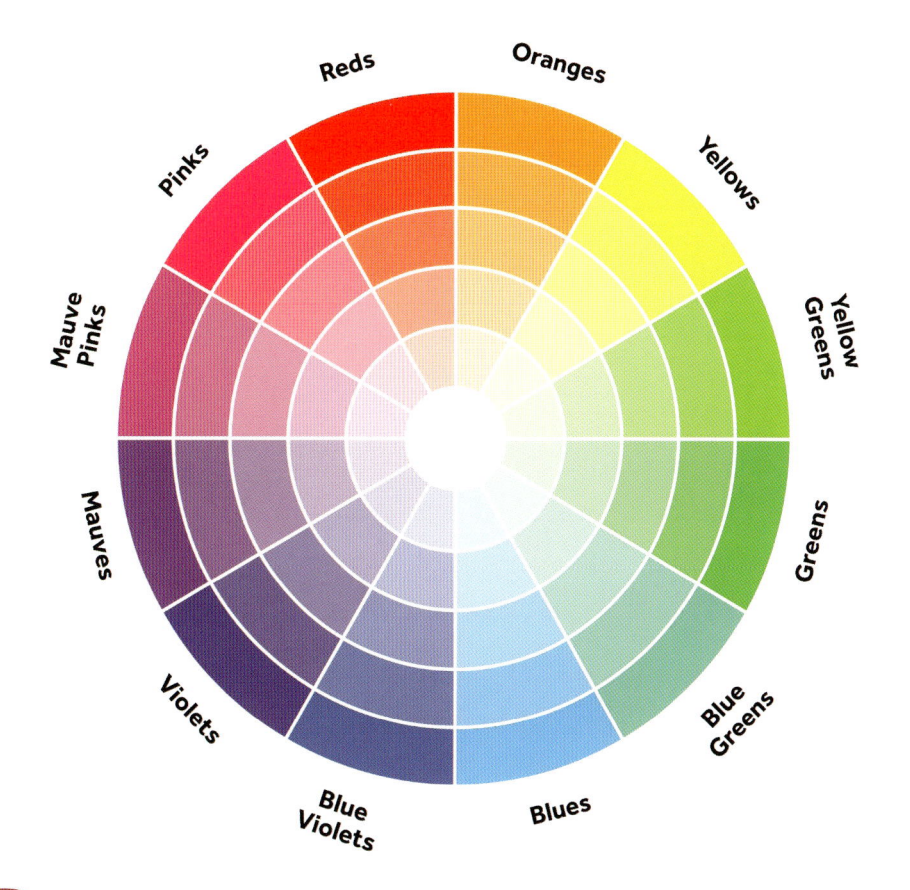

Reds · **Oranges** · **Yellows** · **Yellow Greens** · **Greens** · **Blue Greens** · **Blues** · **Blue Violets** · **Violets** · **Mauves** · **Mauve Pinks** · **Pinks**

It's time to lift the 'lid' on eye makeup! Bad puns aside, there is no place I like experimenting more than through eye makeup. Playing with your peepers is your chance to explore a kaleidoscope of combinations, and when you land the right one – BOOM! – you have a makeup moment to remember.

The idea of play is so important! One may argue that play is best saved for at home at the risk of looking like Heath Ledger's Joker, but if you are going to take it to the streets, wear it with confidence.

In case you haven't heard, I hate rules! And I also hate being told what to do! So many people ask me, 'What color would look good on my eyes?' Now while I am a firm believer in the idea of 'if it feels good to you it will look good on you!', there is one very simple guide to start you off on your eye makeup (and general makeup) discovery: complementary colors will enhance each other!

Complementary colors sit opposite each other on the color wheel. When they are used close together they give life to each other. That is why Christmas colors of green and red are so happy and perfect together. We also see so many vibrant examples of this in nature. Use the colors here as a fun guide to picking your next favorite colors!

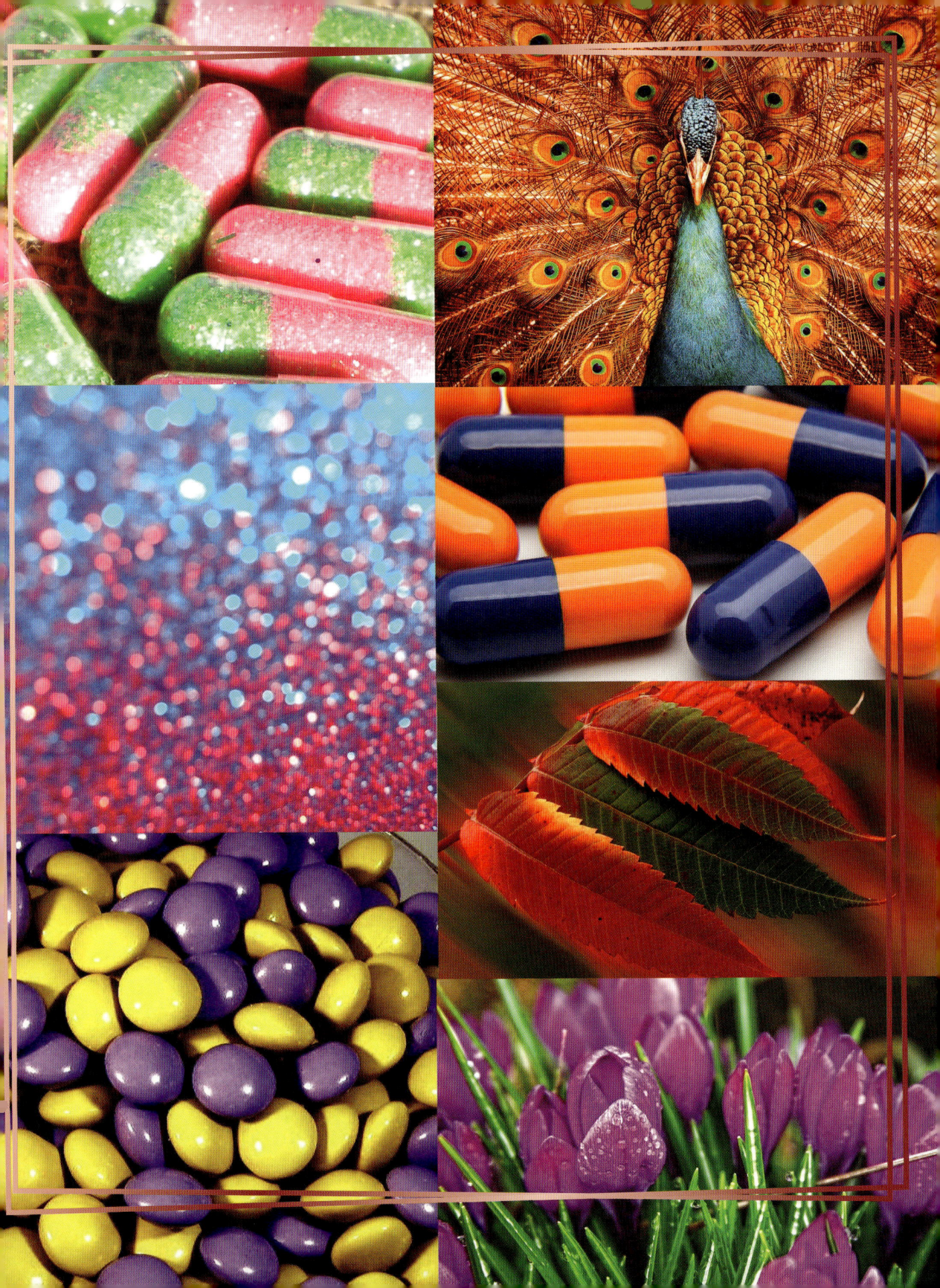

NUDE CONTOURED EYE

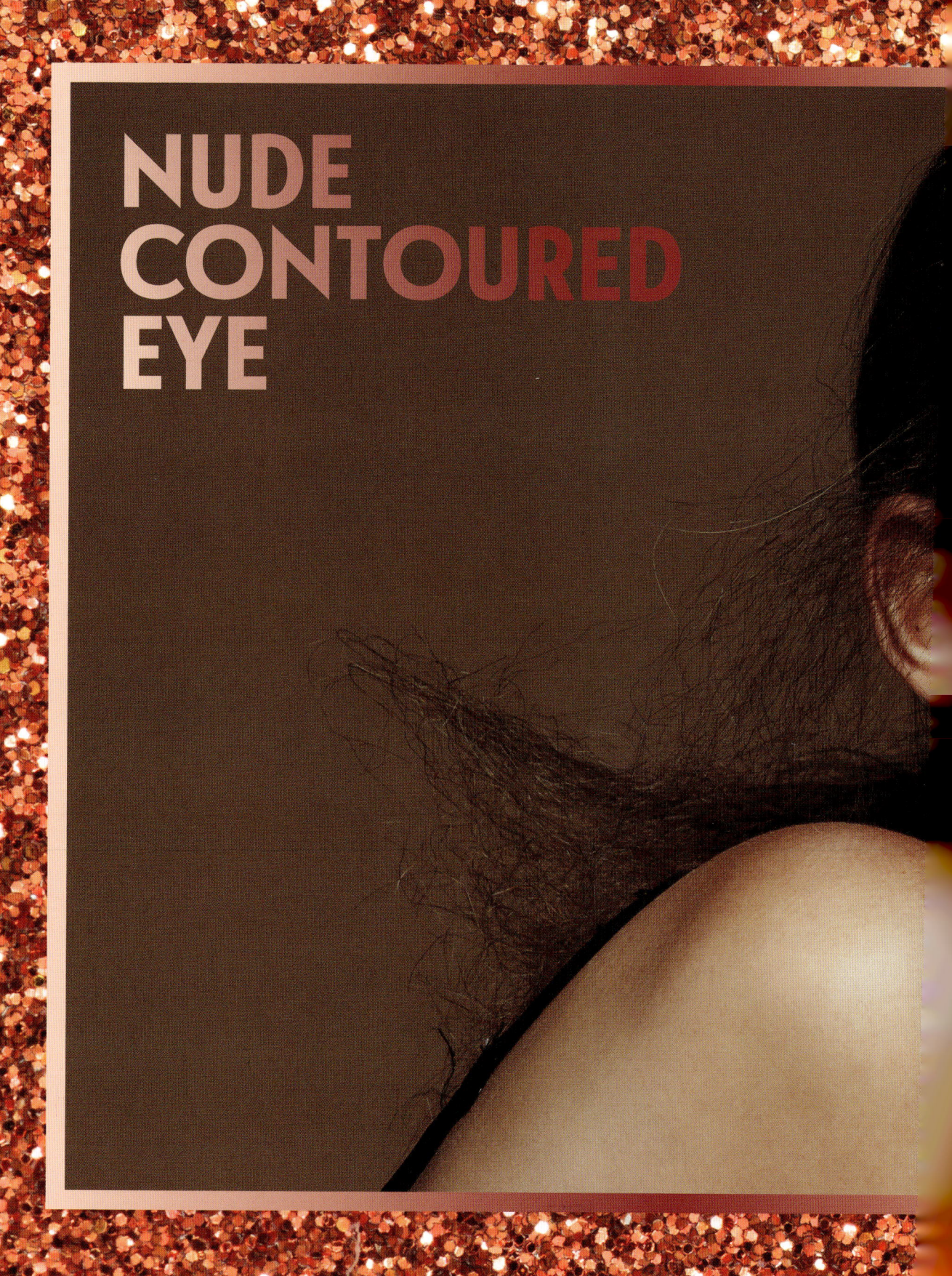

EYE SPY WITH MY SMOKY EYE

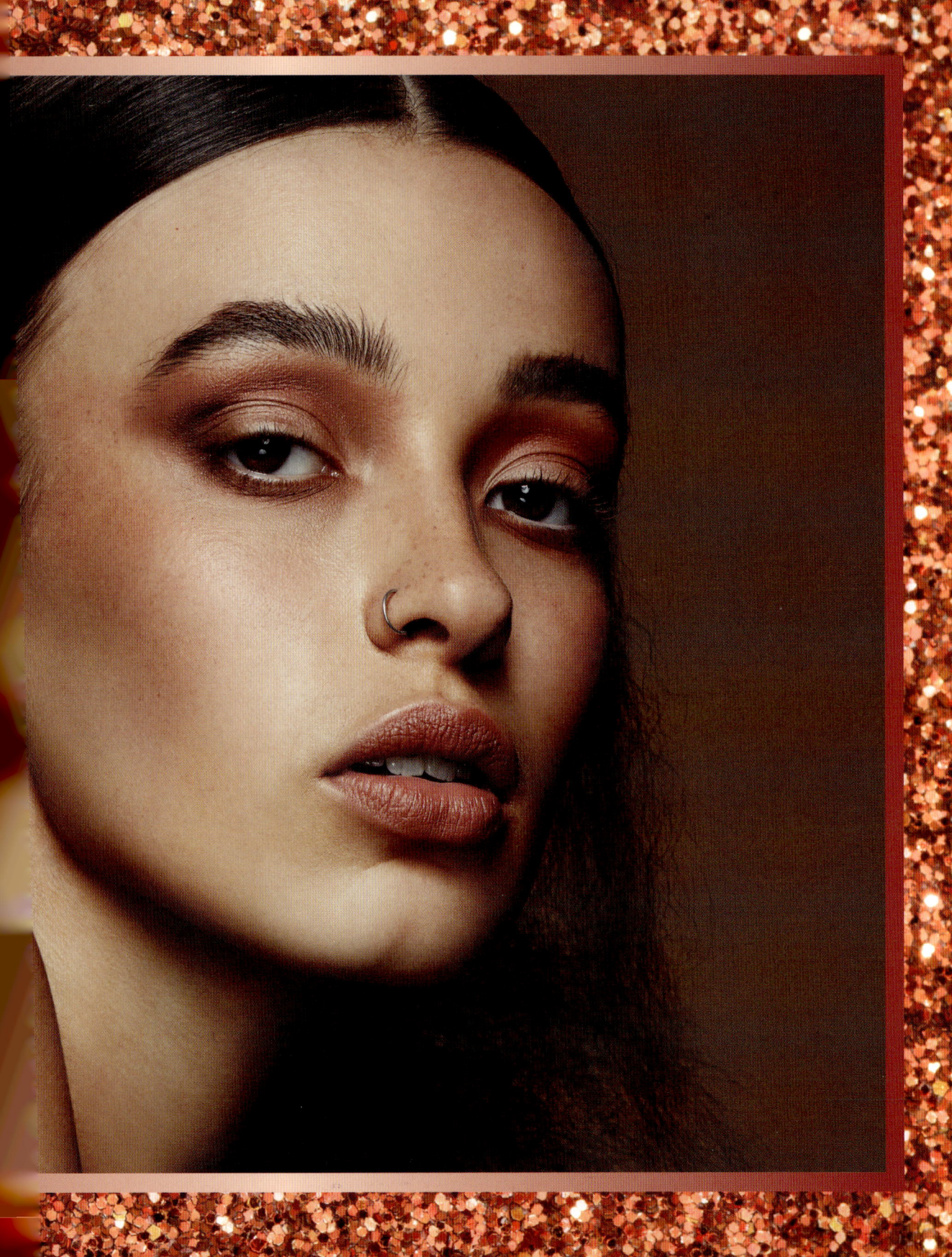

H

ell yeah, you contour your eye! Having eyes appear in the shape of perfectly symmetrical almonds is the holy grail. Through makeup artistry you can achieve that upward and outward swooshing we all desire.

It is a huge misconception that to make a statement with your eyes you need to turn the color dial up to music festival fluoro glow stick! Your eye makeup can make as strong an impact if you nail the nude contouring. In my experience, perfection beats pop, when the pop isn't perfect.

STEP 1

Prime those eyes! Spread the primer out over the lids and right up to the eyebrow. No edges here please. You have a few choices when it comes to priming the eye and it all depends how much makeup you like to buy! I really like an eye primer that is clear so I can use it under *any* shadow situation. Even though it is clear, you want to make sure you can see a texture difference on the skin – skin should look and feel smoother and shine should be muted.

The other choice is going in with a bulletproof cream shadow in a natural color you love. This can do a few things at once, with color and staying power, and on days when you have one minute to get ready it's a quick swipe and go color!

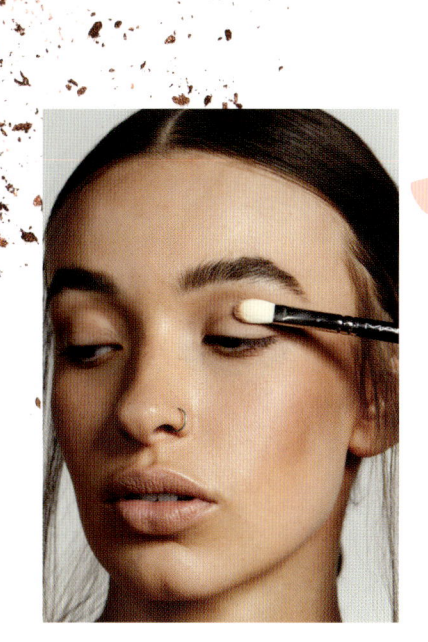

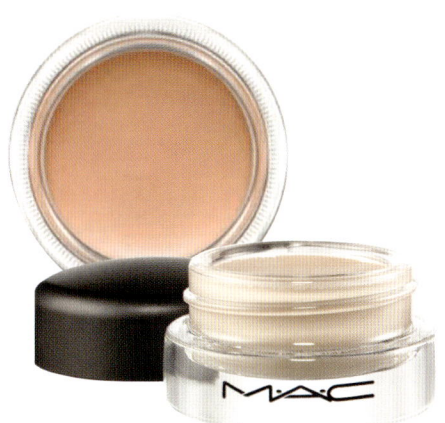

MAC Painterly or Layin Low Pro Longwear Paint Pot

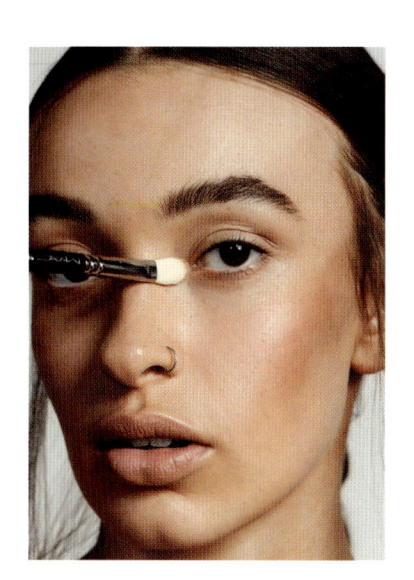

STEP 2

Use a light nude eye pencil or shadow to highlight the inner corners of the eyes. This is a great starting point with color, as often when you highlight first to clarify your eyes, you don't need as much of the deeper colors to define.

STEP 3

A lot of people will start with eye shadow here, but I love to use pencils to shape and sculpt the eyes. I am too impatient to use 10 different eye shadows or do all that blending, not to mention the eye shadow fallout! I have such control with a pencil and can get the color and shape on *quick*.

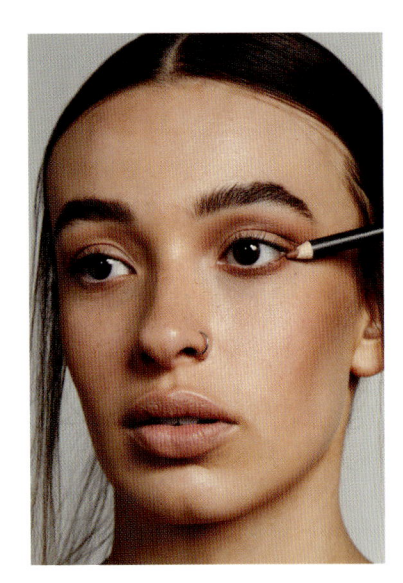

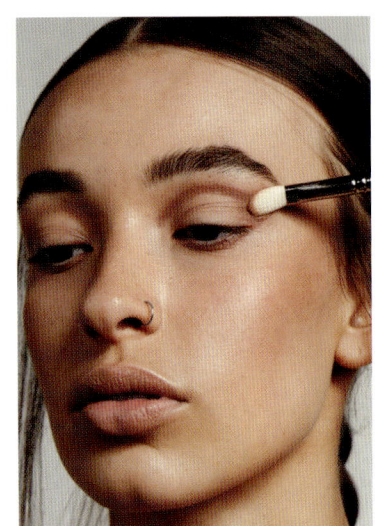

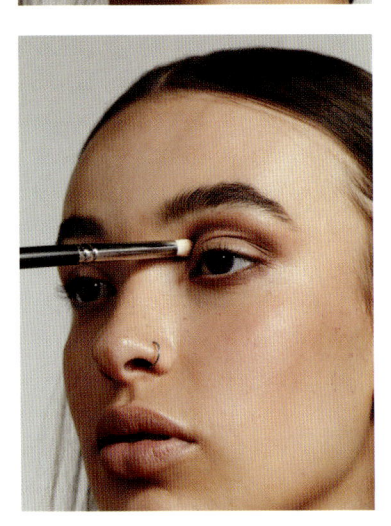

Okay, so pencils don't sound too out of the ordinary around the eyes, right? I'm actually using a lip pencil! Yep that's right. I adore using all my nude and tan shades of lip pencils around the eye for much more subtle definition that doesn't instantly turn into a dark smoky eye like a brown pencil would. Also lip pencils have strong color pigment and are designed to last on the lips so there is no reason why they wouldn't do the same on your lids!

For a monochromatic look, use the same lip pencil as the base to your lip and eye look. This is a great way to focus on both features in a sexy, balanced way.

> **TIP!** Now that you have warmed up to this lip products on eyes business, get crazy! Branch out to your plum shades for the base to a violet eye, a peach pencil for a fresh summer look and a magenta pencil under a cranberry shadow for a punchy party eye.

STEP 4

Add and blend, add and blend with the pencil and a soft fluffy brush. To really lift the eyes, sit the color just above the crease of the eye, and sweep it up and out towards the temples. Try to keep your eyes open during this step so you can really see where that color is going.

Draw and blend the pencil underneath the eyes as well. We are avoiding the top lashline with the pencil for this look as I don't want to deepen or close the eyes. We are going for bright eyed and bushy tailed here!

> **TIP!** Stop at Step 4! If you want the caramel-toned contour but would like it to remain more on the subtle side, stop here, at the point where you use the pencil to blend over your eyes. To set you can use a much paler nude matte shadow quickly, or some translucent face powder.

STEP 5

Set and enhance with a matching nude matte shadow. Use a smaller fluffy brush to add the color with precision and less fallout. Matte shadow is best here as it will recede and refine, providing shape to the eye.

EYE SPY WITH MY SMOKY EYE

TIP! Add some shimmer shadow or glitter to the eyelids to glam up those eyes and open them up even more.

STEP 6

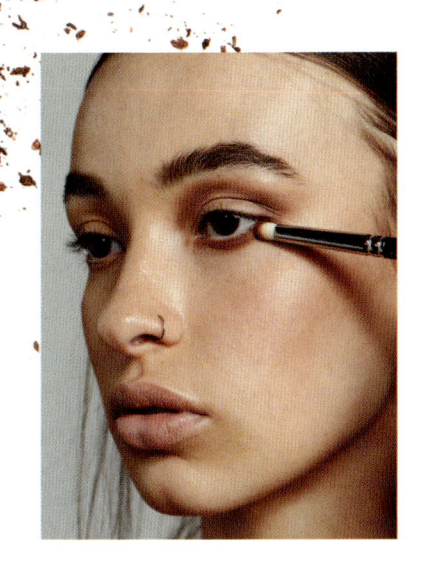

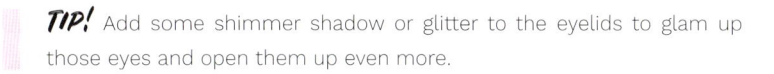

We are all guilty of over-blending! We just love to blend so much, we often blend it all away. Crazy! Press the color down on the skin and *only* blend the outer edges. The smaller, rounded, fluffy brush underneath will add shadow in a controlled way without dropping too low under the eyes.

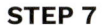

STEP 7

Continue with this shape, now with a larger fluffy brush, and drag the shadow out towards your temples, with your eyes open. I like to use a slightly lighter version of the shadow I used earlier and lightly glaze over the whole eye makeup – this can fuse the eye look together.

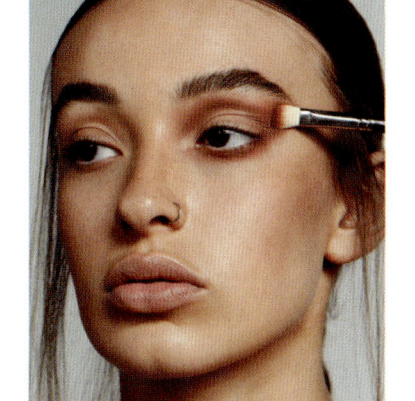

STEP 8

Get in close with your larger fluffy brush and make sure to blend all the way around to create one unified shape, no gaps, patches or wobbly edges.

If the caramel color got a little low beneath the eye and started invading your cheek clean up the shade and give the eye makeup more of a defined edge by using a sponge and some of my superhero product, MAC Prep + Prime Fix+. Sponges naturally absorb, so will pick up that fallout of shadow. Dampen the sponge lightly with MAC Prep + Prime Fix+ and glide over the edge you want to clean up. With Fix+ being a moisturizer not a remover, it will soften the skin, producing a suppler, welcoming surface to help you correct your look with concealer and powder without the edges.

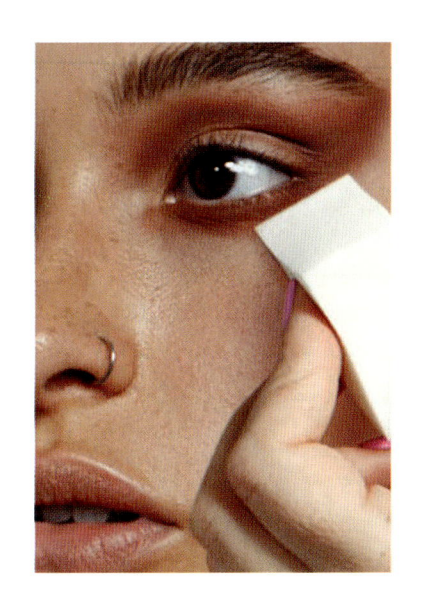

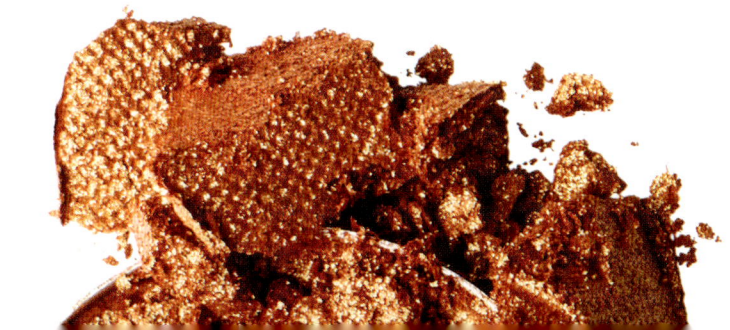

ELLA FROM PRISCILLAS

Products Used In Step By Step

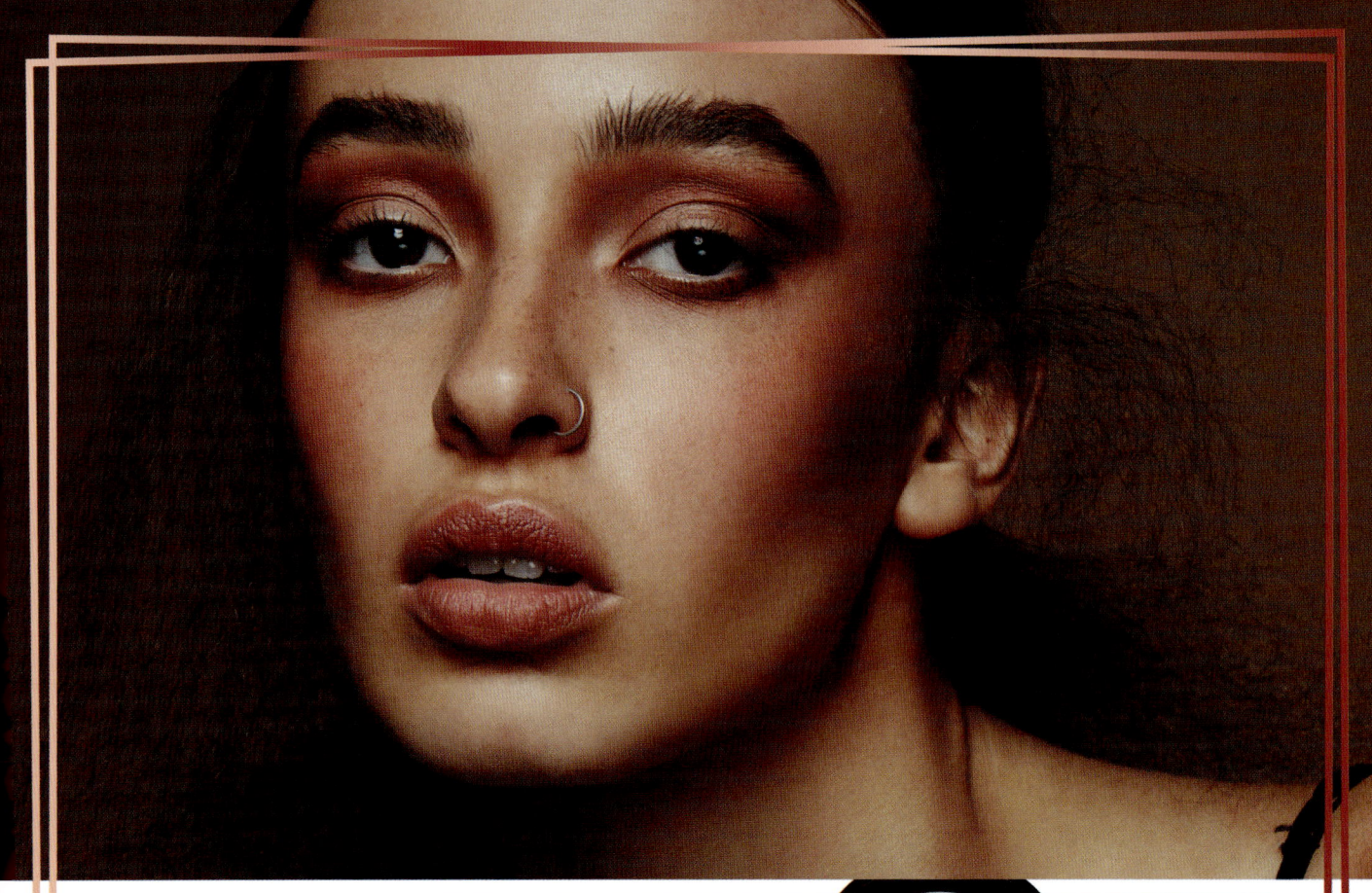

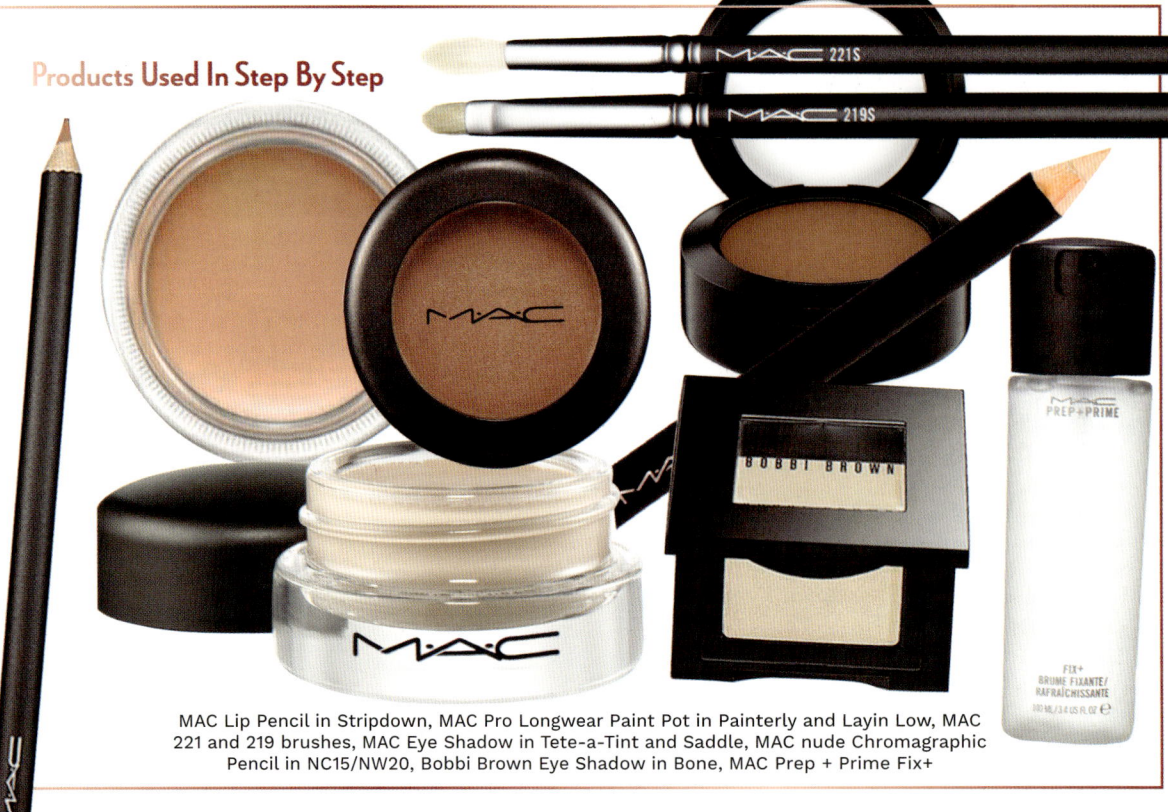

MAC Lip Pencil in Stripdown, MAC Pro Longwear Paint Pot in Painterly and Layin Low, MAC 221 and 219 brushes, MAC Eye Shadow in Tete-a-Tint and Saddle, MAC nude Chromagraphic Pencil in NC15/NW20, Bobbi Brown Eye Shadow in Bone, MAC Prep + Prime Fix+

EYE SPY WITH MY SMOKY EYE

THE NOT-SO-SMOKY EYE

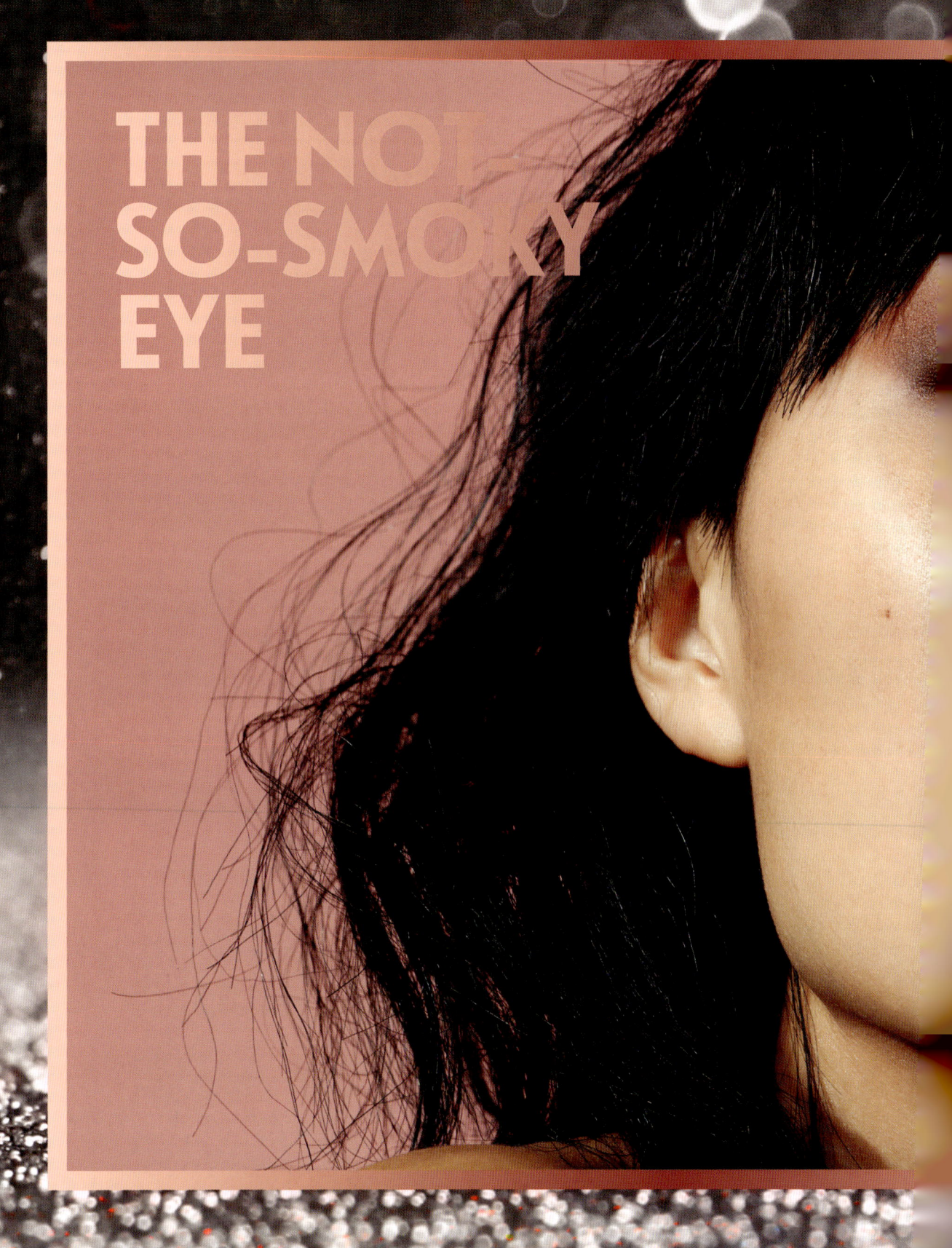

EYE SPY WITH MY SMOKY EYE

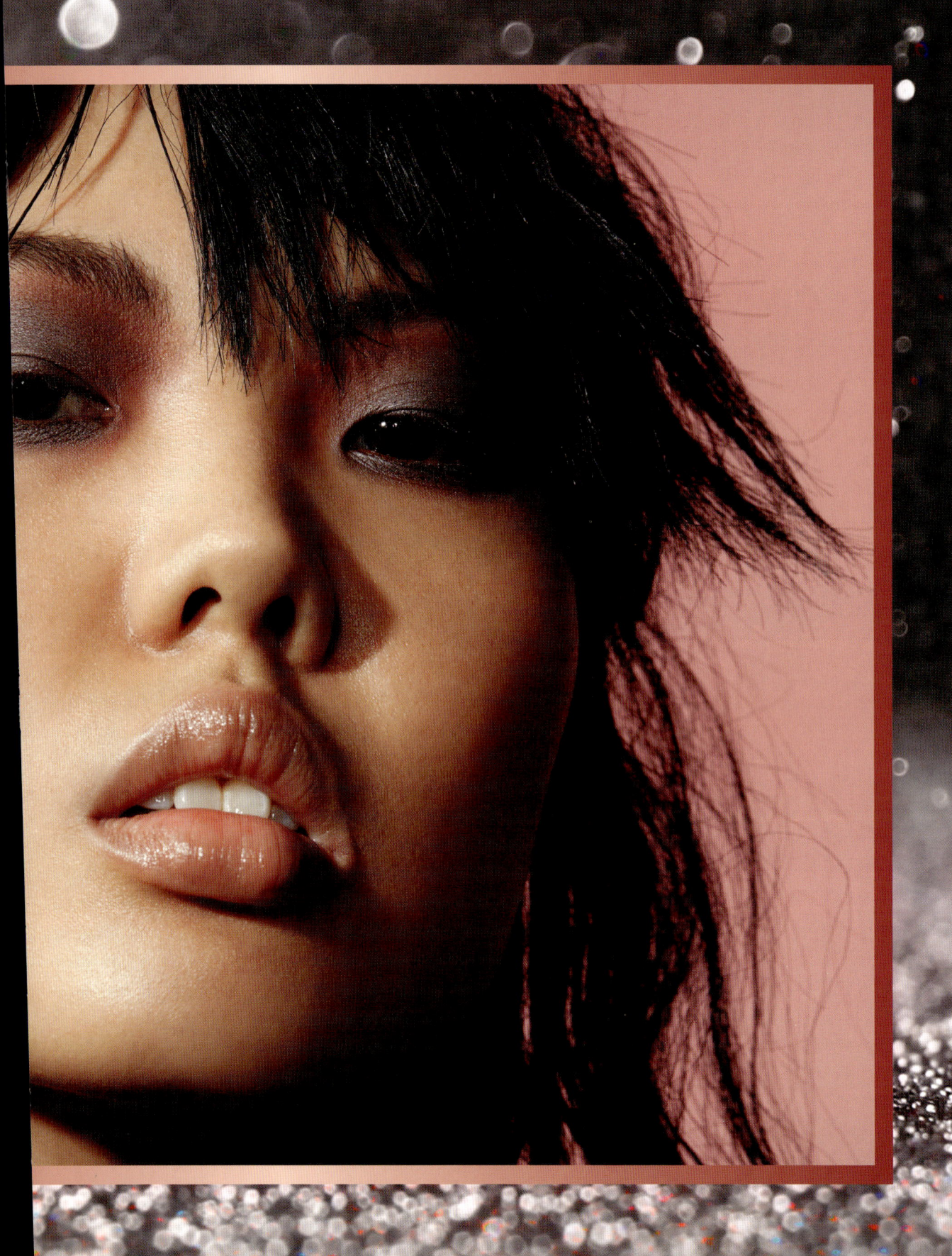

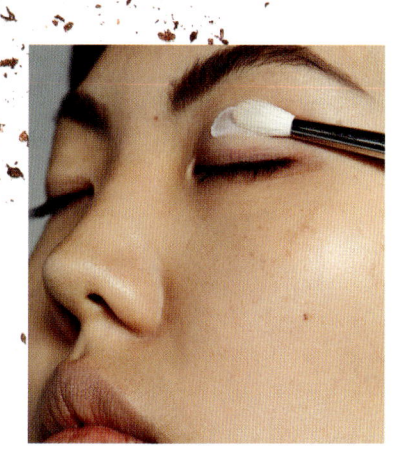

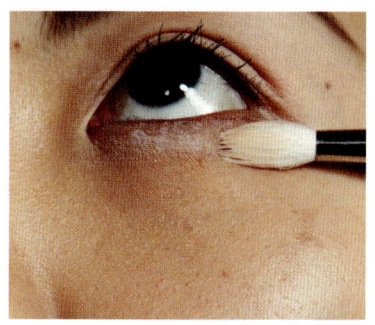

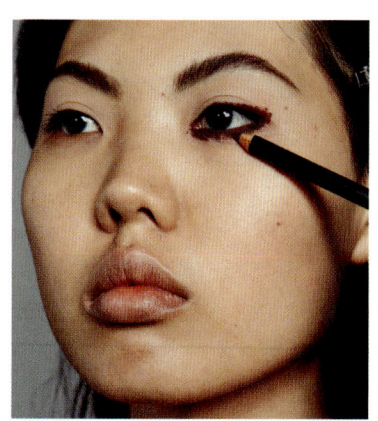

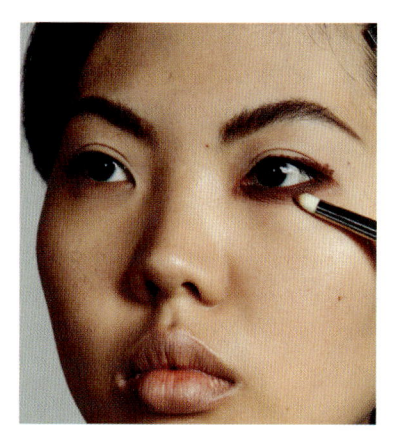

It has been the go-to eye makeup at weddings and formals for the best part of the last 30 years. But for all these years of popularity, there has been a huge misconception when it comes to this artistry staple. Smoky eye is a description of the shape, not the color!

Mind blown, right? Probably not, but all the same, this look has the capacity to be recreated in so many different forms, and you have the power in your shadow palate right now. Yes, the dark grey tones still have a place in the smoky eye spectrum, but don't be afraid to spin that color wheel and see where it ends up.

I have done more smoky eyes than I have had glasses of bubbles, and let me tell you, that is a lot. This has become my go-to technique, but the color and where you take it is entirely up to you. So go forth you crazy cats – explore and experiment!

STEP 1

Primer, yes! Me again! (By the end of this book I am going to need a new word for primer – undercoat anyone?)

So you could skip this step, but then your smoky eye may be at risk of looking like the bottom of an ashtray in an hour or two. It really does make a huge difference. Here I have used my favorite MAC Prep + Prime 24-hour Extend Eye Base. I love the smoothing effect and how it actually intensifies the color you add on top while ensuring it doesn't budge for 24 hours. (I was part of the testing panel for this product which is why it's close to my heart. Also why I am so confident in the results!)

STEP 2

Whichever primer you pick, don't forget to prime under the eyes. Even if you aren't taking color under the eyes at all, the primer will help to stop the concealer from moving or, worse still, falling victim to my old nemesis, panda eyes, thanks to your mascara smudging.

STEP 3

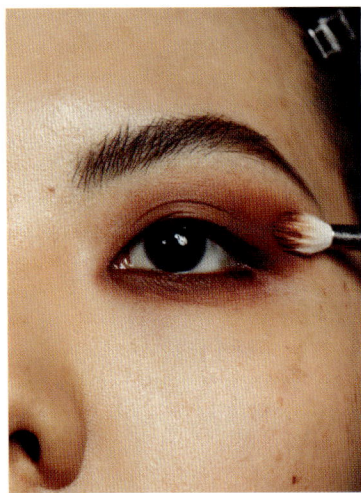

Grab your thick, crayon-like eye pencil, and create a generous line all the way around your eyes. Don't be wuss! Forget about precision and be plentiful in your application of this product, remembering you will be blending it in once you are done.

STEP 4

Use a small fluffy brush to move and blend the liner as you go. For me, the under-eye area is not an afterthought; it's not the part you hurry when you realize you have just spent 35 minutes blending your crease! Often I will start a 'classic' smoky eye by adding the color underneath – this is the part of the eye you actually see first!

> *TIP!* I never really understood the idea of prepping the lids with a super-light shadow before you pile on a dark smoky eye. I won't say *don't* do it, as it's your choice, but really think about what is going to make your job easier! I like to get straight to the goods. If I want dark, I prep with dark, If I want light, I prep with light – whether it be a pencil or cream shadow. If I want it all, I prep clear! I do *not* have the time it takes in all those sped-up YouTube blending montages to build up that color and painstakingly take a white eye all the way to charcoal.

STEP 5

Use a fluffy brush to buff all the way around your eyes in a windscreen-wiper, circular motion.

STEP 6

Add. Blend. Repeat. Concentrate the strongest amount of color along the top and bottom lashlines, then hugging the outer corners. This will extend and shape, creating an illusion of bigger eyes.

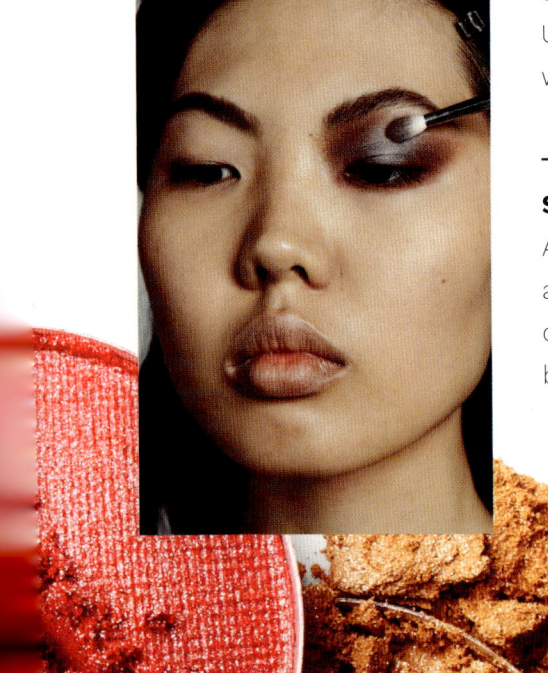

EYE SPY WITH MY SMOKY EYE

STEP 7

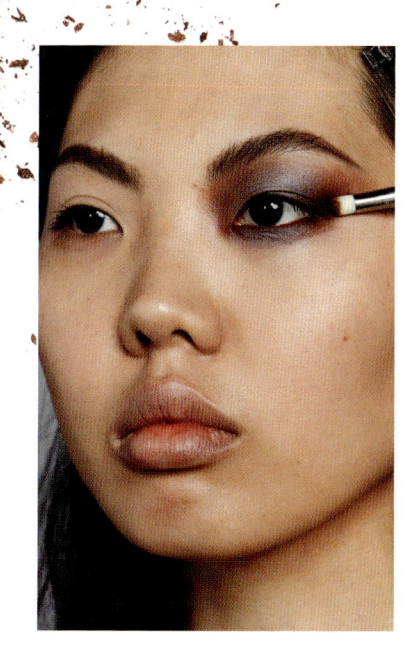

Set the shape with your eye shadow! First apply the cool toned shimmer eye shadow over the whole eyelids and blend it outwards. For beneath the eye, do the same, except I want you to start from the center working outwards.

> **TIP!** To get the most out of your shimmery shadow don't forget to spritz your brush with Fix+ to grab the color and have it glide on with an opaque and smooth finish.

STEP 8

I like to play with opposing tones of color and texture to build a multidimensional eye. I love using shimmer with cool tones through the center to enlarge the eye. Then take your pressed matte powder (I'm using a warm-toned dark-brown here) and work it into the outer corners before softly dragging along the lash line. This will strengthen the shape and really push that 3D effect!

You can get creative with colors and textures and easily use the same chocolate-brown pencil base and then switch up the colored shadows you set with. I hate to break the illusion, but smoky eyes are pretty much the same shape, different colors!

STEP 9

One last blend! Open and close eyes while giving them one last blend to tie it all together.

> **TIP!** To do eyes first or not to do eyes first? That is the question! Truth be told, there is no right or wrong here. They both have their advantages. I prefer spending a moment getting my skin polished and perfected as it makes me feel *so* much more confident, I find the same thing with my clients – once our skin looks good, we feel good. Having your foundation done first also means you have something to blend your eye makeup into, so it can look more finessed as a completed look. Doing your eyes first means you can go in balls to the wall with your eye makeup, and then clean up any remnants of your work after.

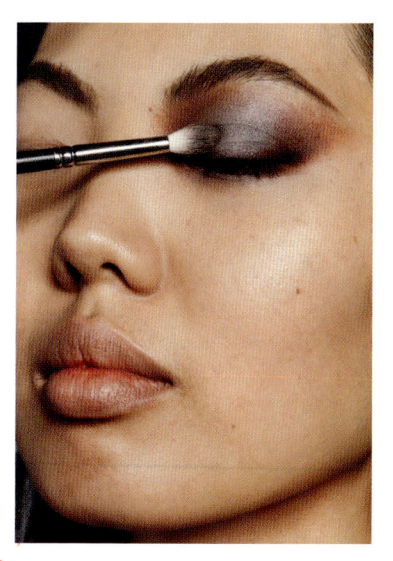

Products Used In Step By Step

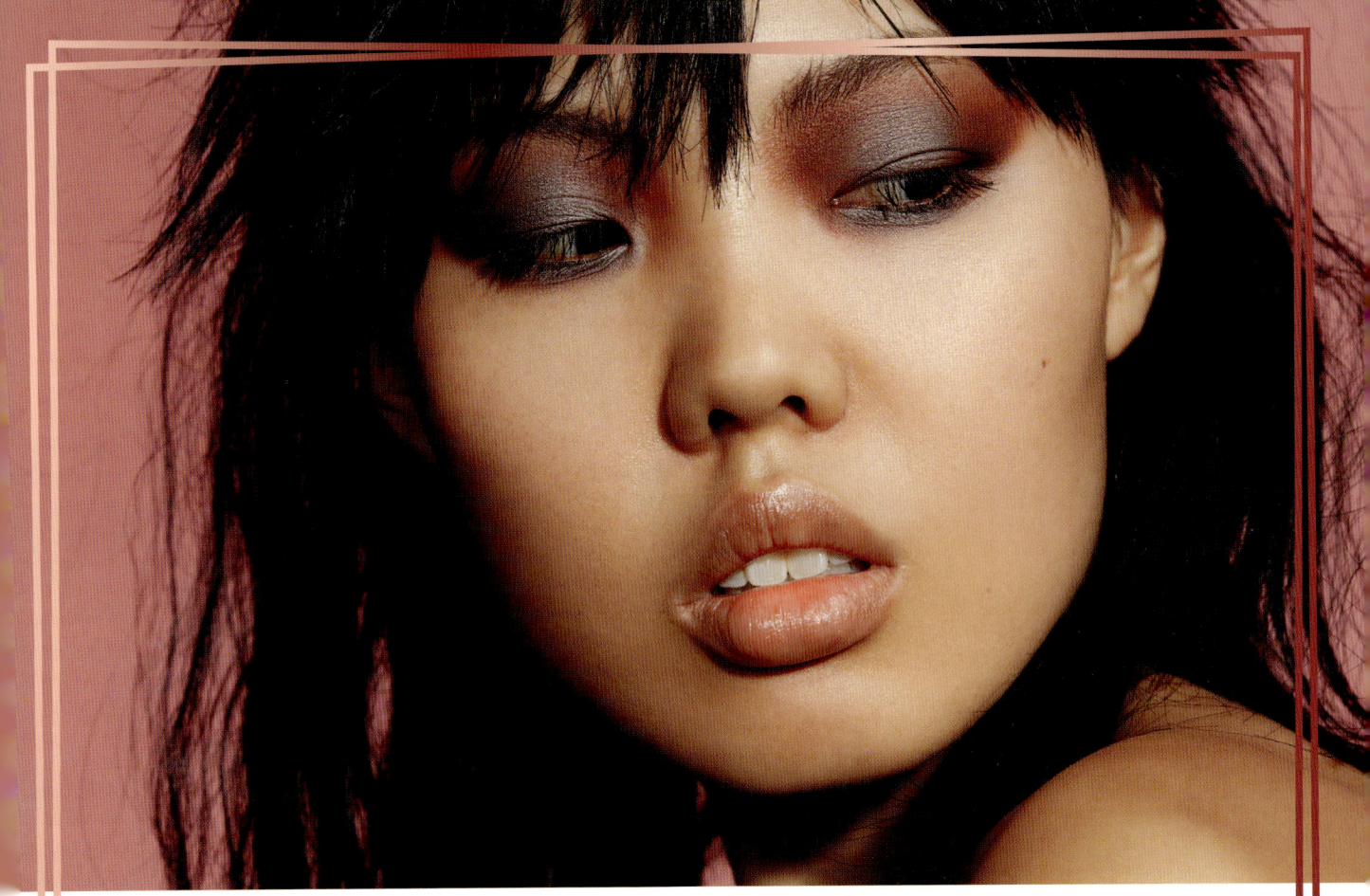

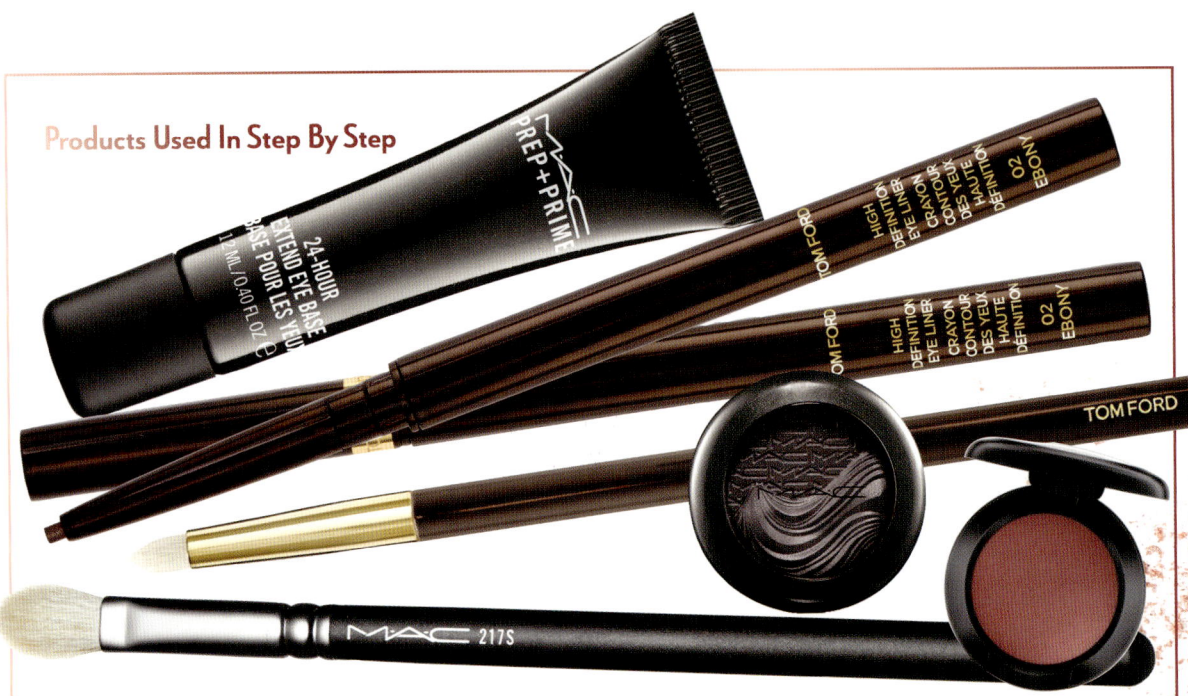

MAC Prep + Prime 24-Hour Extend Eye Base, Tom Ford High Definition Eye Liner in Ebony, Tom Ford Smokey Eye Brush 14, MAC 217 Brush, MAC Extra Dimension Eye Shadow in Fathoms Deep, MAC Eye Shadow in I'm Into It

EYE SPY WITH MY SMOKY EYE

METALLIC EYE

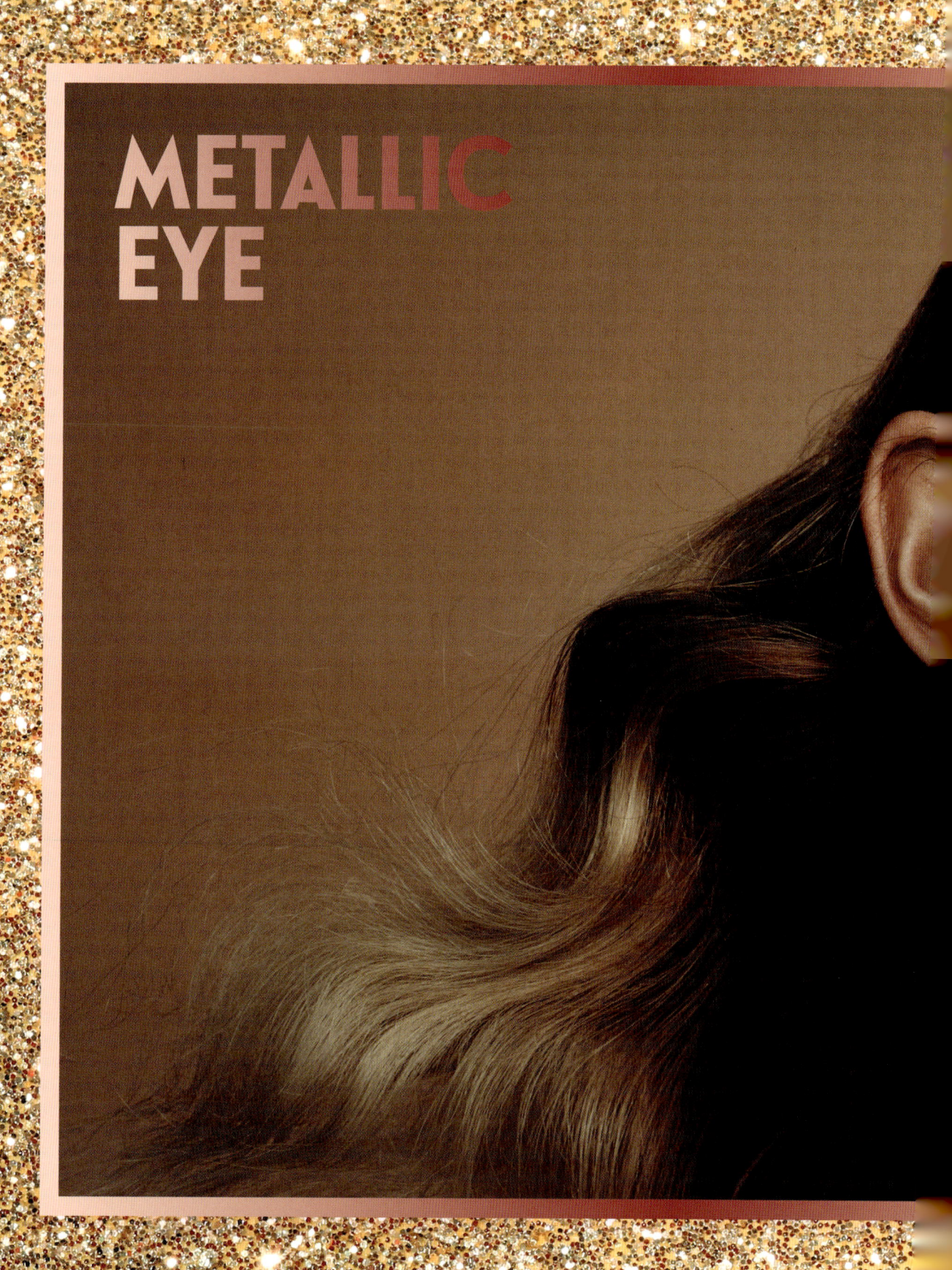

EYE SPY WITH MY SMOKY EYE

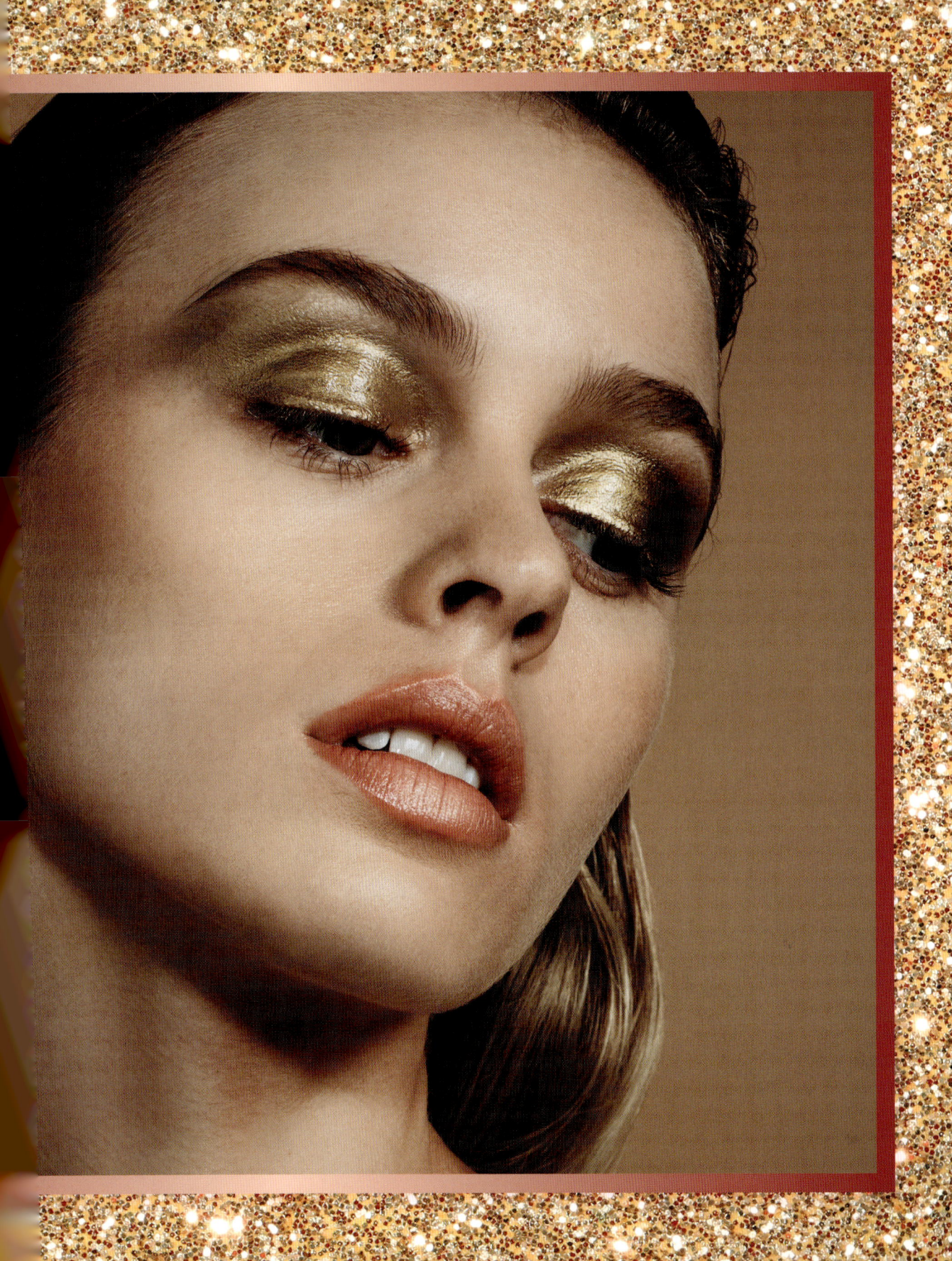

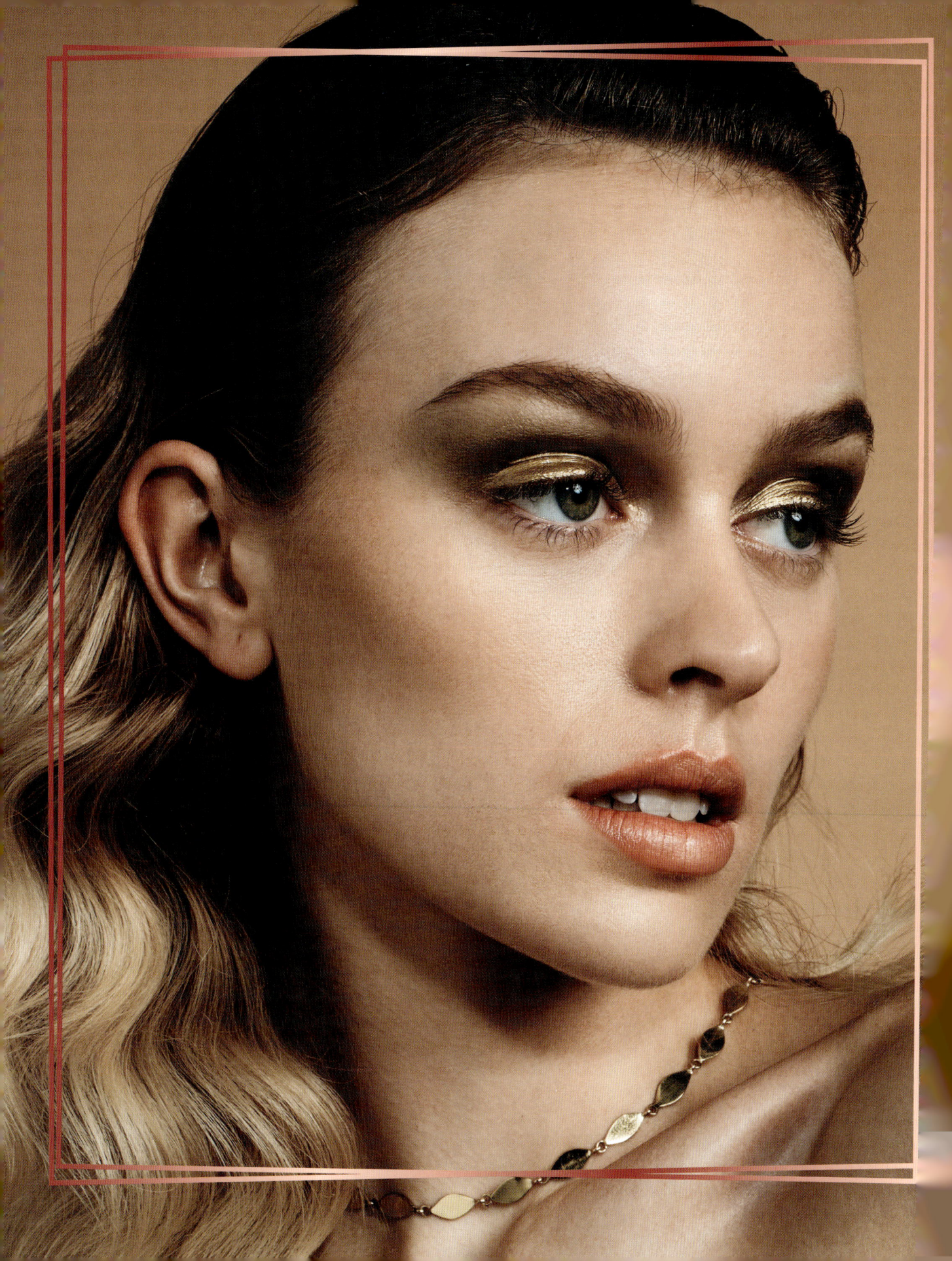

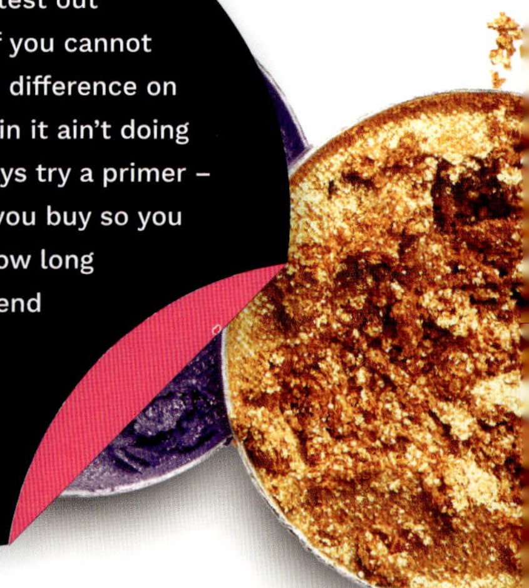

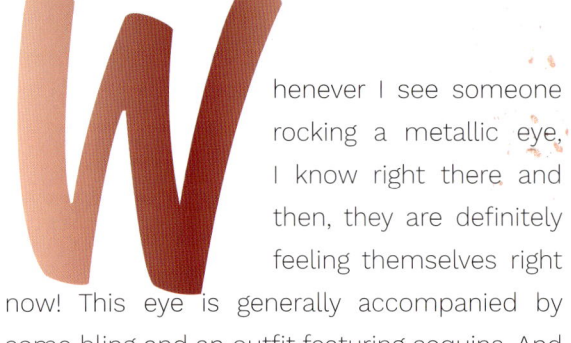

Whenever I see someone rocking a metallic eye, I know right there and then, they are definitely feeling themselves right now! This eye is generally accompanied by some bling and an outfit featuring sequins. And why not? If you're going to do it, go full Tina Sparkle, right? Apologies kids for the *Strictly Ballroom* reference.

Multidimensional eye shadows look intricate and tricky but the technique to achieve a stunning foiled eye is not as hard as you think. Trust me! That said, there are a few factors that will change how intense and metallic your look will be.

What Are You Using as a Base to Your Metallic Eye?

Nothing? Well you are not under arrest, but you will find the shine doesn't last and the eye shadow will move within the hour. Boo.

Eye cream? Nice one governor! This is amazing for anti-aging purposes (future you says thank you), however, this will do *nothing* for the longevity of your makeup, In fact, if it's really nourishing and creamy it may lead to the makeup sliding away! I suggest using eye creams heavily overnight to get max hydration. Then during the day when you do your makeup opt for a primer instead.

Primer? FAB-U-LOUS. You must have heard me mention primer 3000 times already! Gold star coming your way. Clear primer will work under anything from your peach eye, to your silver shimmer or your gold metallic look. A colored primer will amplify your metallic moment further, if you dare…

Concealer? Coolio, your skin tone is even-steven, great! There are approximately one million types of concealer out there and they definitely don't all do the same thing. Concealers are designed to give you perfect, correcting coverage for all areas of the face, not to be an eye-shadow primer. Yes your skin will be a bright, blank canvas to paint on, but it may crease, and therefore move your eye makeup. If you are determined to use a concealer, make sure you try a waterproof concealer that sets and stays – test it out!

Translucent powder? Great! You are eliminating moisture form your lids so you can blend eye shadow smoothly on top. This is my prepping method of choice for this look.

> **TIP!**
> Make sure to test out your eye primer. If you cannot see or feel a texture difference on the surface of the skin it ain't doing anything! You can always try a primer – grab a sample before you buy so you can see for yourself how long it lasts before you spend your dosh.

EYE SPY WITH MY SMOKY EYE

What Are You Mixing It With?

For loose powder pigments and metallic pressed shadows, you can use them wet or dry. Dry will be easy to blend and deliver a more subtle version of the metal finish. Mixing with a cream or liquid to apply will give you a more silky and shiny finish.

Water? Okay cool, you will see instant shine with that pigment straight away, but I hate to burst your bubble. Unfortunately, because there are no cosmetic ingredients or adhesive qualities in plain water, by the time you find your phone and keys and walk out the door your metallic eye would have lost much of its shine.

Face mist? Test it and try it! I have played with a few and have found mixed results. Face mists that have a setting quality (stated and advertised) should mix well, while hydrating at the same time, and the mix should stay put. Try your metallic pigment with a small spritz of the spray you have used to set your makeup and see how long it lasts.

Mixing mediums? Here. We. Go. These guys are made specifically to mix, amplify, and set your makeup. TICK, TICK. TICK! I used the MAC Eyeliner Mixing Medium here; it has been a kit favorite of mine through 10 years of fashion week and color mixing. Mix with pigments to make into a precise liner, mix with powder to make into an easy to blend liquid shadow that is water resistant.

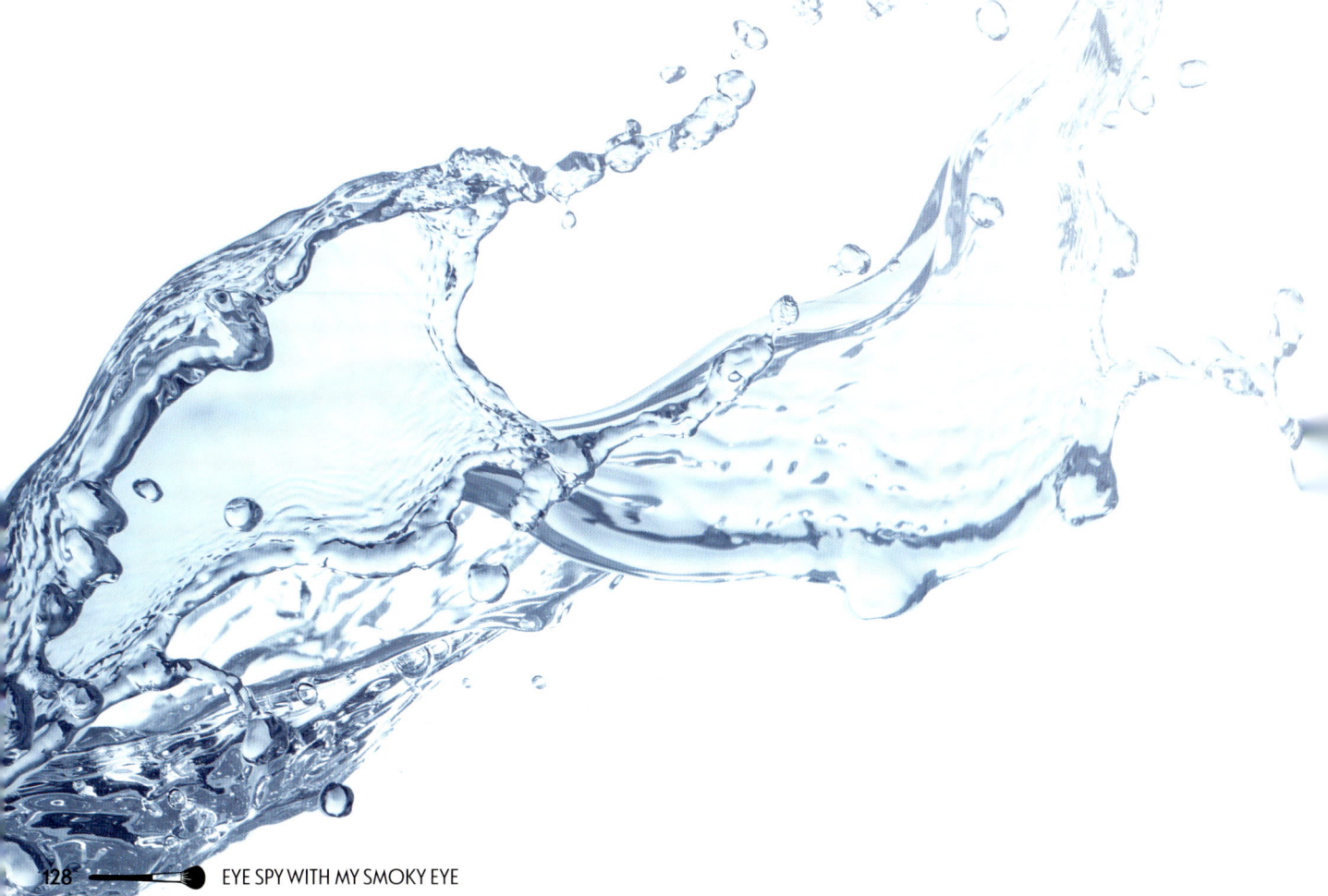

STEP 1

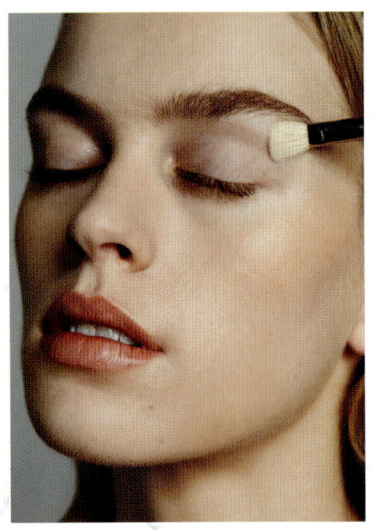

Remove any excess oil from the lids by pressing a good amount of translucent powder over them, then brush the excess away so you are left with super matte, smooth lids to start. I used a powder because I am going to be painting a liquid shadow on top and liquid will sit well on a dry surface. If I was using a dry metallic pigment or shadow over a dry powdered lid, I would find that they would not stick together, meaning it would be super hard to build up color or shine. You would need to lay down something for the powder to grab onto, which is why you would use a cream shadow or primer underneath.

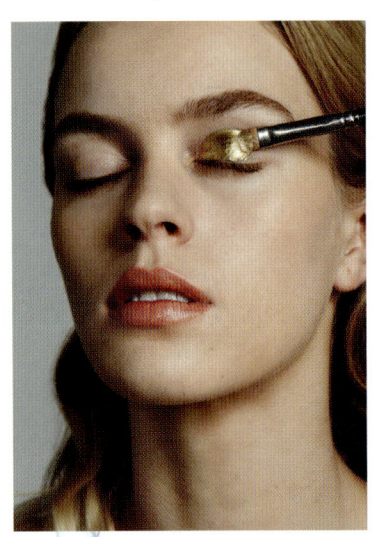

STEP 2

Mix the metallic pigment with a gel mixing medium on the back of your hand or on a little dish. Tap the powder down first, then slowly mix in the gel, little by little, so you don't add too much and dilute the color. Paint the mix across the eyelids from lash to crease with a soft, flat small brush

Don't pile on the color straight up! A liquid can be quite deceiving with how far it can spread. If you add too much, it's quite hard to blend it away. In fact, if you add too much you'll end up blending that gold into a gold face mask! Instead *build* the look one stroke of color at a time.

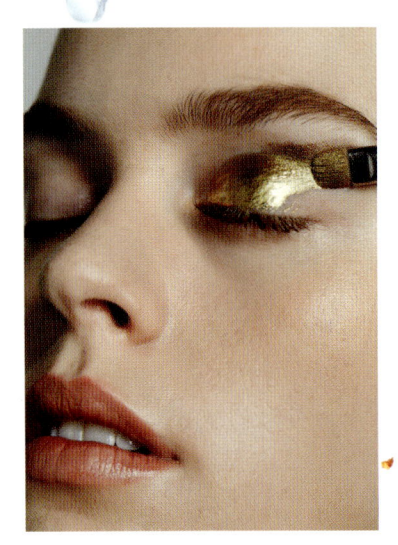

> ***TIP!*** Don't mix liquid shadows, especially waterproof ones, on the back of your hand if you are wearing fake tan! When you scrub to get rid of it with waterproof remover, you will also remove your tan, leaving you with a lovely blotched hand before your night out.

STEP 4

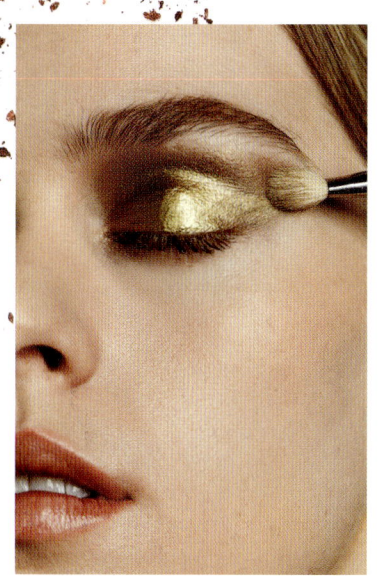

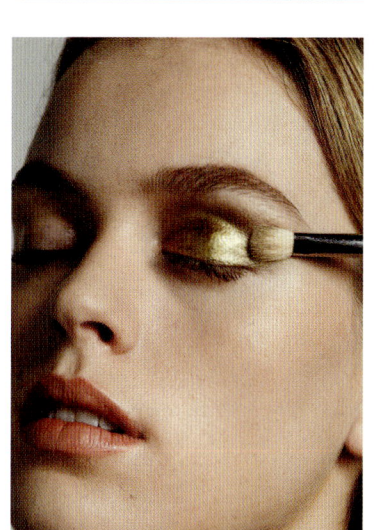

Use a separate brush to blend. This makes all the difference and will help you blend what you need to without adding more and more color. Adding and blending with the same brush can easily become a hot mess before your shiny eyes.

STEP 5

Metallic shadows are wonderful as they contain multiple tones – this one shadow looks like three! Applied wet over the lids it sets like one color, but once you buff it out it honestly seems like you are using another product all together.

If yours doesn't do the same thing, use a matte shadow through the crease. It will shape the eyes in a similar way. Make a final stamp of the metal liquid along the lids with the same small brush. You want to be sure that the strongest amount of color is just behind the lash line so your eyes twinkle when you walk.

STEP 6

When the eye shadow makes this much of a statement, I really like the idea of keeping most of the color on top, and just doing a small amount of mascara or nothing at all underneath. However, this look can be customized so easily by tweaking the shape and the brushes. Use an angle brush or pointy eyeliner brush to paint this gold mix on as an eyeliner – clean and subtle or full-on cat flick! Keep the shape smaller on top then continue it around the eye with a smaller fluffy brush, in an almond shape.

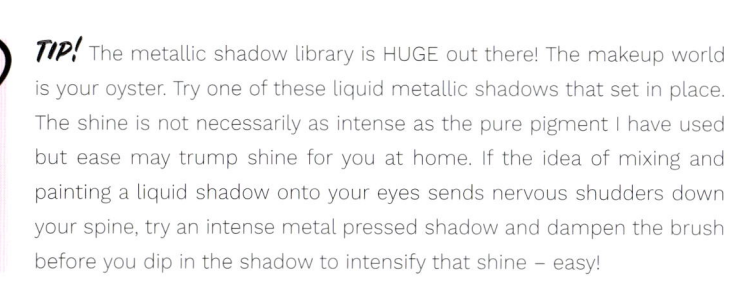

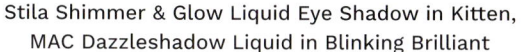

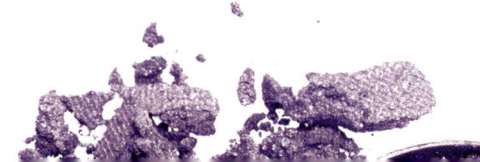

TIP! The metallic shadow library is HUGE out there! The makeup world is your oyster. Try one of these liquid metallic shadows that set in place. The shine is not necessarily as intense as the pure pigment I have used but ease may trump shine for you at home. If the idea of mixing and painting a liquid shadow onto your eyes sends nervous shudders down your spine, try an intense metal pressed shadow and dampen the brush before you dip in the shadow to intensify that shine – easy!

Stila Shimmer & Glow Liquid Eye Shadow in Kitten,
MAC Dazzleshadow Liquid in Blinking Brilliant

TIP! Mix your pigments together to make your own custom color. I like to tap some of a few different colored pigments into the center of a tissue, then I gather the corners making sure it is enclosed, and I shake the tissue to reveal a new color. Get creative with your mixes!

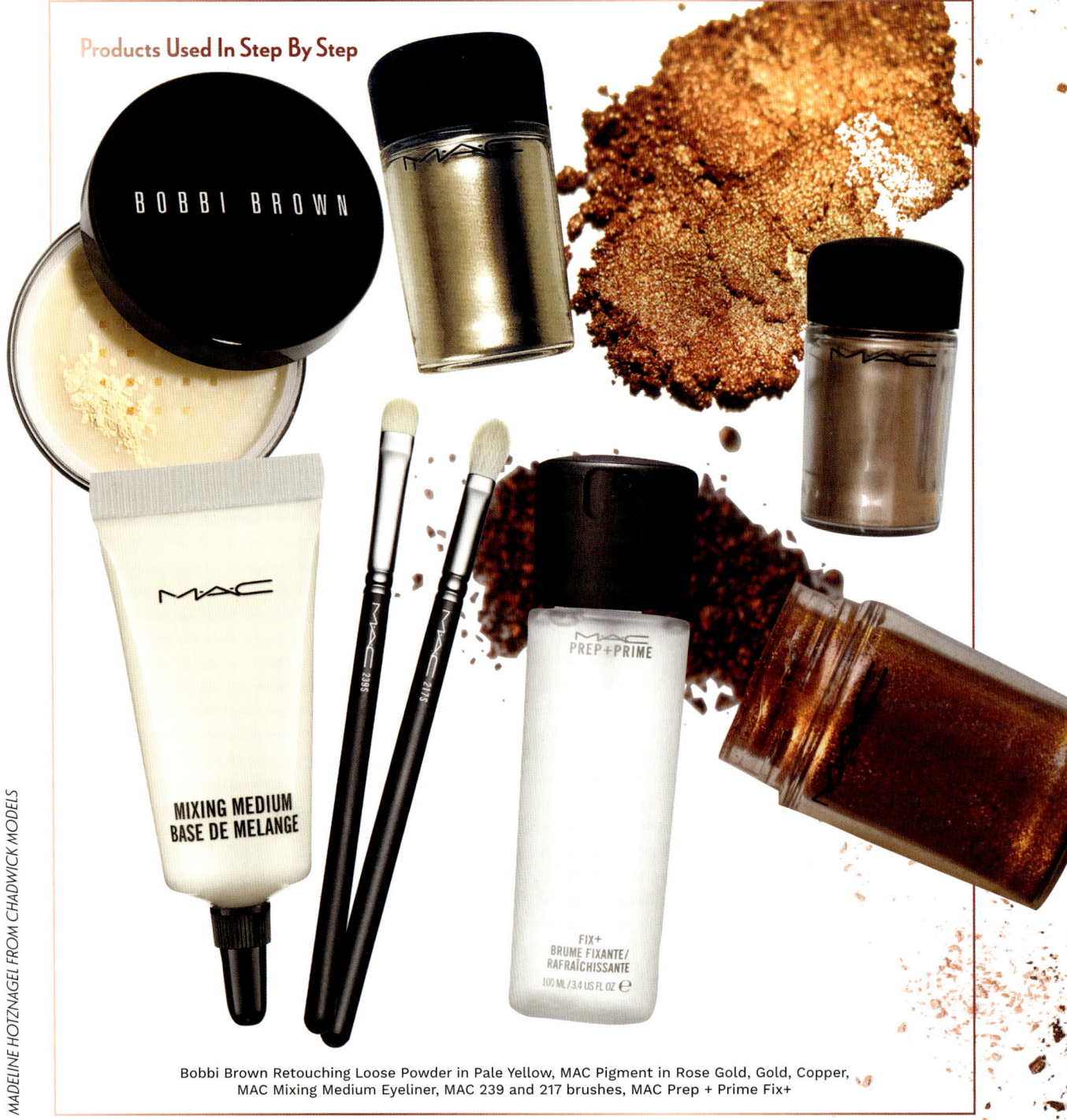

Products Used In Step By Step

Bobbi Brown Retouching Loose Powder in Pale Yellow, MAC Pigment in Rose Gold, Gold, Copper, MAC Mixing Medium Eyeliner, MAC 239 and 217 brushes, MAC Prep + Prime Fix+

MADELINE HOTZNAGEL FROM CHADWICK MODELS

EYE SPY WITH MY SMOKY EYE

PASTEL LAVENDER GLOSSED EYES

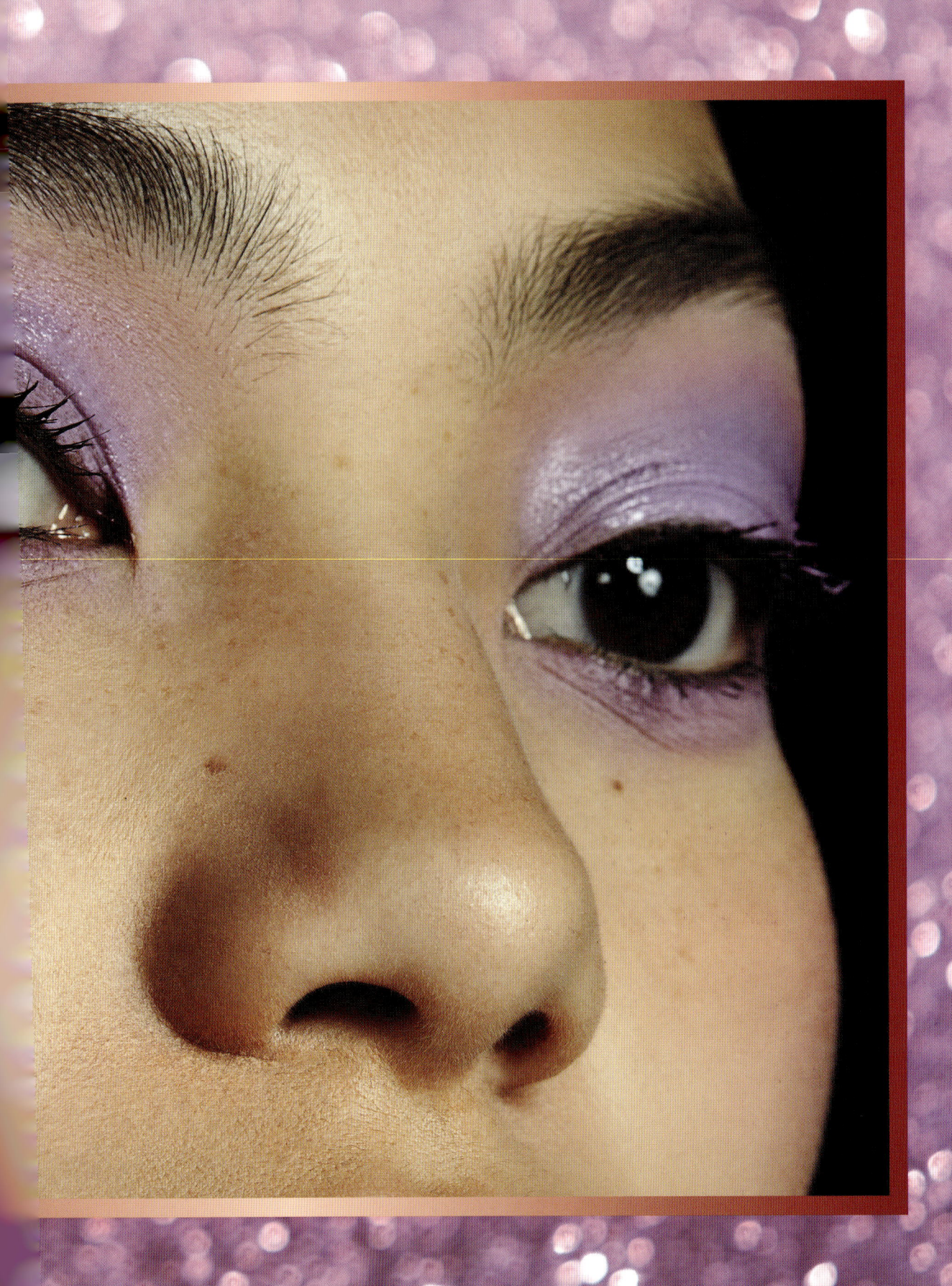

It doesn't even have to be metallic at all when it comes to shiny washes across the eyes! With this look being a matte shadow, it will mean that the color pigment is quite strong, so if you want some extra crease security, lay down a long wearing waterproof primer or concealer first!

The main difference between this and the metallic eye is instead of using the press powder and the mixing medium I used a matte cream lipstick as the base. Using a lippy on the eyes makes it really easy to blend; simply swipe straight from the tube and blend with your fingers or a fluffy brush. Then set with a slightly lighter colored eye shadow, so you can blend to your heart's content without it looking too heavy.

For a glossy finish you can fake it or make it.

To MAKE it, use a shiny gloss without any stickiness so it can be easily slicked across lids. Apply onto the lids just behind lashes for that sheen to pop in photos, but remember, less is more! If you are daring, slick it all the way over your lids.

To FAKE it use a high-shine eye shadow just through the center and wet your brush while applying to really smooth the shine and imitate gloss.

TIP!
Lip products are the secret weapon! If it claims to last for 12 hours on the lips, where else can you use it? Forget what your product is supposed to do, be led by what color you want to see, and try it out in unexpected areas on the face!

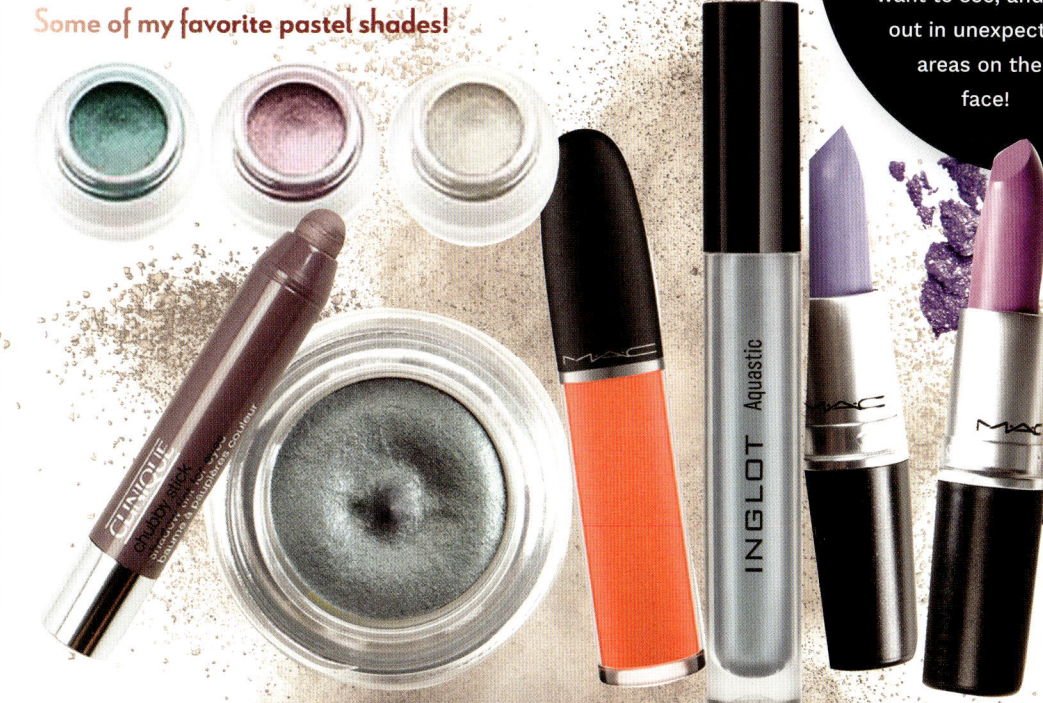

Some of my favorite pastel shades!

NYX Professional Makeup Holographic Halo Cream Eyeliner in Killing It, Cotton Candy and Frost, Clinique Chubby Stick Shadow Tint For Eyes in Lavish Lilac, Tom Ford Cream Color For Eyes in Siren Blue, MAC Retro Matte Liquid Lipcolor in Rich & Restless, Inglot Aquastic Cream Eye Shadow in 19, MAC Matte Lipstick in Flatter Me Fierce and Lavender Jade

MARLO FROM CHADWICK MODELS

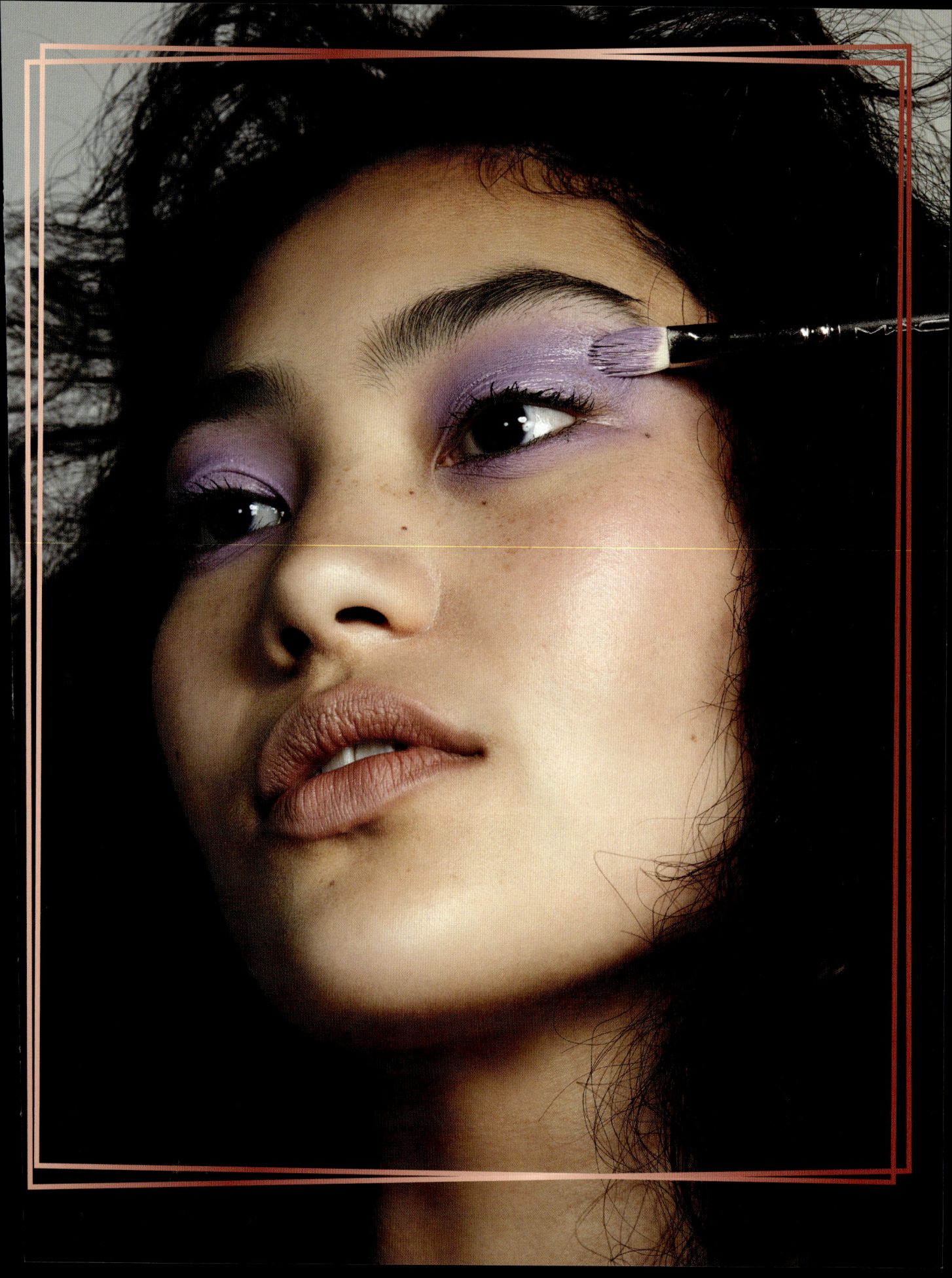

GLITTER EYES

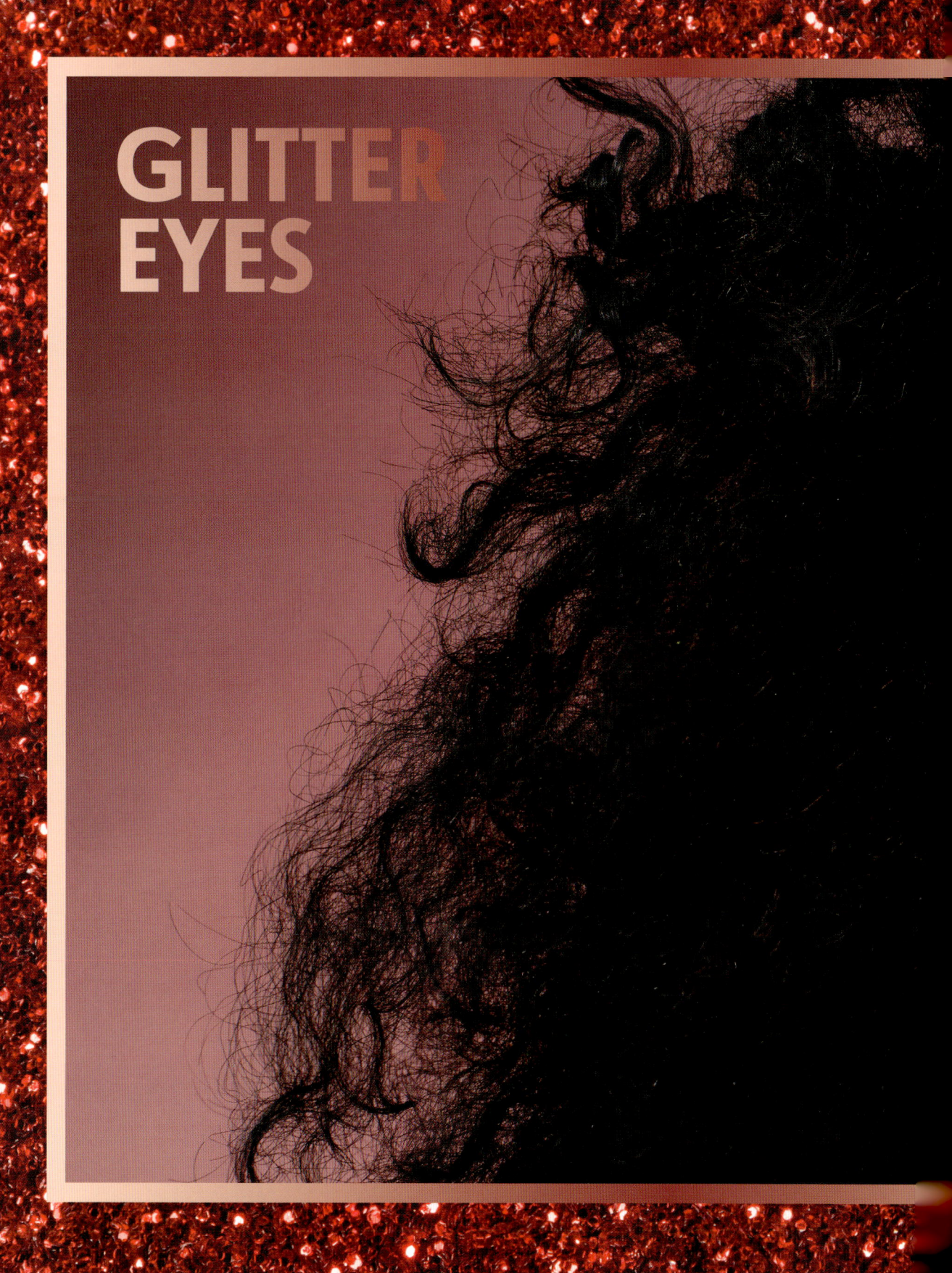

EYE SPY WITH MY SMOKY EYE

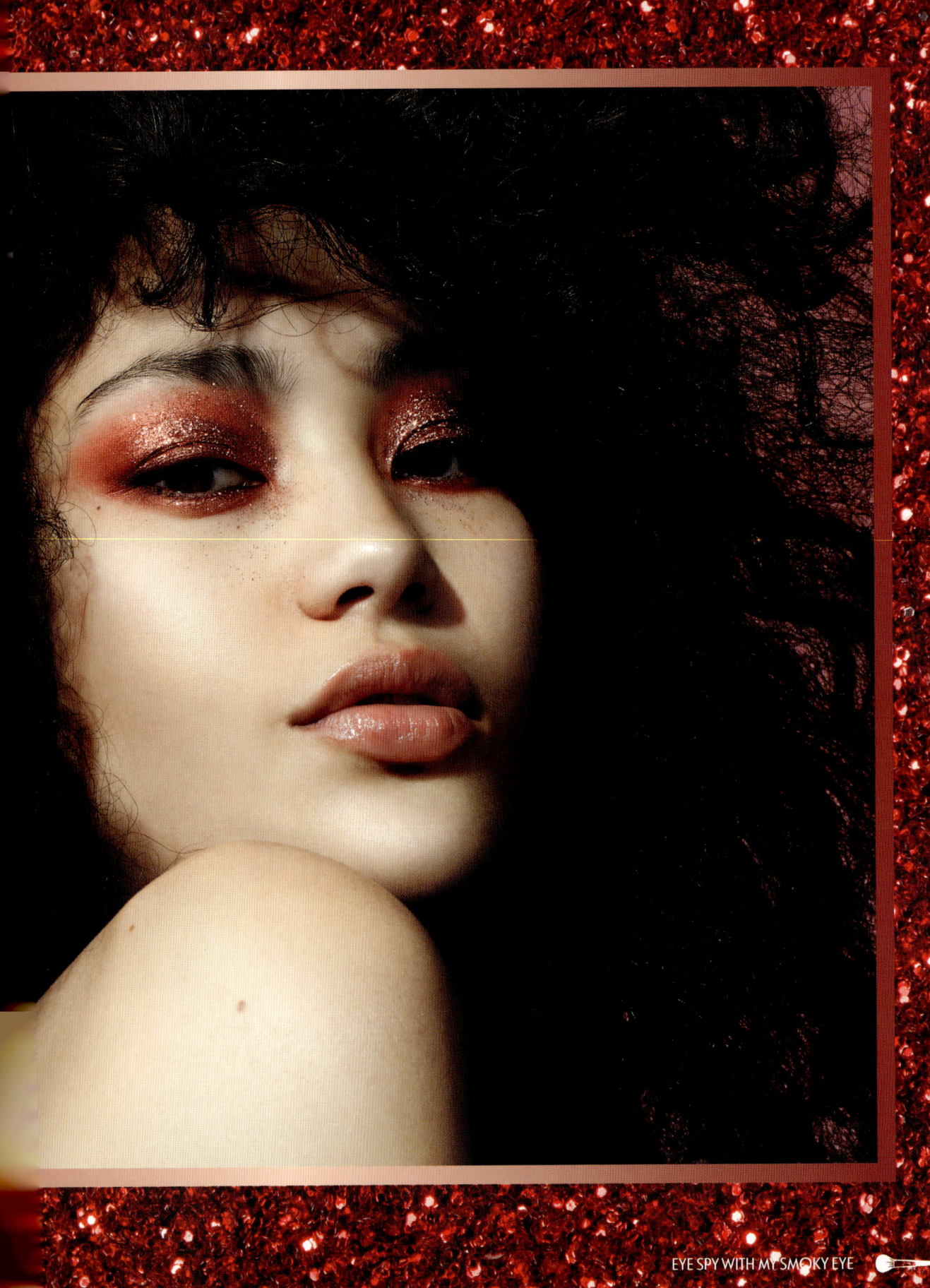

There are certain things in this world that simply make you smile. Rainbows, puppies, the popping sound of a champagne bottle opening in the distance and glitter! All the glitter. So, it is no surprise that nothing makes me happier than when the trends in beauty swing back to glitter! When is it appropriate to wear a glitter eye outside of attending Mardi Gras, you ask. Um, always, obviously!

STEP 1

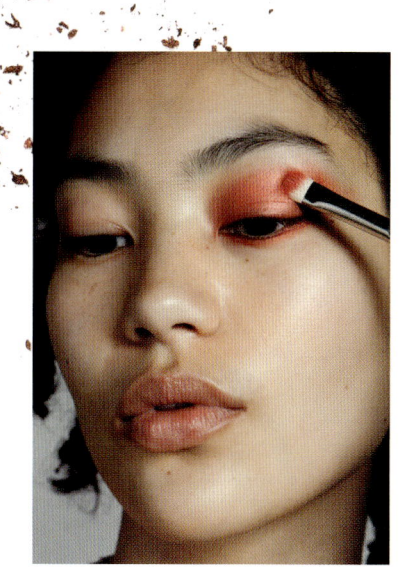

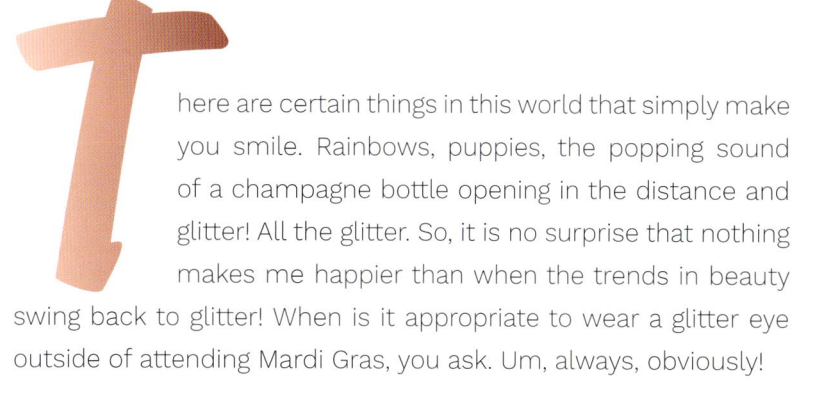

Glitter can have a mind of its own when you are applying it. Sometimes it can be patchy, then sometimes it can apply so perfectly you don't know how you did it. I like to give myself a security blanket so it looks good *all* the time – get your eye makeup on first! Whatever glitter color I am using I love to add a similar color shadow underneath to conceal holes in the glitter and make the look more dramatic over all.

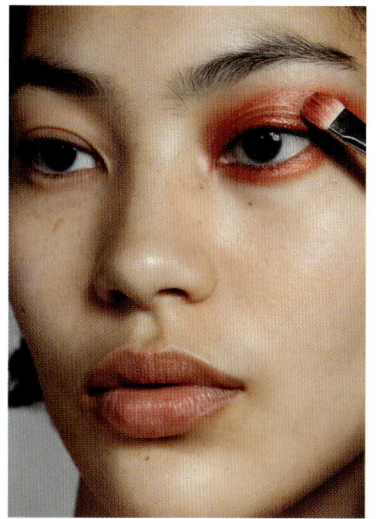

STEP 2

For longevity, tap on mixing medium or glitter glue wherever you want to see the glitter attach. I like to take it just inside the eye shadow shape so I have something to blend into – going all the way to the edge will make this look more superhero than sexy.

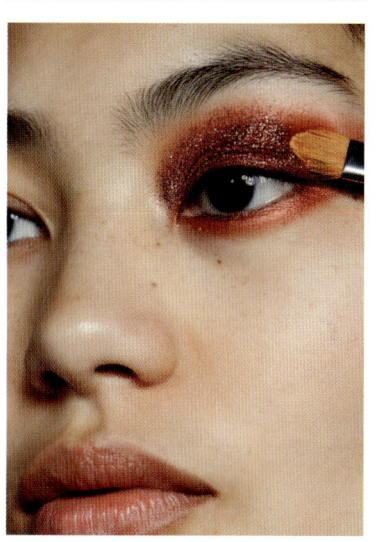

STEP 3

Tap that glitter onto the lids with a flat brush or your finger tip – either way you need something flat and dense to really press this sparkly goodness into place! A fluffy brush will drop those particles everywhere – leave that brush for blending.

STEP 3

Glitter fallout clean up, or as it can sometimes be known, the never ending story! Urgh. If you have ever worn or used glitter you will know that it can live on long after your night out. On

your clothes, in your carpet or in your hair. Now in all my years I'm still yet to find a way to completely eradicate glitter run off in those places but I have learnt some ways to minimize the sparkle explosion across the rest of your face and body. My favorite is to use a small lint roller to roll away stray glitter. This is a trick I saw backstage and I have kept small lint rollers in my kit from then onwards. Roll along under your eyes and cheeks. The stick is so strong it will pick up heaps of the fallout! If you don't get it all, peel off that layer, and keep rolling!

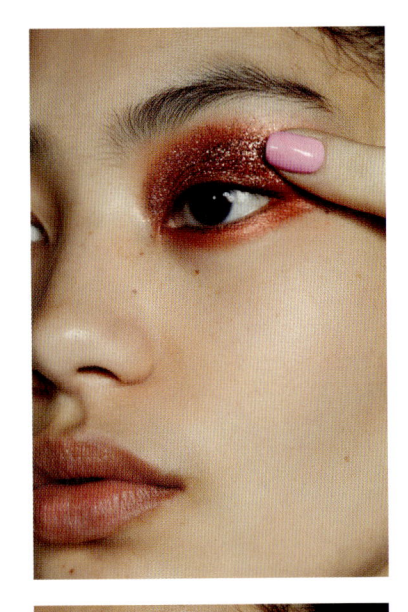

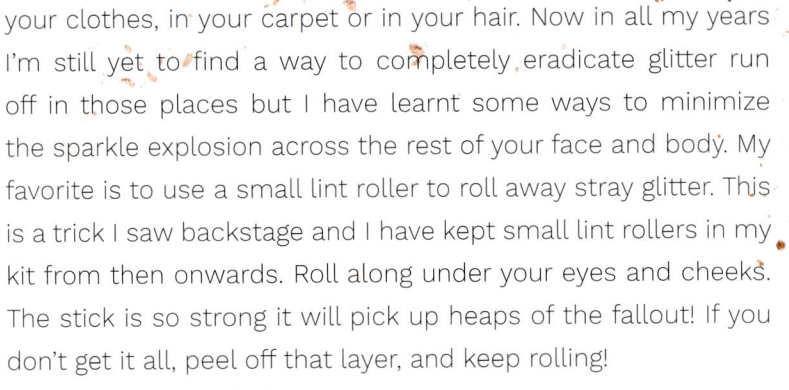

Some other hacks include:

- A little roll of craft tape can be wonderful for pickup on the skin.
- Surgical tape can do the same thing, and can be more sensitive on our skin and perhaps not make you feel like a school project.
- A spoolie can be great to flick away stray glitter (too much of this and you can feel like you are at the pet groomer's).
- Powder. This one I love – it works especially well when you are using large, chunky glitter. Layer that powder on *heavy* wherever the glitter has fallen. It will absorb the moisture that is holding it on your skin and you should be able to brush the particles away. Keep powdering and brushing, then any remaining flecks you can flick away easily with your fingernail or spoolie brush.
- Just don't use glitter (clearly I don't recommend this *at all*!).

TIP! Important! If you are using a glitter glue, do not use a brush to apply! All the hairs will be glued together and removal of glue out of brush hairs is about as enjoyable as pulling a tooth. The reality is you will likely have to throw the brush away – drama! We want drama on our eyes not in our brushes! If you are using a mixing medium like I did, or a cream, you can use a brush or fingertips, as the product will wash out of brushes easily.

EYE SPY WITH MY SMOKY EYE

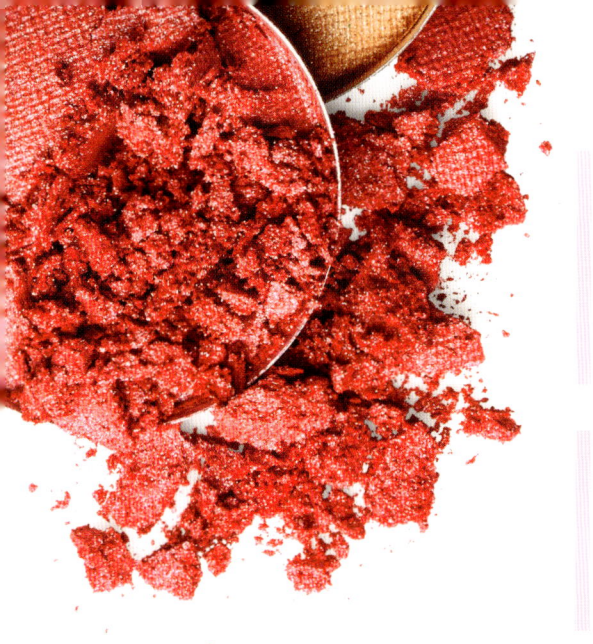

TIP! Another common dilemma is whether to apply foundation before or after the glitter. I totally agree with people doing their foundation afterwards, especially if they are going straight up DISCO with their glitter. If you are like me, and like to see something on your skin to make you feel better before doing your whole face, do your base first. The key is to keep it light on coverage and hydrated under the eyes, as this will make it easier to remove any excess glitter that has made its way to your cheeks.

TIP! Gravity and a tissue can help you! Apply glitter while holding a hand mirror, with your chin up as high it can go without putting your neck out. Then the fallout is only falling back onto your eyes instead of your cheeks! If you are looking into a hand mirror, chin right up again, this time hold a folded strip of tissue about 3 cm wide under your eyes or lips as you apply, catching the jumping glitter dust.

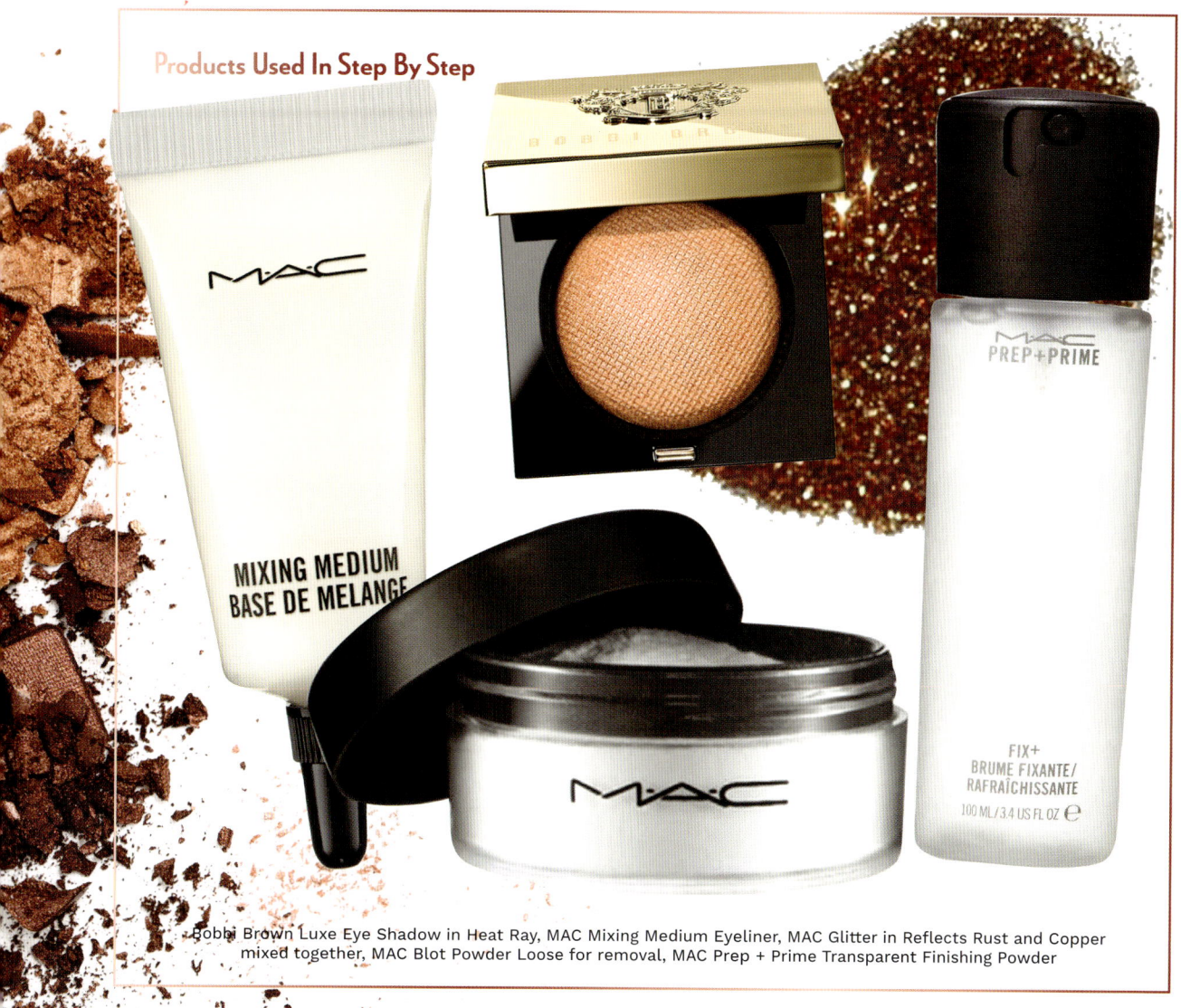

Products Used In Step By Step

Bobbi Brown Luxe Eye Shadow in Heat Ray, MAC Mixing Medium Eyeliner, MAC Glitter in Reflects Rust and Copper mixed together, MAC Blot Powder Loose for removal, MAC Prep + Prime Transparent Finishing Powder

MARLO FROM CHADWICK MODELS

EYE SPY WITH MY SMOKY EYE

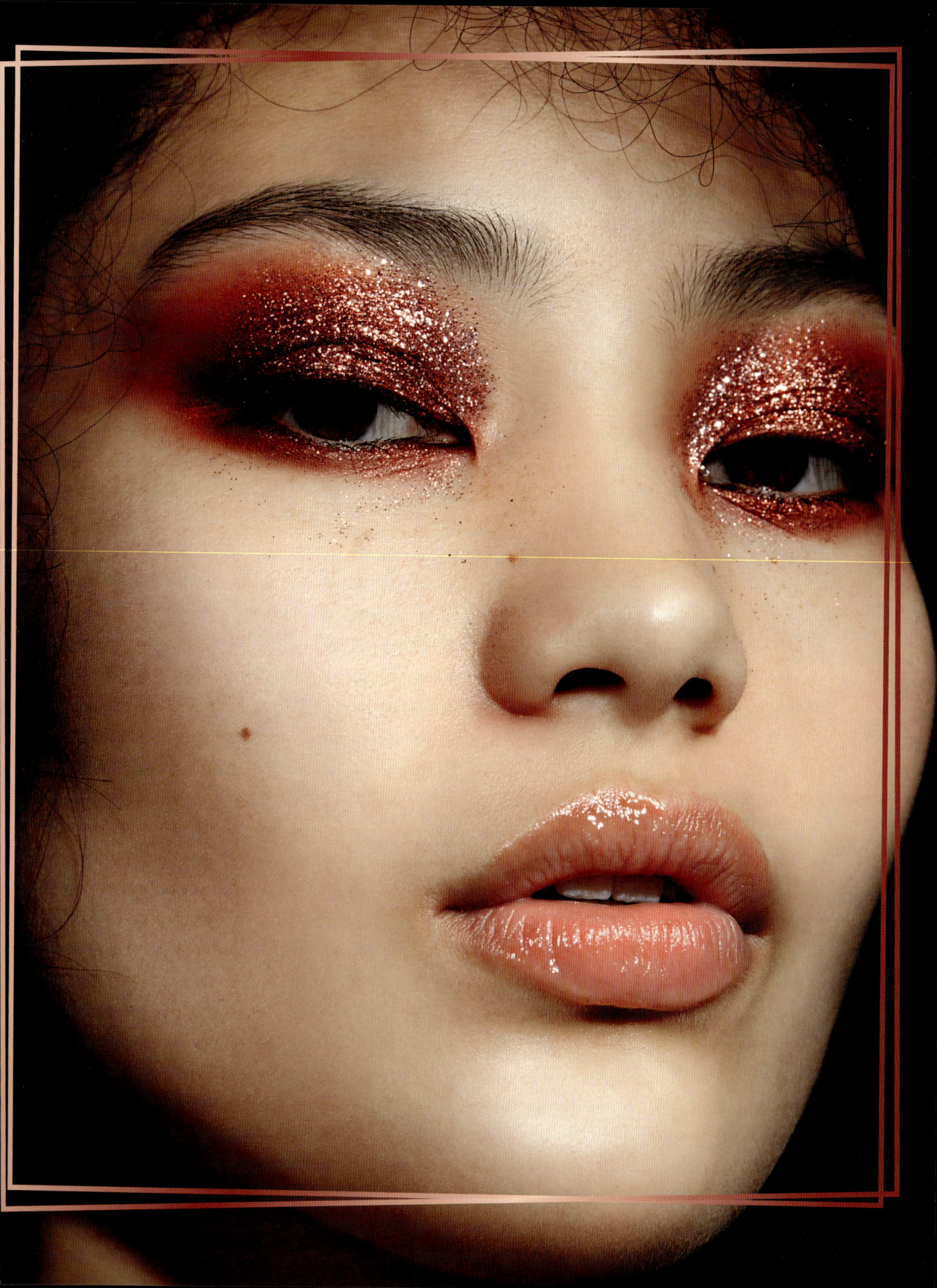

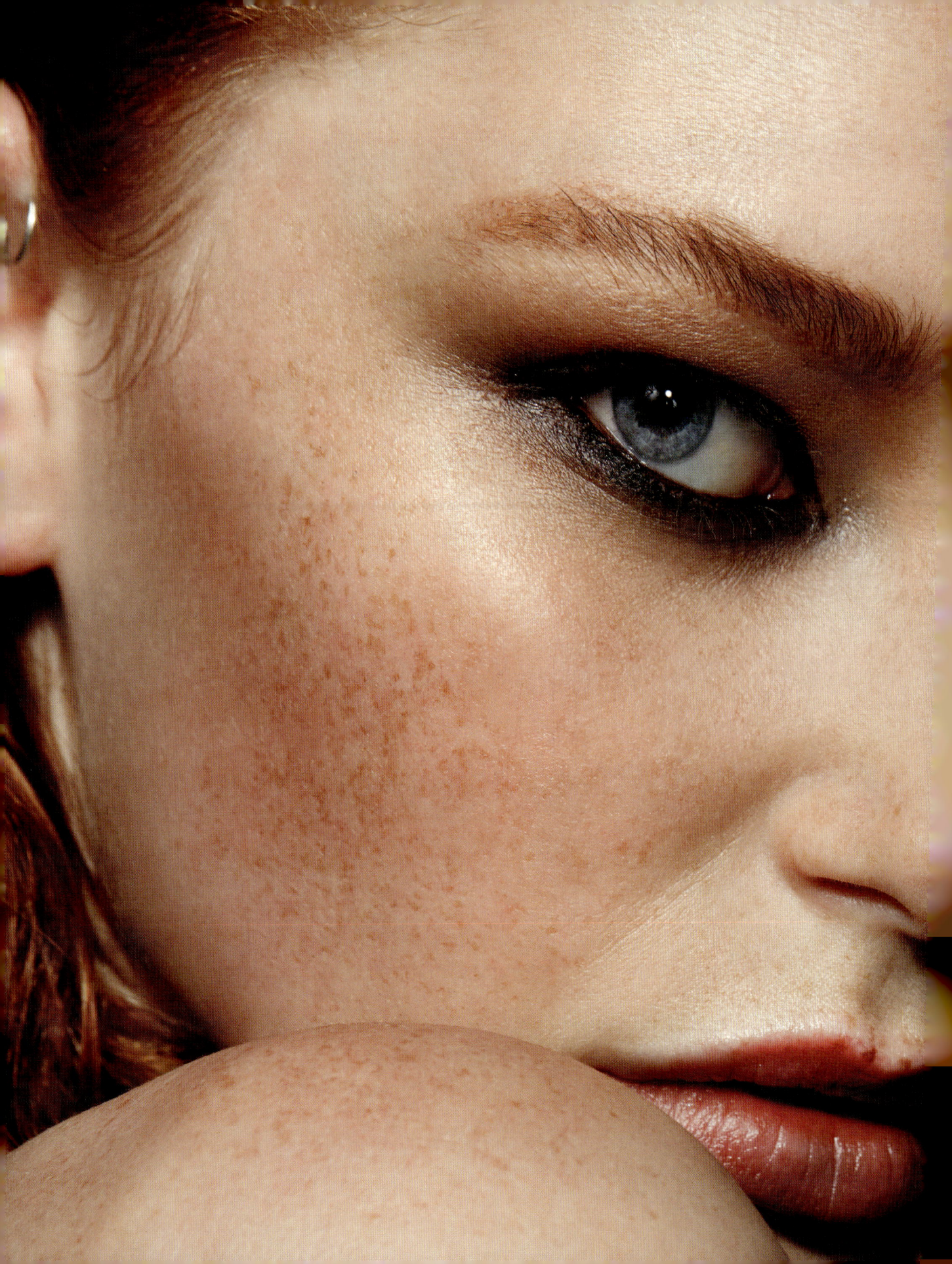

Looking fine ms eyeline

BLACK FLICK LINER

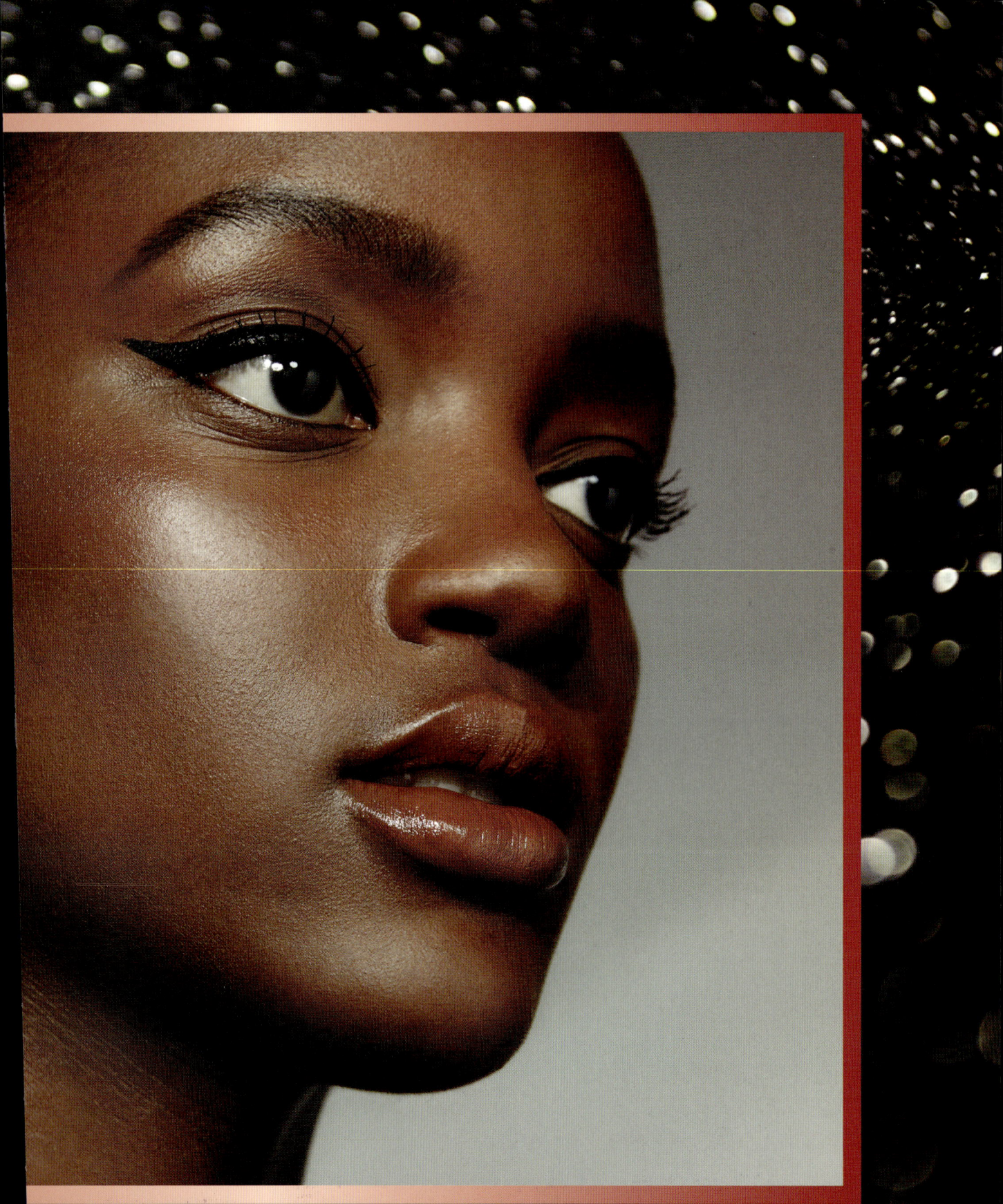

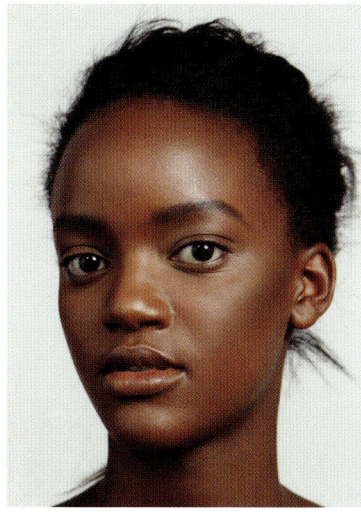

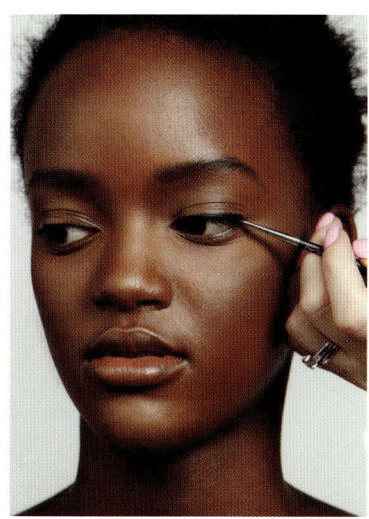

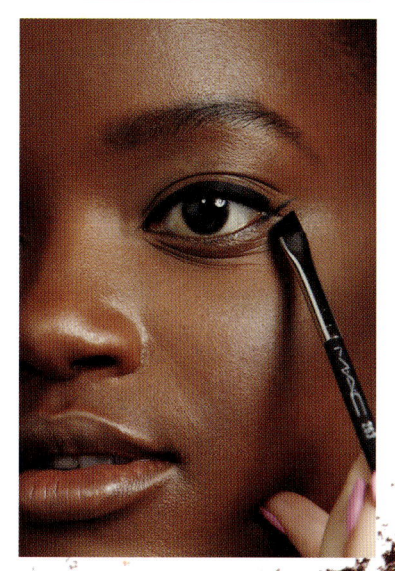

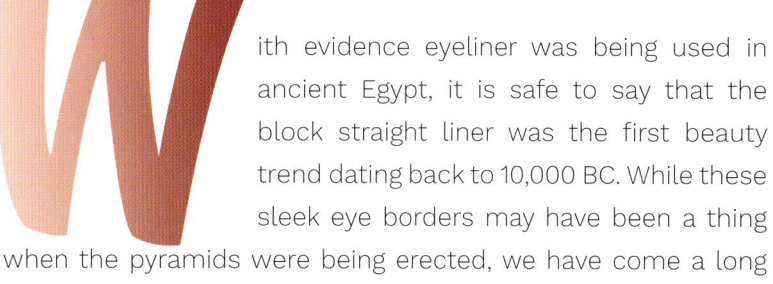

With evidence eyeliner was being used in ancient Egypt, it is safe to say that the block straight liner was the first beauty trend dating back to 10,000 BC. While these sleek eye borders may have been a thing when the pyramids were being erected, we have come a long way since, with many iconic looks along the way. From Marilyn Monroe's liquid liner flick to the smudgy rock look of Kate Moss, liner matters and it makes an impact.

STEP 1

Powder those lids! Take away any of the natural skin shine that will damage the makeup application process before you start your delicate liquid-liner journey.

> **TIP!** Beware the translucent powder that isn't! Many translucent powders will claim they are translucent, the reality though is the majority of them aren't, unless of course you have white, porcelain skin. Make sure you try these out in store before forking out your hard earned for them, because on dark or tan skin a bad powder can really hijack your look.

STEP 2

Put down the liquid and start with something easier! Going straight in with a liquid liner can be nerve-racking. I much prefer a crème gel eyeliner; they are easier to blend within your comfort zone and build color while also drying waterproof. Paint the liner across the top lash line, starting thin and getting thicker at the outer corner. Pull your eyelid up and out in a 45-degree angle so you can get right up *in* that lash line. Start slowly, and keep adding color until you are happy with your thickness. Stop at the end of your eye (important for next steps!).

> **TIP!** Does the idea of creating this shape straight up with black crème or liquid freak you out? Don't worry, me too sometimes! When I am not having a good makeup day, or I have had too many coffees, I will use the angle brush and map out the shape first with a black or brown shadow stamping of color, then I can confidently add my liquid straight over the top. So much less stressful!

STEP 3

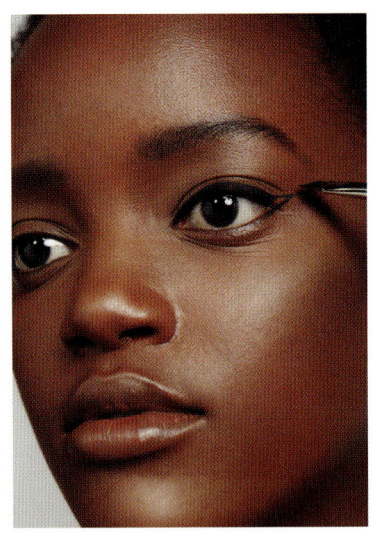

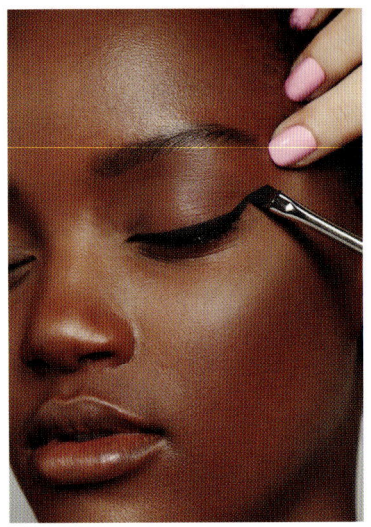

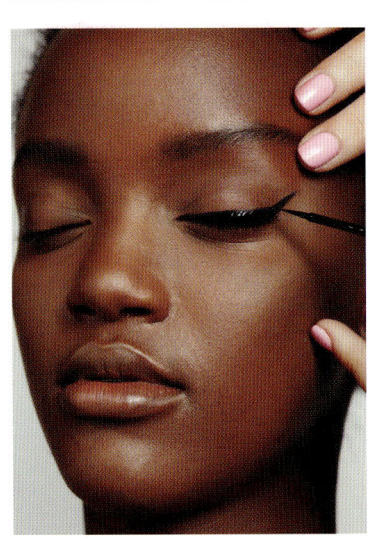

For this next bit, you *must not* tilt your head, you *must not* stretch out the skin next to your eye and you *must not* close your eyes! Very dramatic I know, but I had to make the point. Doing any of these will give you a false idea of where you need to draw your line, resulting in disaster. Geez eyeliner is dramatic!

With your eyes looking straight ahead into the mirror, use the your angle brush to do a light stamp of the liner from the bottom outer corner upwards – the angle of this stamp depends on the shape of your eye. The line needs to follow the same angle as the bottom of your eye: imagine you are drawing it straight out from the bottom of the eye. This will ensure the flick suits your eye regardless of its shape.

> **TIP!** The thinner the angle brush the better for this technique. Make sure you are not applying liquid liner with a hardened, chewed-up angle brush. Avoid this by cleaning it after every use. Please see (page 236) for how to clean your angle brush to keep it defined for each application.

STEP 4

Now, with your eyes looking straight ahead, make another stamp with your angle brush covered in crème liner, connecting the outer line with the line you painted along the top of your eyes. You are creating a triangle shape.

STEP 5

Now color in!. You have your outline, now go for it! You can close your eye and fill that bad boy in.

> **TIP!** Nothing worse than loving it all while your eyes are closed, laboring over the edges and correcting the shape only to then open your eyes and be surprised that the line is now suddenly on your jawline! Anyone who has done this put your hand up with me! Our faces are not symmetrical so sometimes there will be a difference between both shapes when your eyes are closed. But fear not friends, when your eyes are open, it all falls into place! Keep opening and checking, opening and checking, and make final adjustments to the line when your eyes are open.

STEP 6

Is anyone else like me and likes their liquid liner to hold all its rich blackness without the need of touch up until the end of the night? Well have I got the trick for you! Layer a waterproof proof and smudge proof liquid liner over the top. It is so much easier to paint on a liquid liner as a topcoat when the shape is already there!

STEP 7

Ever tried to perfect that sharp edge but added just that *little bit more* and you have slipped and drawn a line straight into your hairline? No? Just me?! Sometimes, the easiest way to get the perfect knife point to that liner, or clean up any rough edges is to *remove* color, not add color. Use a flat brush with a little remover on it and drag along the rough edge! Tadah! Then if you want to take it that step further, use the same flat brush to press some skin-toned face powder on that same edge and blend outwards to make crisp and clean.

> **TIP!** Don't even think about an oil based remover to clean up liner mistakes! The oil is amazing for breaking down waterproof makeup at the end of the day, but this could possibly melt the liner away if you are just correcting. Water based remover is best.

> **TIP!** I have layered two different liners here for ease of application and for longevity. If you are in a hurry, do the same technique but go straight in with your liquid liner.

> **TIP!** If liquid liner still makes you hella nervous, try practicing and gaining confidence in the technique of creating the shape with pencil instead.

SAMEERAH FROM CHIC MODELS

Products Used In Step By Step

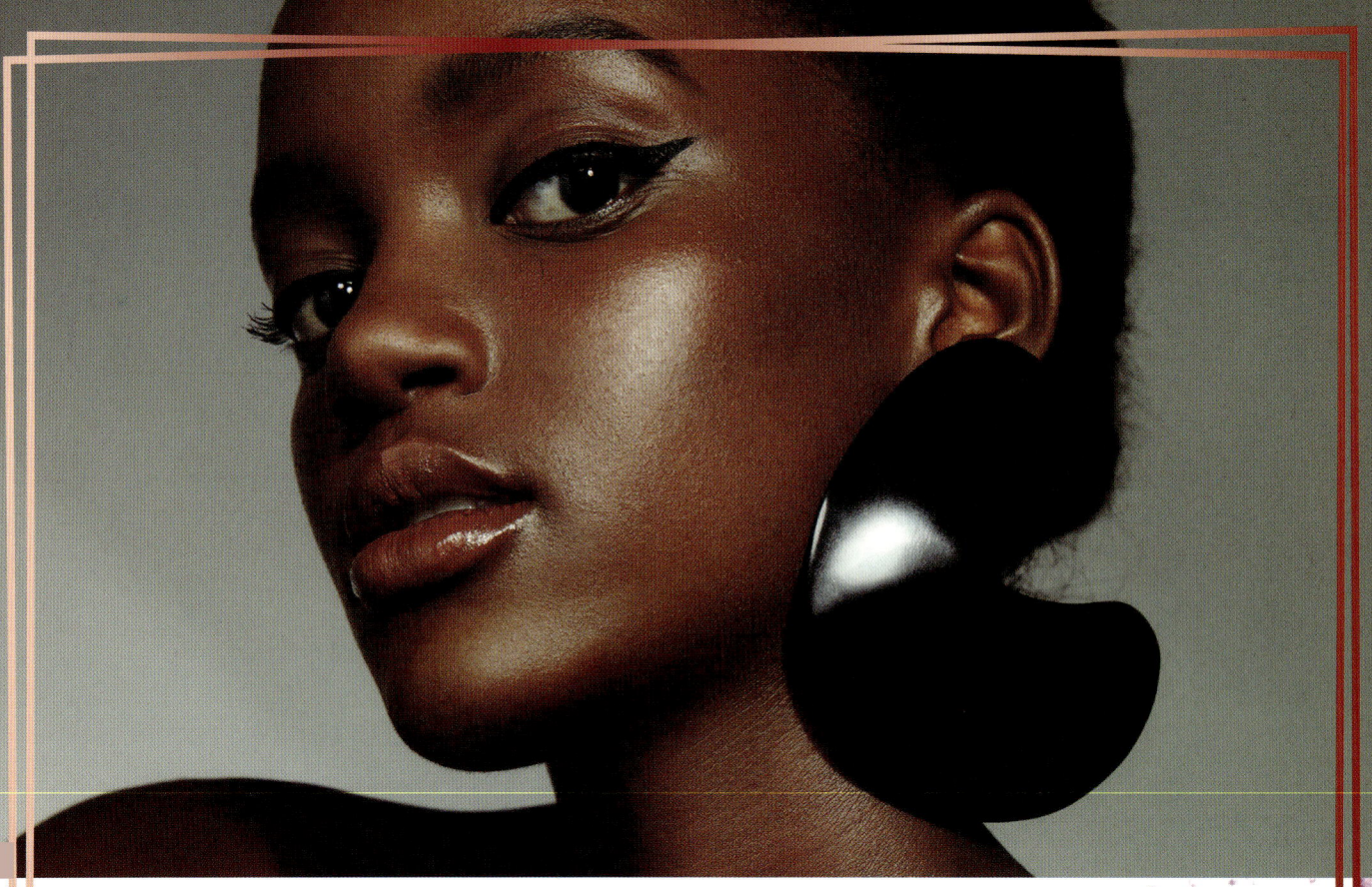

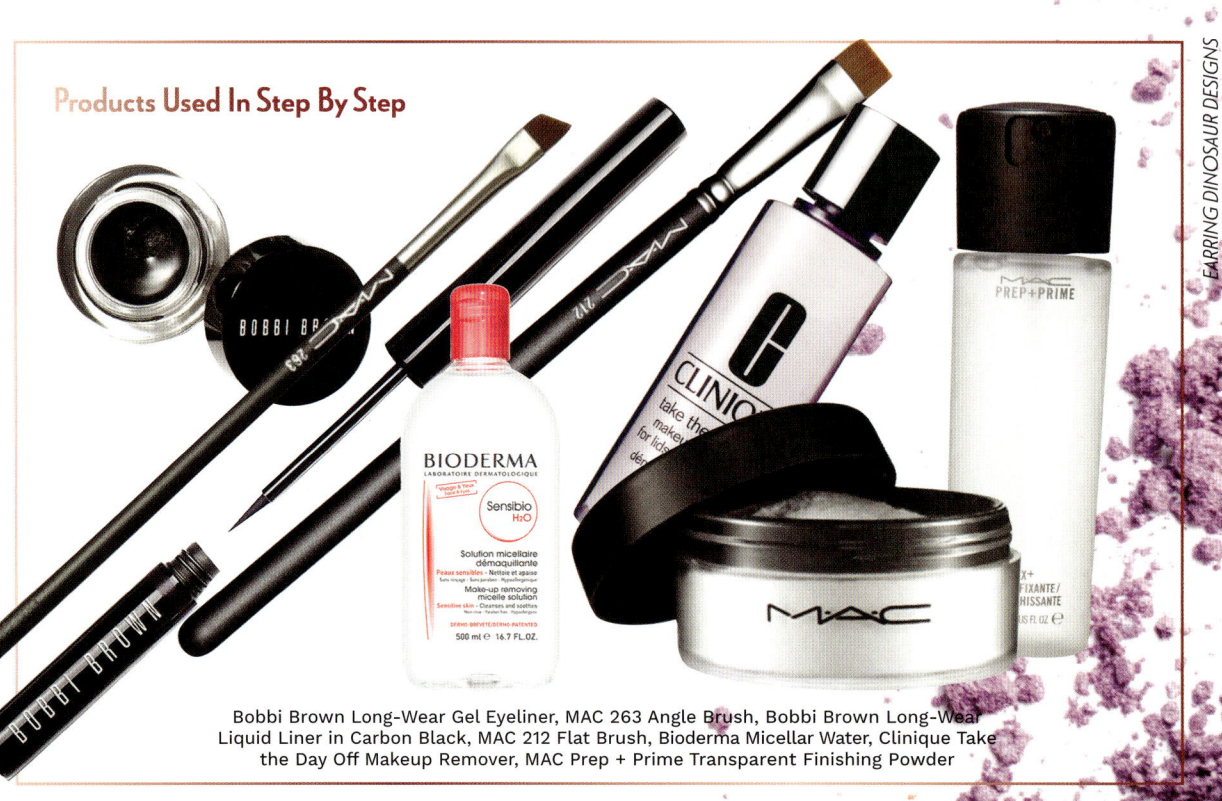

Bobbi Brown Long-Wear Gel Eyeliner, MAC 263 Angle Brush, Bobbi Brown Long-Wear Liquid Liner in Carbon Black, MAC 212 Flat Brush, Bioderma Micellar Water, Clinique Take the Day Off Makeup Remover, MAC Prep + Prime Transparent Finishing Powder

EARRING DINOSAUR DESIGNS

POP COLOR LINER

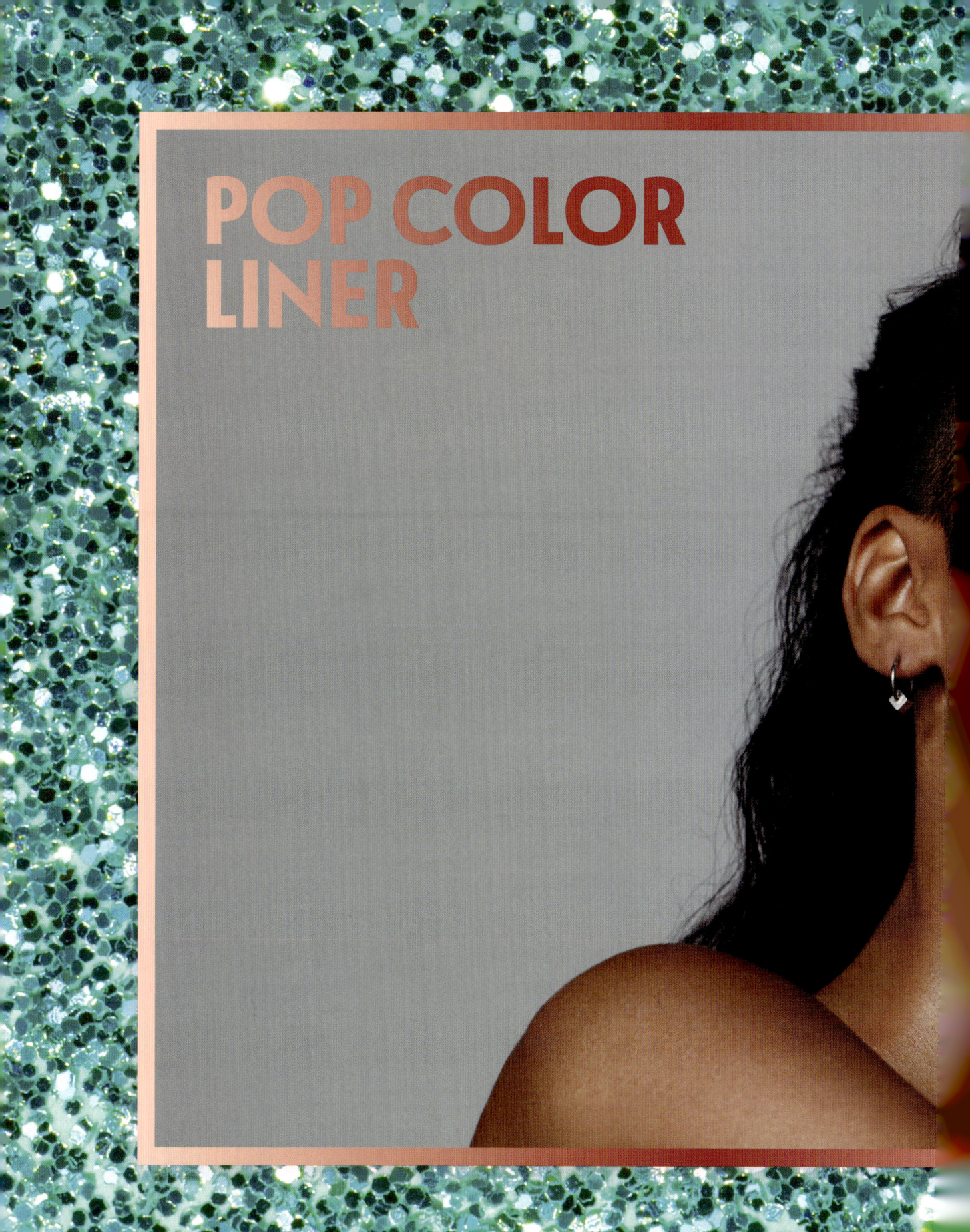

LOOKING FINE MS EYELINE

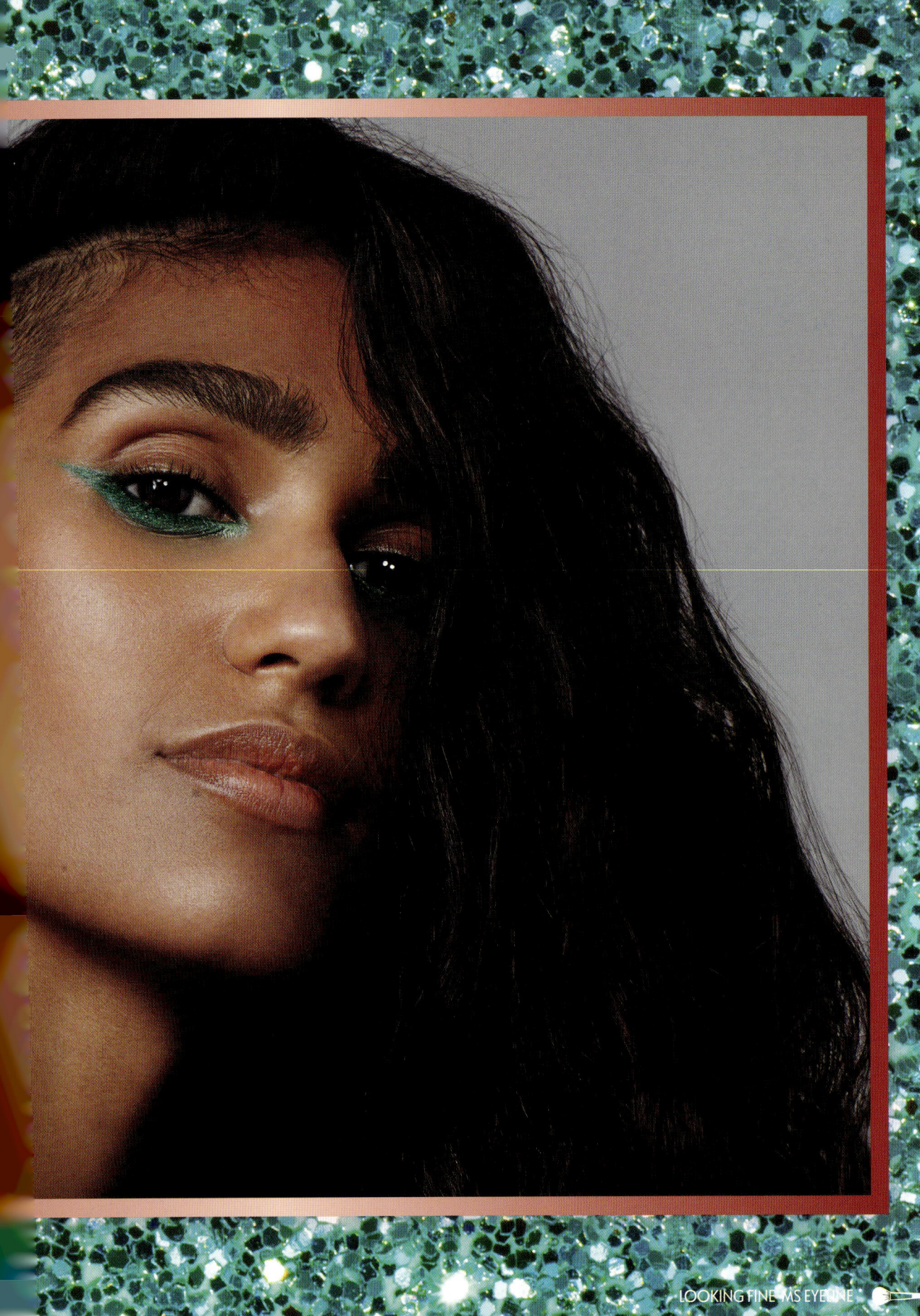

STEP 1

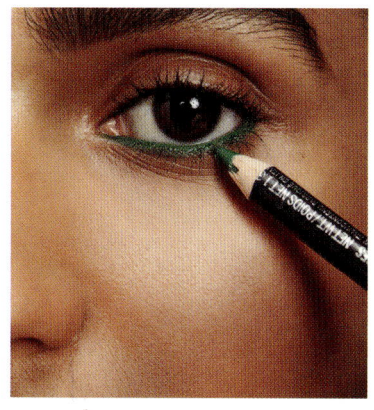

Starting on the waterline of your eye, scribble this pencil like your childhood crayon. Be brave when drawing on the color! An ample amount of liner is much easier and more efficient to blend into the shape you want. The alternative is adding and blending over and over again.

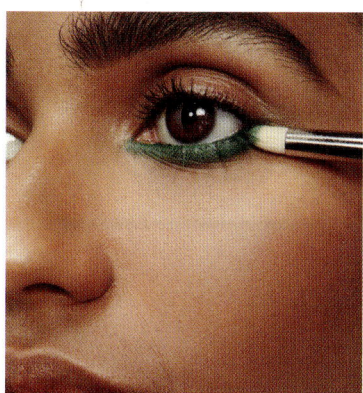

STEP 2

Using a small and soft pencil brush, give the product a good smudge, concentrating the smudging action on the outer edge. By doing this you won't blend all your color away as you go.

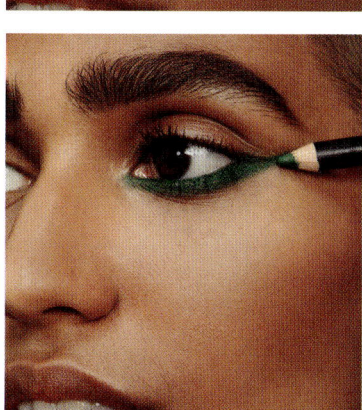

STEP 3

Looking straight ahead into your mirror, drag the color out towards your temples. Do you see a theme here? Look straight ahead while creating a liner shape. Not only is it super important to achieve the most flattering shape for your eye but you can see where you are going.

> **TIP!** For a more low-key pop liner look, pump up that waterline. Draw your pencil hard onto the water line and pair it with your favorite safe-zone tan brown eye shadow.

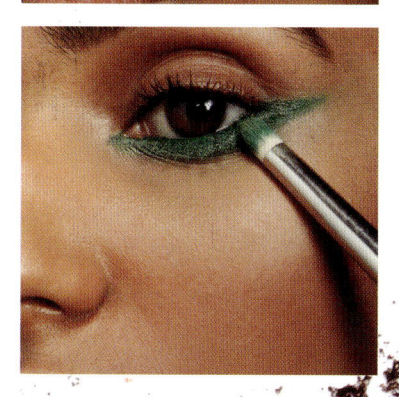

STEP 4

Dip the same small pencil brush you used to smudge your liner into a matching shadow and press along the lash line to set the color in place. Doing this will also smooth over any patchy bits and deliver you a flawless finish.

Matte or shimmer eye shadow? Matte shadow will intensify and deepen the color. Shimmer eye shadow will pop the color and be light reflective!

STEP 5

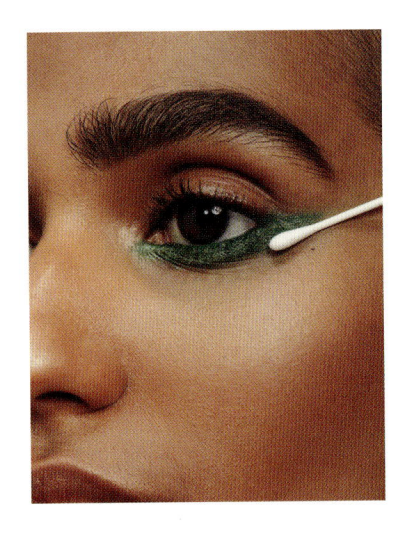

Give a cotton tip a spritz with some MAC Fix+ and gently soften the edges of your liner cleaning up the shape as you go. Soft edges work so well for this look so it doesn't look like you are preparing for your solo performance in Cirque du Soleil!

Using a remover to clean up edges will wipe away all your eye cream, primer, foundation, concealer and whatever else you popped on around the eyes! Fix+, as a hydrator, used with a delicate touch, will just erase your fuzzy line without removing all the essentials.

TIP!

Teal green is certainly not your only option. Have a play with some flattering jewel-toned liners and shadows to update your look. Some of my favorites include:

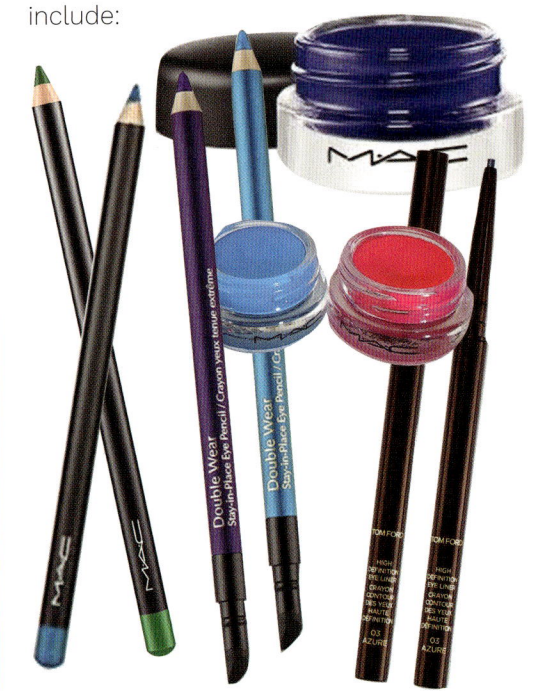

MAC Chromagraphic Pencil in Landscape Green, High-Def Cyan, Marine Ultra Bright, Process Magenta, designer purple, Estée Lauder Double Wear Stay-in-Place Eye Pencil in Night Violet and Teal, Tom Ford High Definition Liner in Azure

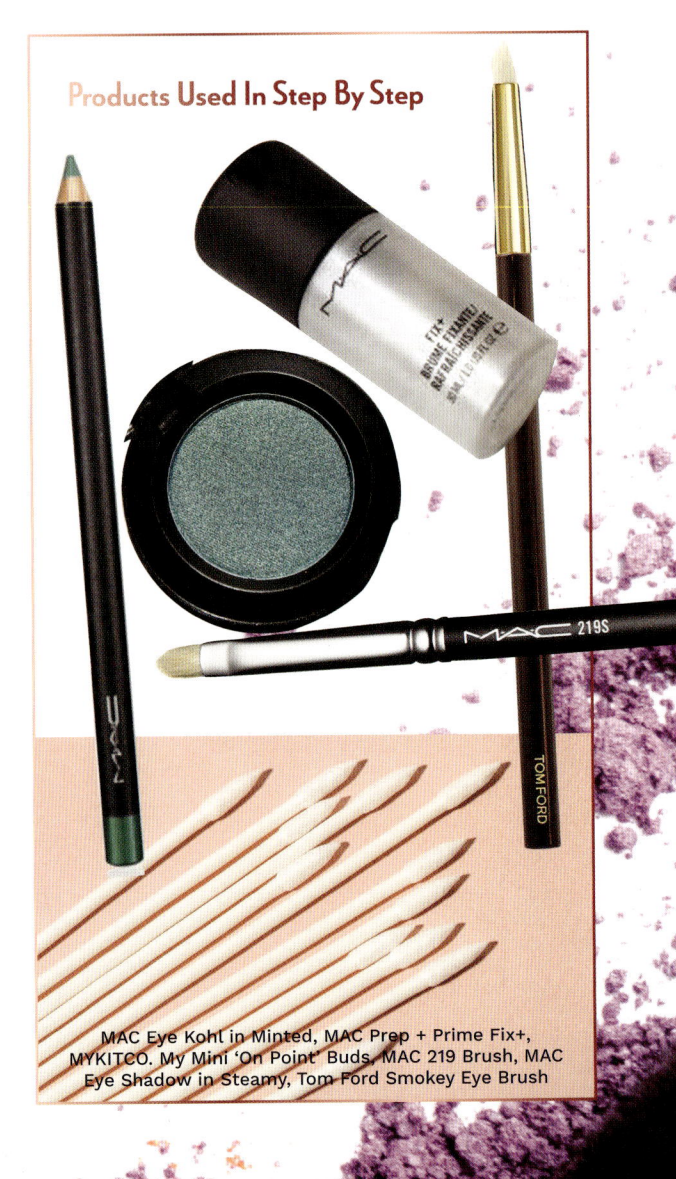

Products Used In Step By Step

MAC Eye Kohl in Minted, MAC Prep + Prime Fix+, MYKITCO. My Mini 'On Point' Buds, MAC 219 Brush, MAC Eye Shadow in Steamy, Tom Ford Smokey Eye Brush

HANNAH FROM CHIC MODELS

THE PERFECT SMUDGE

LOOKING FINE MS EYELINE 155

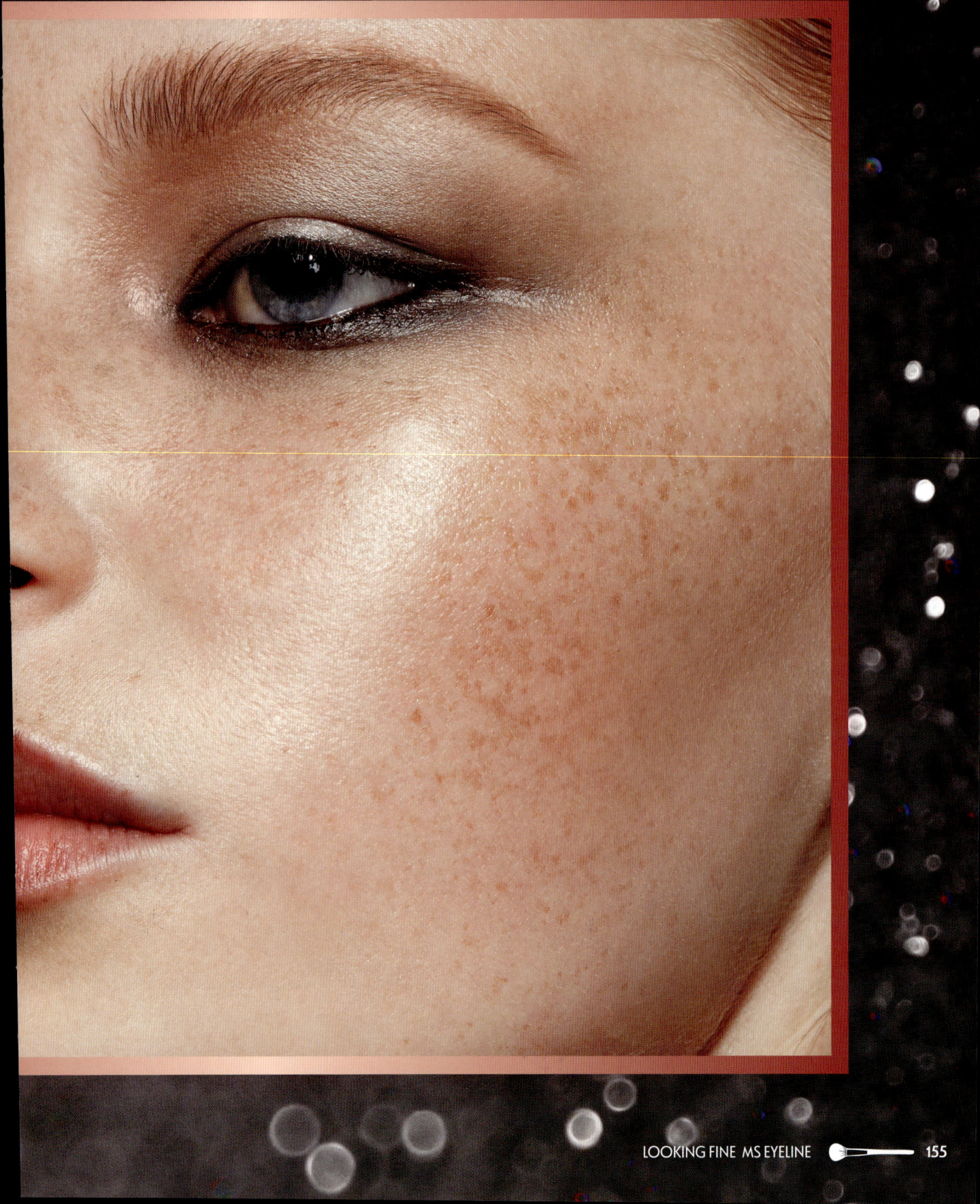

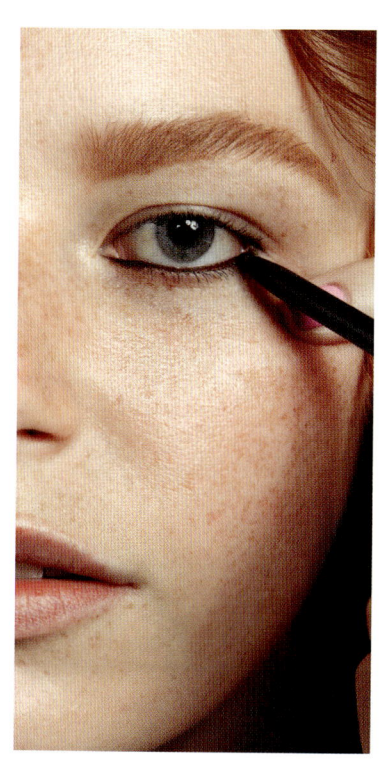

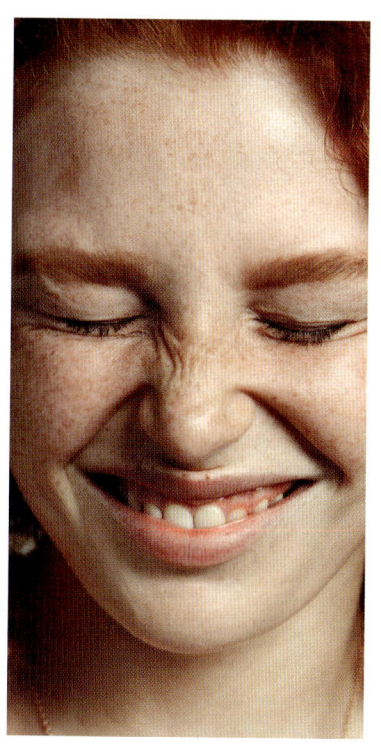

As a child of the nineties (born in the eighties) the grunge look was everything. From Kate Moss walking out of a London nightclub at 4 am to Billie Jo Armstrong fronting a concert for Green Day, the smudgy liner look defined this moment in time. It was feminine, it was masculine and it could even be androgynous but most importantly it was timeless.

This look is a fashion week favorite and is as relevant now as it was when Keith Richards was rocking it back in the day with the Rolling Stones. Follow these tricks to have it looking like a (hot) mess, not just a mess!

STEP 1

Start by drawing a pencil along the bottom waterline of your eyes – otherwise known as a tightline. Just like the pop color liner, do not be shy with your application! The more product you apply here the more you have to blend with!

The texture of your pencil is super important. Make sure the pencil you use has strong color pigment. One swipe and you should see full color payoff. If you have to scribble or press super hard to see color then chuck it away.

> *TIP!* A tightline is often seen in magazines and fashion shows as *the* liner look! It looks amazing on its own with plenty of mascara and highlighted skin. You can easily stop here and pop your mascara on for a defined eye look in a hurry!

STEP 2

If you can, draw the same liner onto the top waterline. If you can't, just scrunch your eyes together to transfer the liner draw from the bottom to the top. This is also why it's important to be generous with your application in Step 1 – so you have color to transfer!

STEP 3

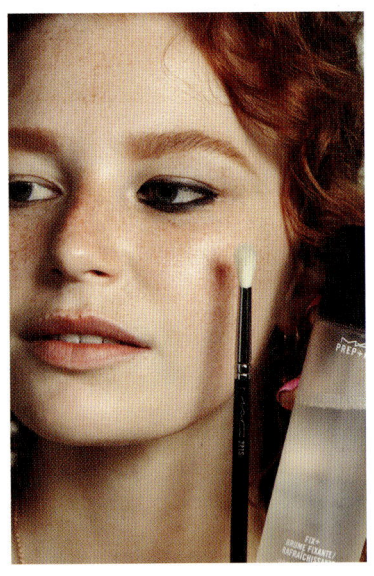

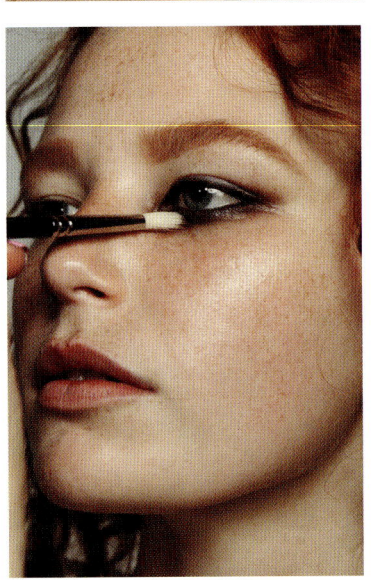

MAC Fix+ and the 100,000th use for it! As a spray moisturizer, it is great to spritz a little on your fluffy shadow brush to give the eyeliner wheels, helping you achieve that perfect blend. It is vital that you don't drown the brush! You only need a little moisture to help the product glide on the skin.

STEP 4

With the same brush or a slightly smaller fluffy brush for closer control, blend on some eye shadow to smooth out the application and perfect the smudge.

Smooth shimmer shadows are the bomb! They are an instant light reflector. Shimmer looks glossy in photos but won't move like gloss. Here shimmery eye shadow will set the liner and add some glam without making the look too heavy and dark. I chose a shadow that is a few shades lighter than the eyeliner color to stop the look from becoming too dramatic or dark.

If dramatic is the name of your game, you get a high five from me! Go and grab a matte version of the liner color and go for it.

TIP! Whether you have chosen classic black, bright teal or a smudgy coffee color to wear around the eyes, just like other areas of makeup, the contrast of what you wear around it can make or break your look. Once you are finished, make sure you take a few secs to clean up the edges, applying concealer where required, and be sure to powder around your eyes.

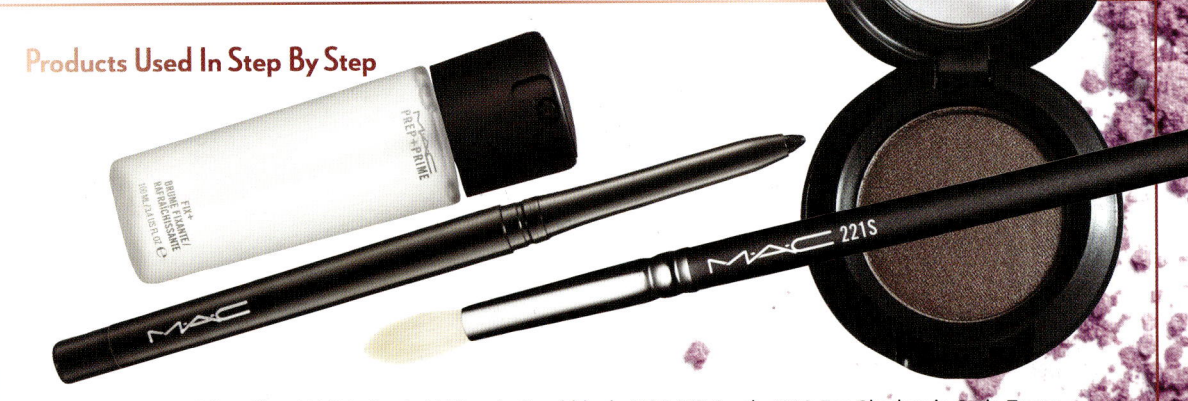

Products Used In Step By Step

MAC Prep + Prime Fix+, MAC Technakohl Liner in Graphblack, MAC 221 Brush, MAC Eye Shadow in Satin Taupe

GEE GEE FROM KULT MODELS

LOOKING FINE MS EYELINE

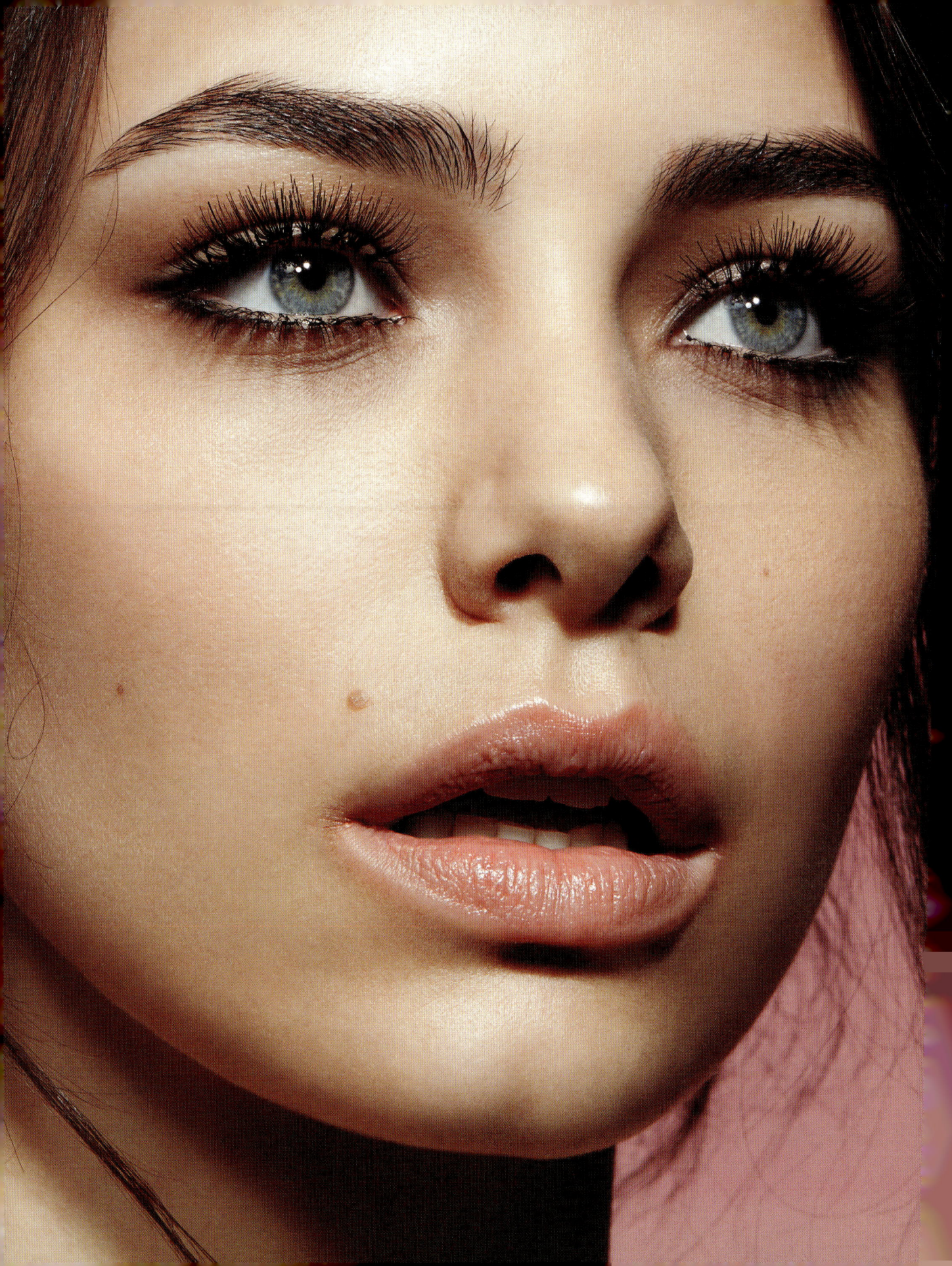

Lashes get pashes

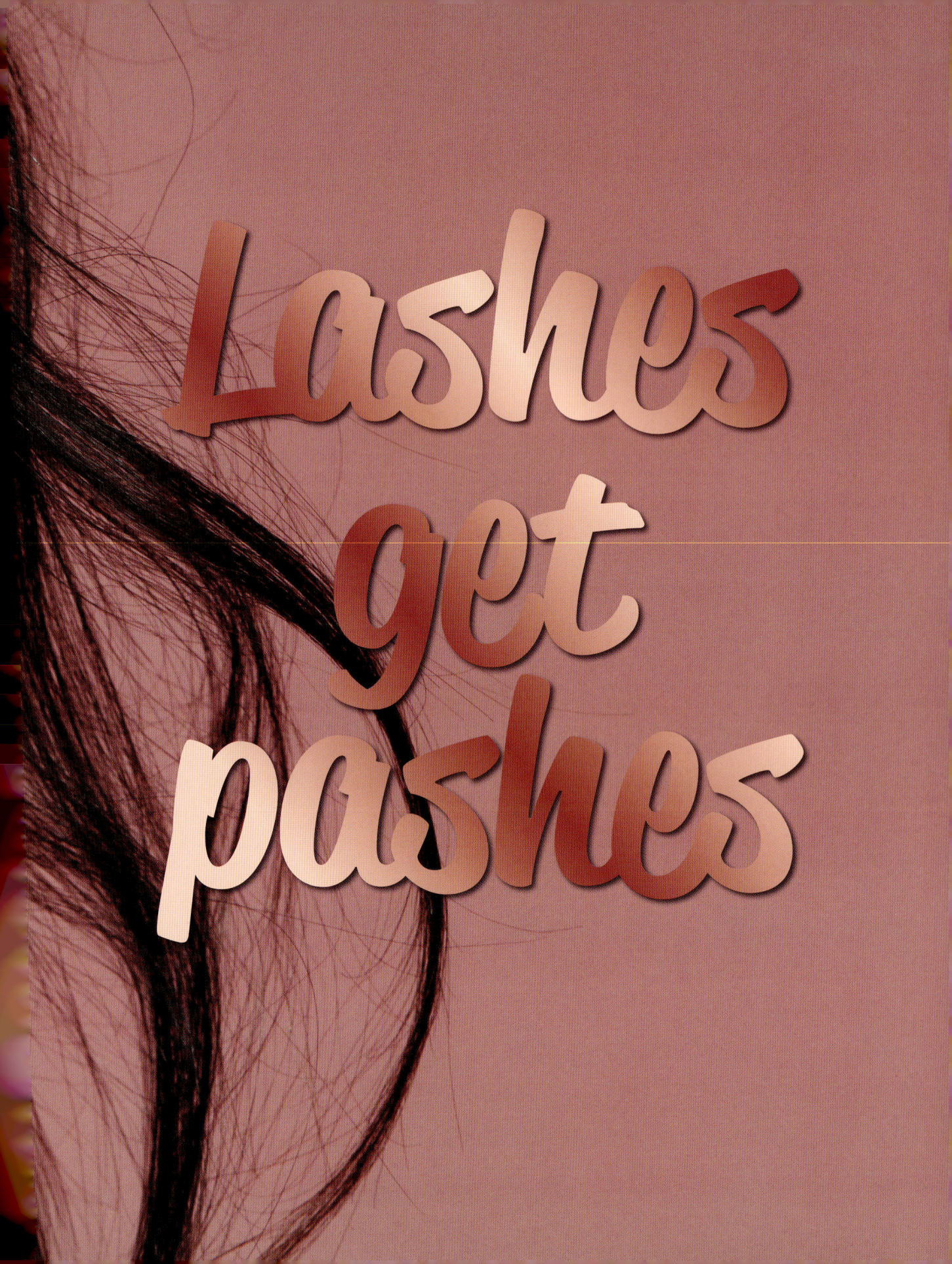

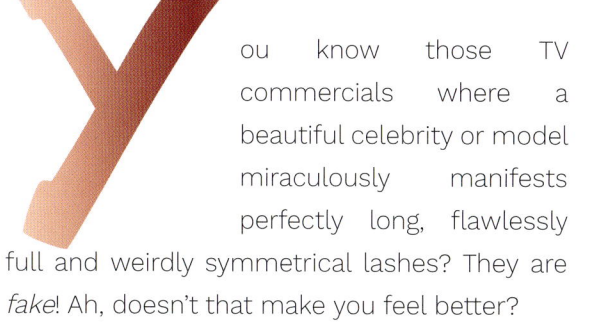

You know those TV commercials where a beautiful celebrity or model miraculously manifests perfectly long, flawlessly full and weirdly symmetrical lashes? They are *fake*! Ah, doesn't that make you feel better?

I cannot tell you how many times over my years doing makeup, in that moment when brush approaches lash, clients have made the same declaration: 'Sorry, I have tiny lashes!' Little do they know that lengthy luscious lashes are just a couple of brush strokes away.

One hundred per cent of the time people cannot actually believe how big their lashes are when I am finished with them; and you know what, it does NOT have to add 30 minutes to your makeup. It just means putting a little more thought and care into your application process rather than chucking it on looking into your rear-view mirror while driving to work! (This book does not endorse applying makeup while driving #rushhourisnotblushhour)

Mascara Types

You have fat lashes but want them longer

If you are one of these lucky people with fabulously fat lashes, first things first, high five yourself. The genetic gods have been kind to you. Grab yourself a fibrous mascara, the Estée Lauder Sumptuous Knockout Defining Lift And Fan Mascara is a good one.

For this type of lash, personally, I trade in the stock brush for a fan brush. The biggest benefit for this is you can really control how much makeup you are applying, ensuring your lashes are a clump-free zone.

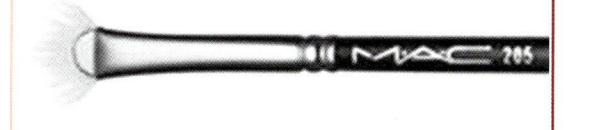

You want to lengthen your lashes

Petite, thinly shaped brushes that advertise a lightweight formula will generally work to give you the length without the flop! Stop giggling. Where were we? Oh yeah, mascara. A slightly tapered end will help you to use the brush in different directions to define and enable you to separate without clumping.

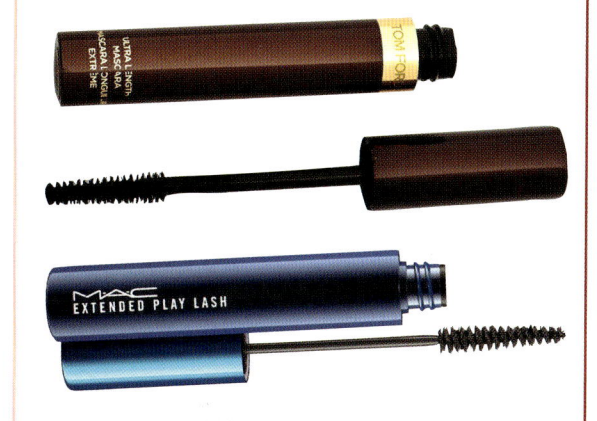

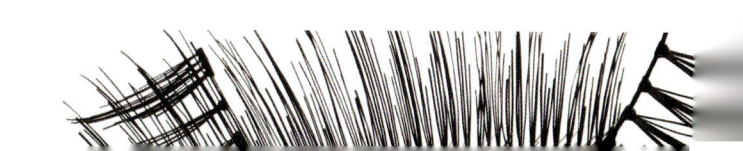

You want to thicken your lashes

Using fat, round wands with oodles of bristles is your best bet.

The big brushes work super well for people who have naturally full lashes already that you are simply trying to get the most out of – but can be tricky for those on the thinner side.

My personal favorite for fattening up your feathery eye frames is the MAC Upward Lash. Don't let the little round brush fool you, the inside is hollow so it holds a bunch of mascara that instantly grabs onto the lashes. You know when you have to dip and dip and dip to get any product out of the tube? Not here mate! The small brush definitely punches above its weight, but its diminutive size makes it ideal to grab every lash and double its thickness.

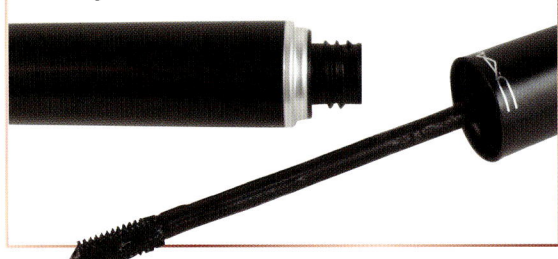

You have damaged or uneven lashes

Using a mascara that contains panthenol or phytokeratin will encourage strength and growth.

Don't forget to prime! Lash primer, which I am going to use in the next few looks, will coat and condition, protect from further breakage and pump up the length and thickness before you even get to the mascara.

You want it all

Go for a mascara wand with split personality. Either a wand with two different sides for two different effects – one to apply volume, the other to separate and define – like the Estée Lauder Pure Color Envy Lash Multi-Effects mascara. Or choose a mascara that holds two different wands in one tube like the MAC Haute & Naughty Lash mascara – then you can have the small brush for those pesky bottom lashes and the fat brush to bulk up the top.

You want them curled

There are *zero* benefits to spending a bunch of money on a critically acclaimed mascara if your lashes are straight and you can't see the results! *Curl, curl, curl!* Immediately, if not sooner.

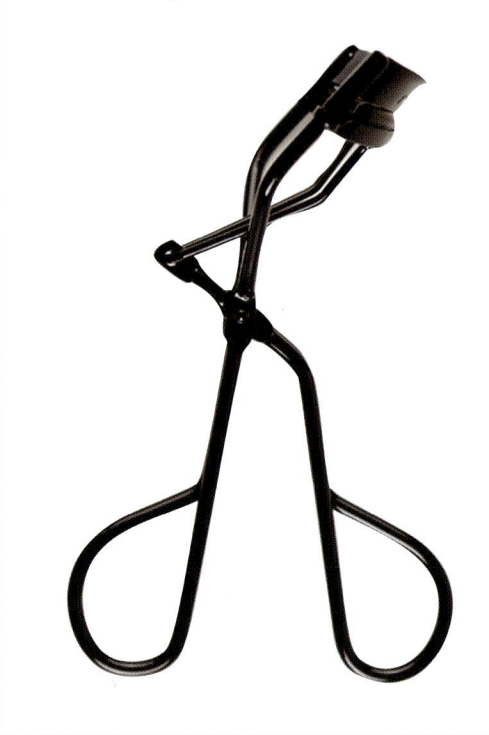

NATURALLY DEFINED (EPIC) LASHES

LASHES GET PASHES

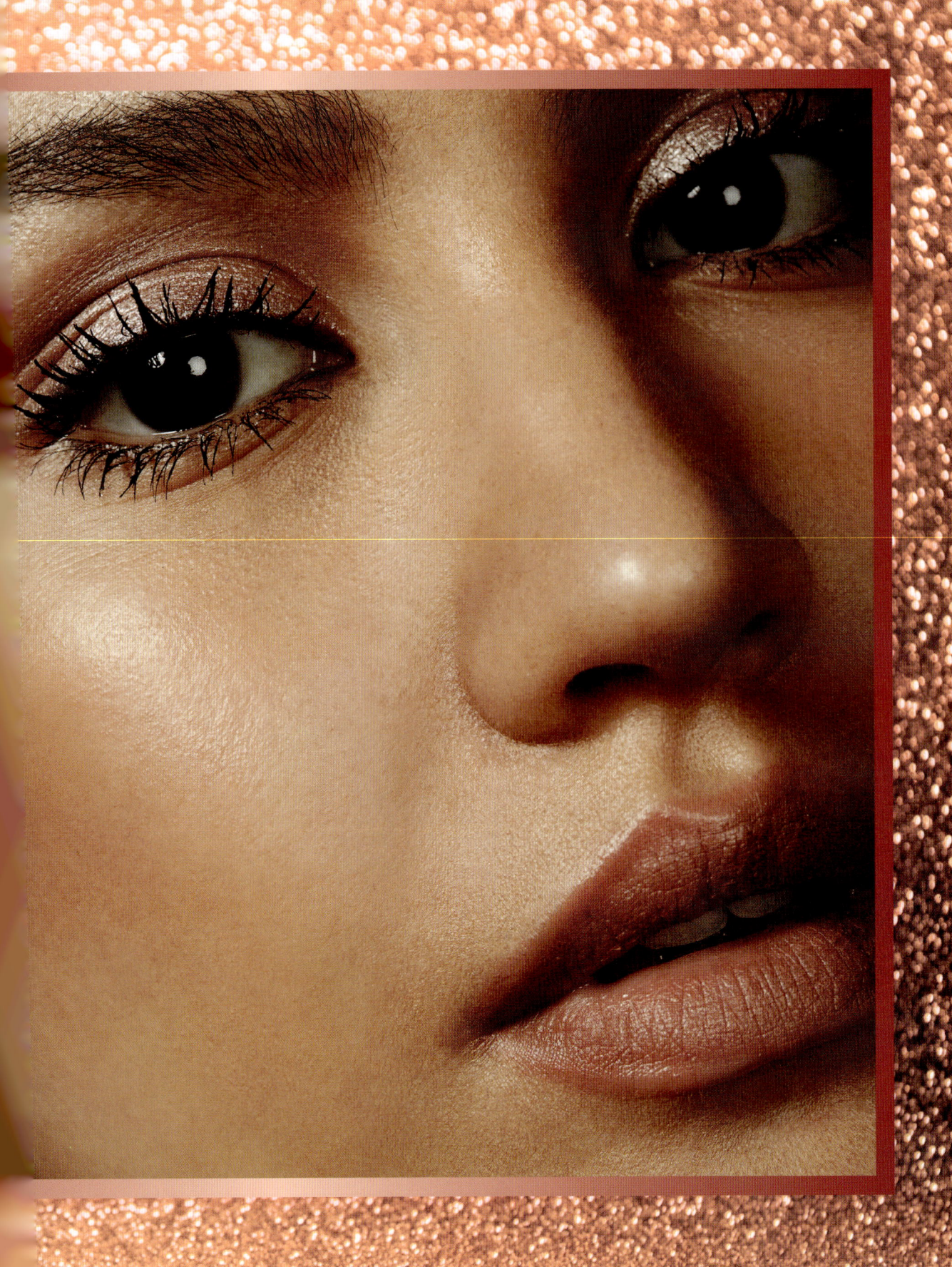

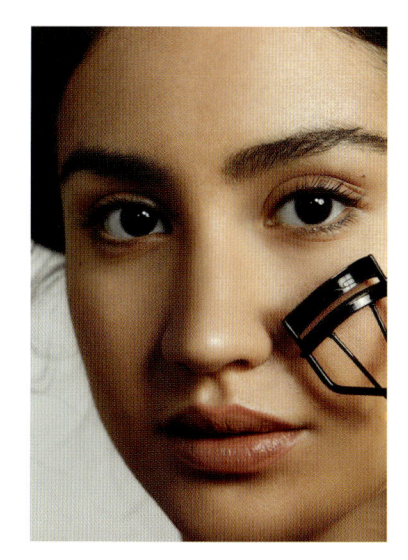

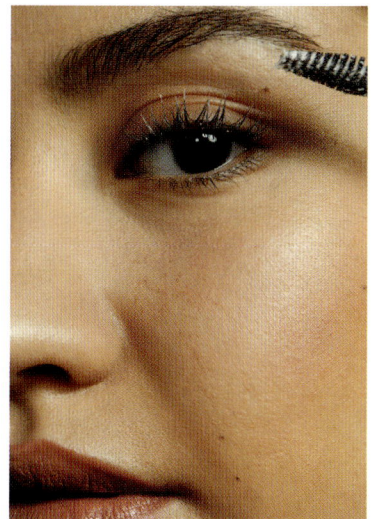

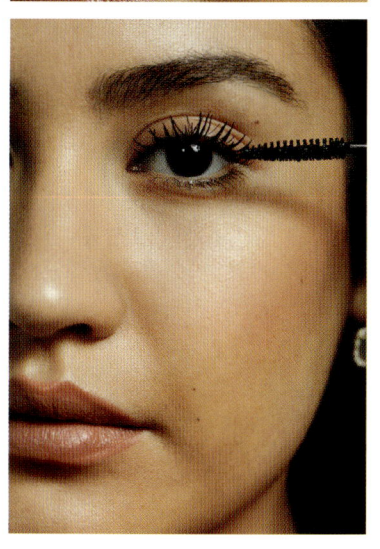

STEP 1

CURL YOUR LASHES! I will say it once and I will say it as many times as people need to hear it – the lash curler is the staple of any makeup bag no matter what you look like! Even if you have long lashes (lucky you!) sometimes they are so long that they flop downwards. Give them a good strong curl – immediately!

Even if you think you have solid seven out of ten lashes naturally (lucky you again!) often a few rebel lashes want to point in different directions. What do you do? Curl, curl, curl! Just a light clamp will have them all heading in the same direction and open up your eyes.

To be honest though, the moral of the story here is if you have lashes, you should have a curler – period.

> *TIP!* Make sure you carry your curler with you at all times. When your lashes need that 3 pm zhoosh, avoid reaching for more mascara as you are more than likely going to get some clumping, which is more akin to a 3 am look. Whip out that curler, and give your look the lift it needs to see you through the day.

STEP 2

Lash primer – I know right, a primer for lashes? I was skeptical too. That was until I saw the results personally and professionally. A lash primer will coat each lash, doubling its size instantly. It will also hold mascara in place and stop smudging under the eyes. I saw this work in real life doing makeup for a close friend's wedding in Greece in the summer. Also, it literally takes five second to whack on before mascara. No excuses; easy peasy.

STEP 3

I adore the MAC Extended Play Lash Mascara for beautifully full, sharp and long lashes. This easy to use brush holds loads of product yet won't clump.

Use the brush flat and give it to a good wiggle at the roots of the lash all the way along your eyes. Wiggle, wiggle, wiggle – you want the roots of your lash to have the bulk of the product.

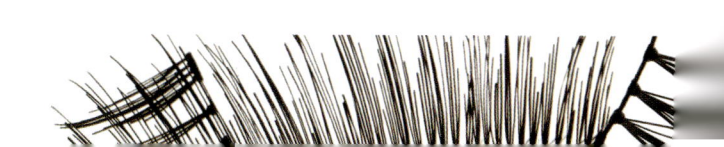

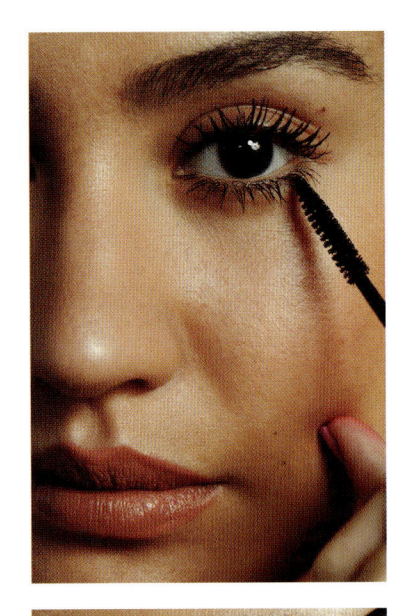

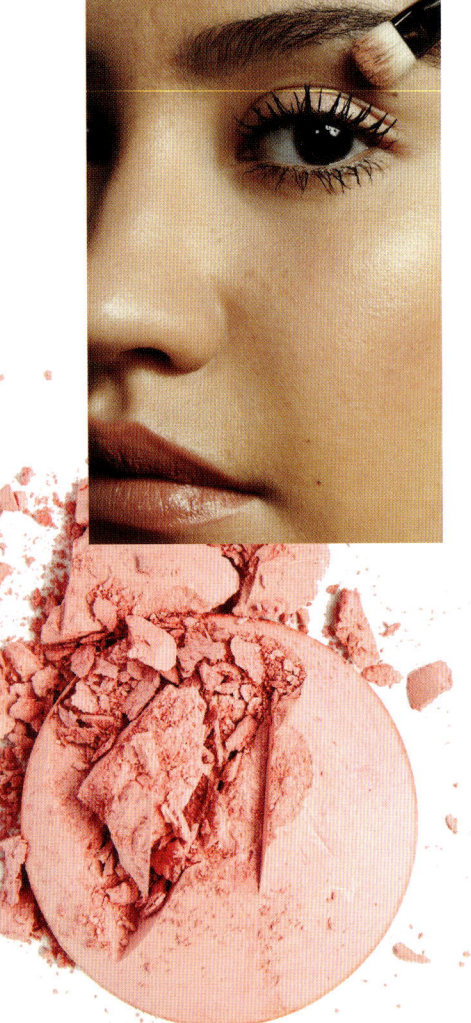

Then wiggle and drag the product up through the lashes. Your instincts will tell you to whip through the lashes at the speed of light; please don't. Take your time sister. By gently applying your mascara you are letting the product grab onto each lash.

> **TIP!** If you have teeny tiny bottom lashes and find it too hard to coat them with color without making a mess, use your tinted brow set. The brows are much smaller and easier to use in this small space!

STEP 4

Switch up your angles! One of the biggest mistakes I see people make is to expect one wiggle of a brush to do all the work. Use vertical brush strokes to divide the lashes, dragging just the end of the brush through your lashes to get more length. Give the outer lashes of each eye a bit more attention to elongate your eye shape. Once those bad boys are well coated from all angles, finish by brushing through again in the direction of your lashes to bring the look together and divide up any clusters of mascara.

> **TIP!** We aren't perfect; I often end up with a random blob of mascara on my nose while doing my lashes! Don't try to wipe it away when wet. If you do it will smudge further and you will end up having to disguise your mistake with a smoky eye. Wait until it is completely dry and flick it away with a small cotton tip. THIS WORKS!

STEP 5

If you are chasing lashes that Kim Kardashian would envy, it doesn't stop at the mascara! What we do around the lash makes *all* the difference. For example, if you spend a lengthy amount of time and effort perfecting each lash only to pop a black smoky eye on around it, I guarantee you'll be asking yourself, where did the lashes go?!

Use a shadow lighter than your skin tone to pop on behind your lashes; it will have them jumping out of your selfie! Using a flat, slightly rounded brush take the color from the roots of your lash up over the eyelids. A matte pale shadow looks great here. To boost your look, use a shimmer shadow and a slightly wet brush for a little extra twinkle at night.

LASHES GET PASHES

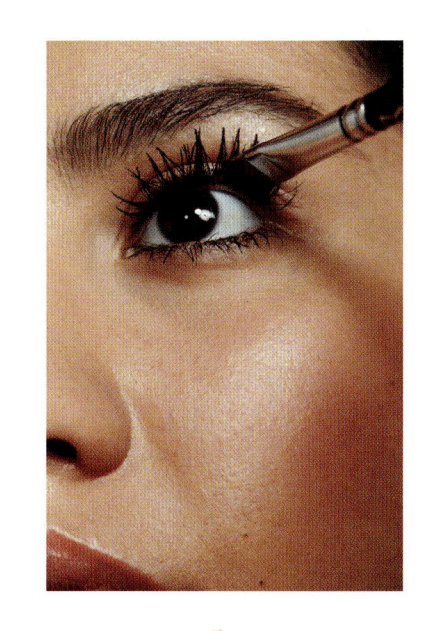

STEP 6

This is a trick I use a lot for photo shoots where the eyes on the model need to look defined without looking like she's wearing a lot of eye makeup. Use a flat brush, and a dark powder or cream shadow and wiggle it just a little bit (yes, that is a 1990s rap reference – google '2 in a Room' kids) just beneath the roots of your lashes, onto the top waterline, while looking straight ahead into the mirror. The flat brush will allow you to get an even amount of color at the base of your lash, which will add length to your look (check out the before picture! Yass!).

TIP! You want waterproof? Go for it! Use the waterproof mascara when you need it, as a top coat to your normal everyday mascara. This will give you the stay-proof color security while also making it easier to remove. Don't use waterproof mascara every day, as it can harden your lashes, which may cause them to break. Save this bad boy for special occasions.

TIP! Mascara does not live forever. There, I had to say it. If you are privately reading this, admitting to yourself that you cannot actually remember the last time you purchased a new mascara, it's time to get one. *Go.* Each time you twist open that tube, you let air in, which effectively dries the mascara out and stops it being the eye saver it once was. Every mascara is the same no matter the price; air is the enemy. Every three to four months, treat yo-self.

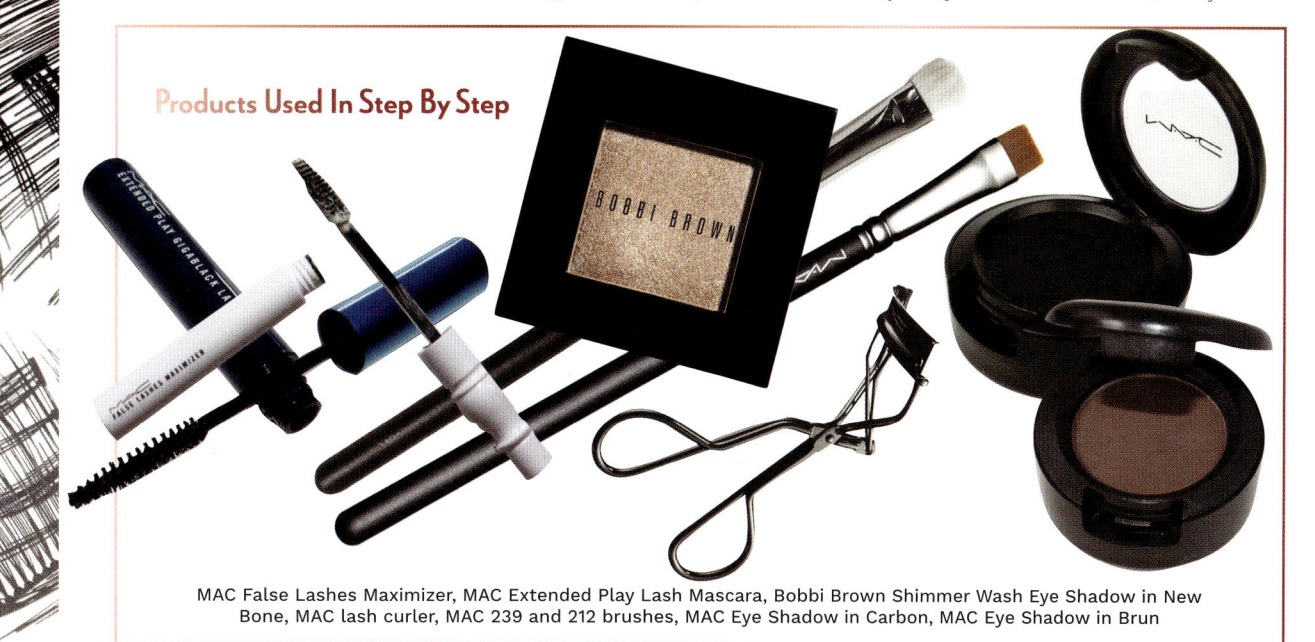

Products Used In Step By Step

MAC False Lashes Maximizer, MAC Extended Play Lash Mascara, Bobbi Brown Shimmer Wash Eye Shadow in New Bone, MAC lash curler, MAC 239 and 212 brushes, MAC Eye Shadow in Carbon, MAC Eye Shadow in Brun

TIARE FROM BELLA MODEL MANAGEMENT

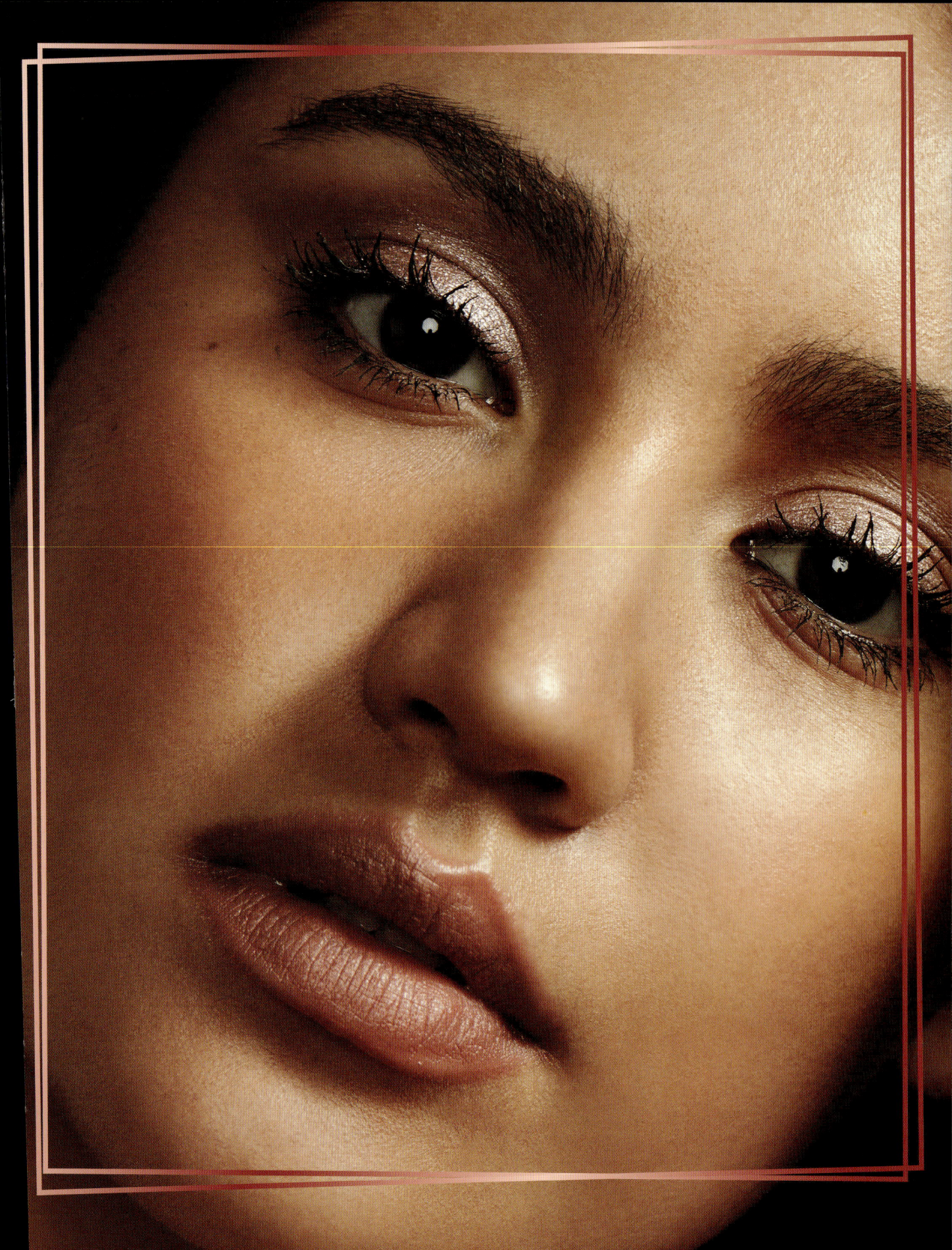

CHUNKY LASHES

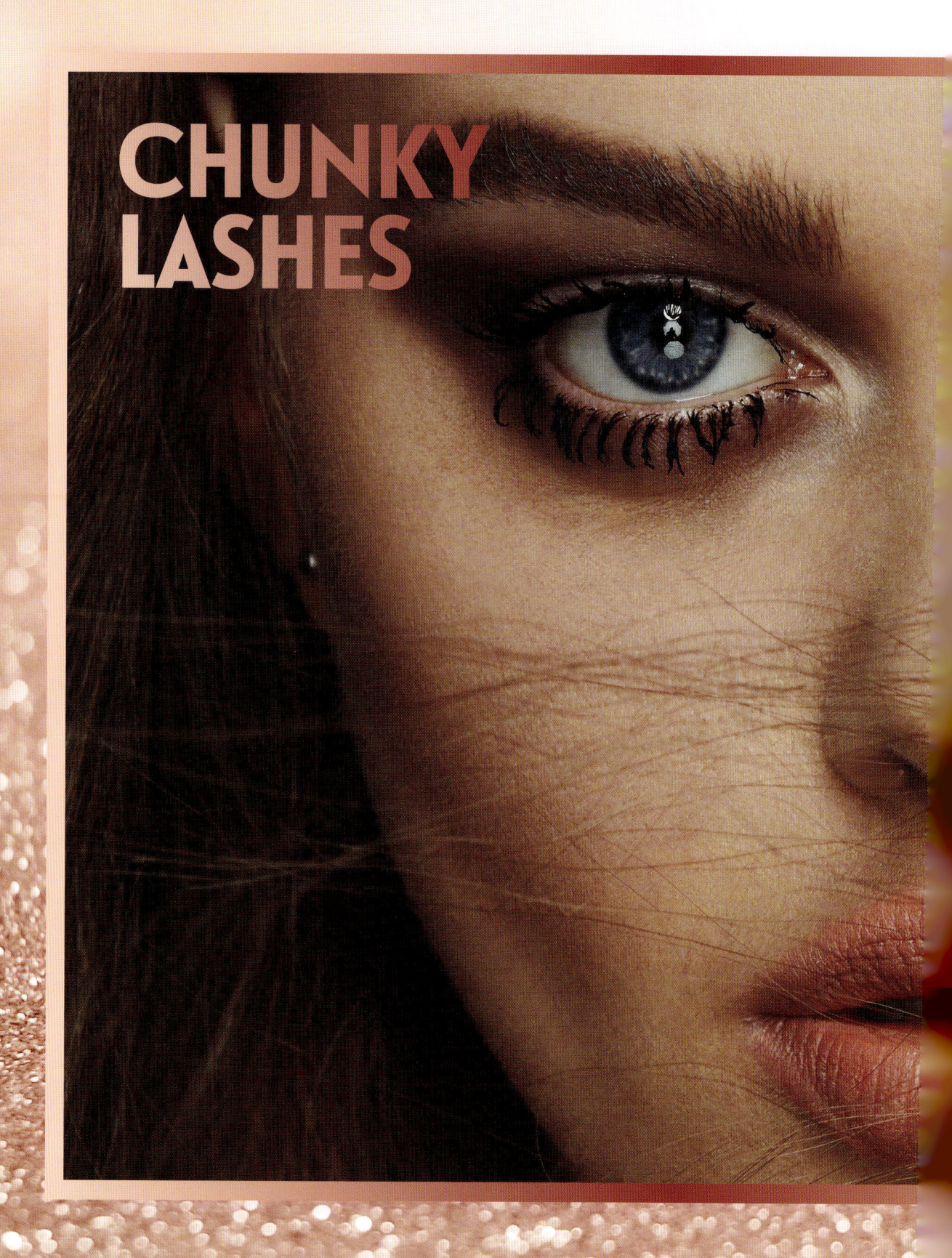

LASHES GET PASHES

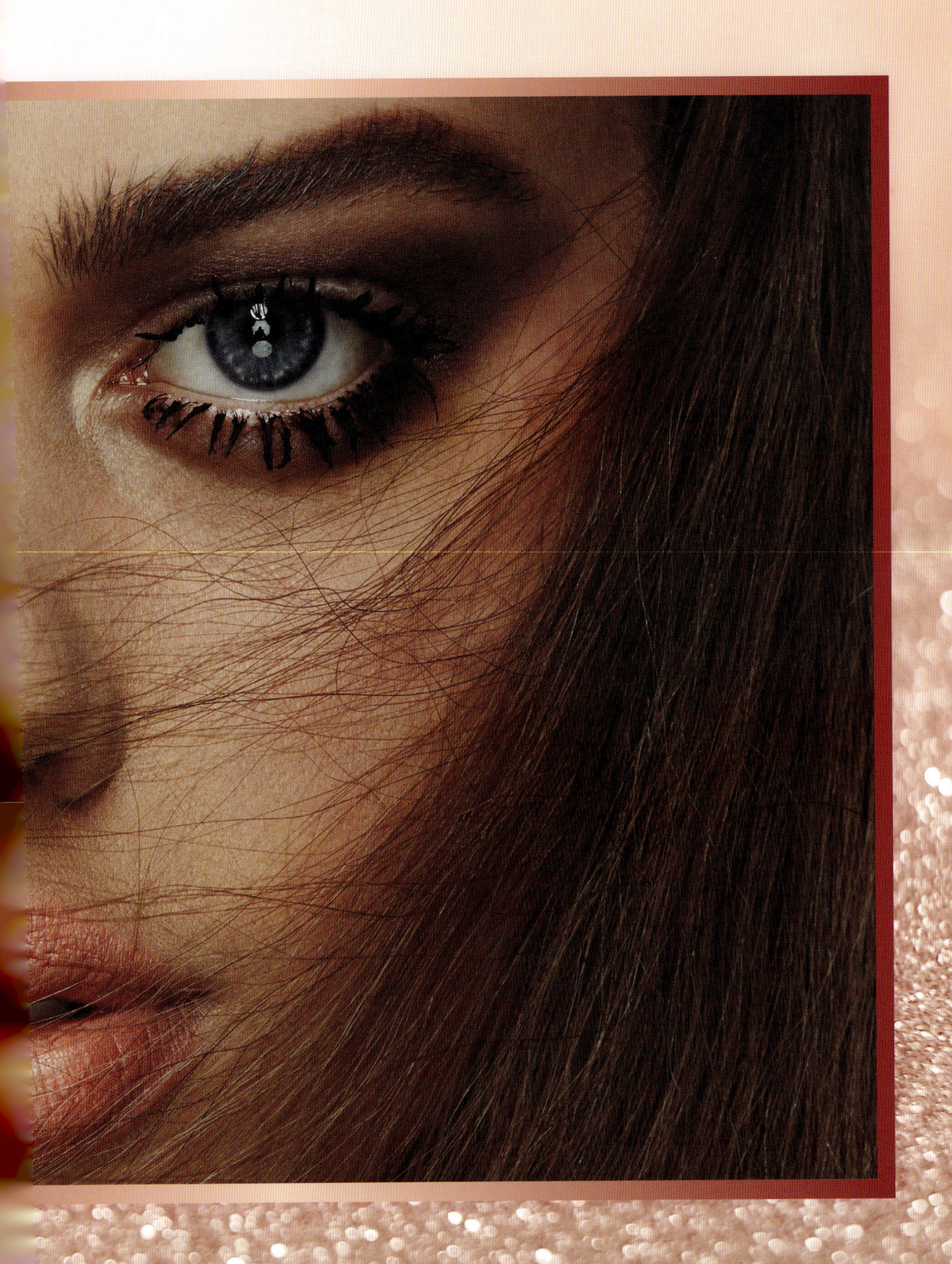

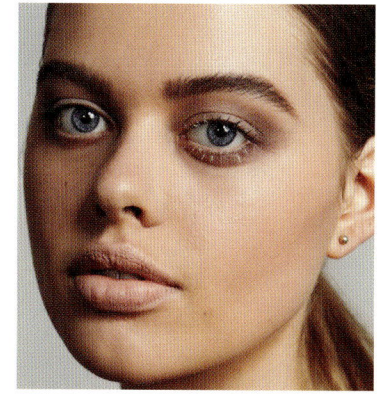

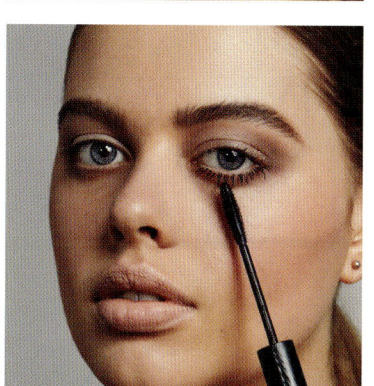

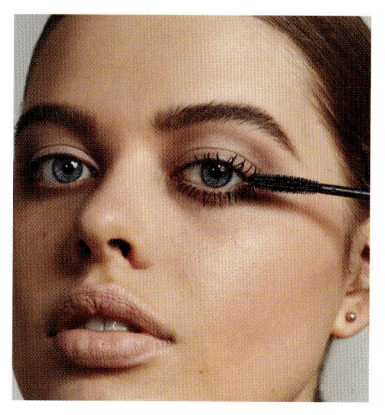

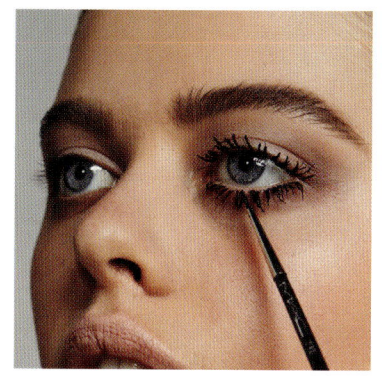

STEP 1

Primer will thicken your lashes and helps hold your mascara in place. This is vital when you are trying to make those lashes thicker than a Snickers. Be careful of being too generous, as primers are generally pretty translucent. A couple of coats will do the trick, ensuring the mascara grabs on to the lash.

STEP 2

If you coat your top lashes first, you risk the wet mascara from on top smearing all over your eyelids when you look up to do the bottom lashes. Save time and clean-up and tackle your bottom lashes first.

STEP 3

Mascara cocktail anyone? I want to coat, define and fan out the lashes to start with, then I want the instant gratification of an extreme volume mascara to really chunk them up. Layer your formulas and brushes. You could also powder your lashes with some loose invisible powder in between layers to really bulk them up.

STEP 4

Not enough length or thickness? Sometimes you need to go beyond the brush. For chunky yet controlled spider lashes, take a small eye liner brush and dip into the mascara wand, wrapping it in a ton of mascara. Then use the precise brush to paint a layer of color onto each lash. The result will be MAJOR fat lashes.

TIP! We all know we *should* take off our makeup overnight, right? The mascara is the most important part to remove because it will get dry and crunchy overnight and is super likely to split and break. It's also scary AF to wake up to.

TIP! Don't just throw away your old mascara willy-nilly! Chop off the old dry wand, give it a wash with dishwashing liquid and keep it as a handy spoolie to brush through any clumps in your lashes or tame your brow hairs.

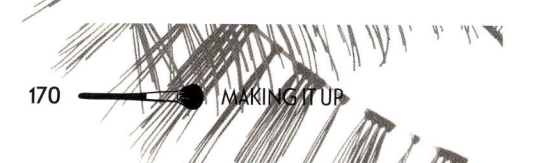

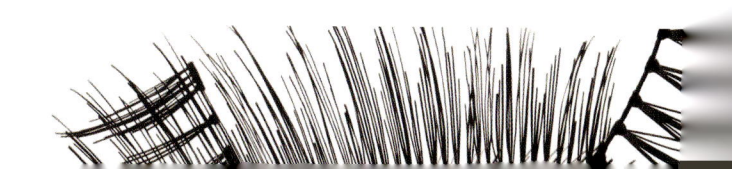

TIP!
Want the perfect pastel that you know will suit you? Mix your favorite bright or rich colored lipstick with a nude lippy to pastelize your favorite hue.

Products Used In Step By Step

MAC False Lashes Maximizer, Estée Lauder Sumptuous Knockout Defining Lift And Fan Mascara, MAC Upward Lash Mascara, MAC 210 liner Brush, MAC Liptensity Lipstick in Bite O' Georgia

LINNEA FROM PRISCILLAS

LASHES GET PASHES

FALSE LASHES

LASHES GET PASHES

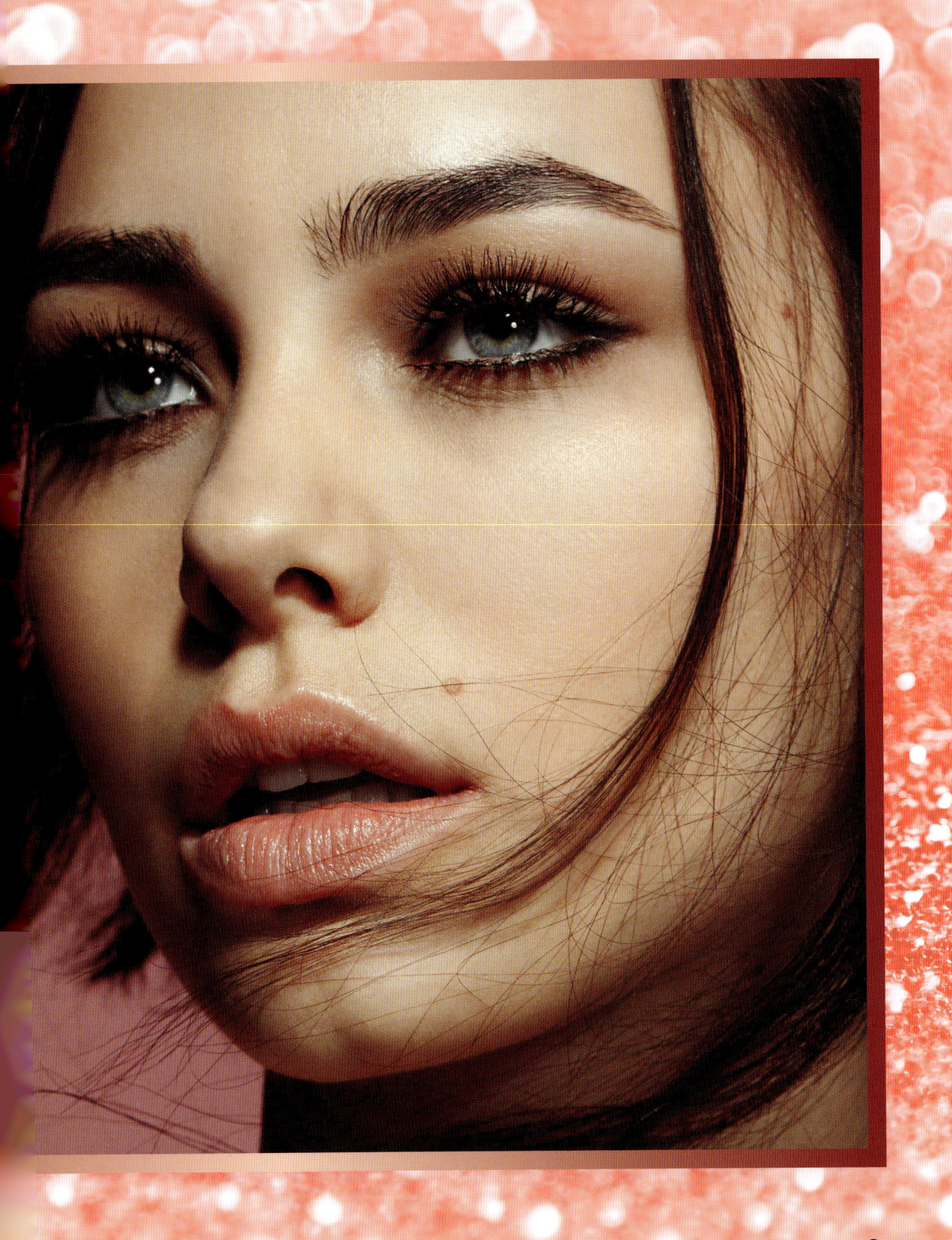

STEP 1

Mascara first! Coating the lashes with a small amount of mascara first will help the lashes sit into the lash line seamlessly. Don't go overboard – you can always add more later on.

STEP 2

Chop up your lashes. Personally I find it *wayyyyy* easier to add my lashes in pieces! They are also likely to stay put for longer. Our eyes are moving all day long and a full strip lash can have a tendency to lift at the inner corners with all that movement. Cutting your lashes up in two or three pieces makes for ease of application and longer wearability as they can move with the eye and not lift.

STEP 3

The easiest way to apply your lash piece is to hold your chin right up, and look down your nose into the mirror, sitting the 'fakey' on top of the lash line. Don't expect it to be perfect instantly! You have about one minute to wiggle that lash into place so take your time. Start with the longest piece at the outer corner and then add each piece, moving inwards along the eye.

> *TIP!* If in doubt, tear it off and try again. If you just can't get the lash right, don't fight with it, tear the lash off, apply a little more glue and give it another go. It will always stick easier the second time!

STEP 4

Now it's time to clamp it all together. When we first apply lashes, they can look and feel a little foreign. Usually this can be fixed with a little pushing and wiggling, bringing the whole thing together. Use your fingers to press your lash together with the false ones all the way along the lash line. This will settle them in.

I love to give it a *light* treatment with my lash curler as this can guide all the lashes in the same direction and make them look a lot more natural! But make sure your mascara is *totally* dry!

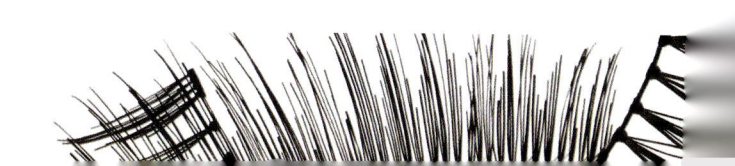

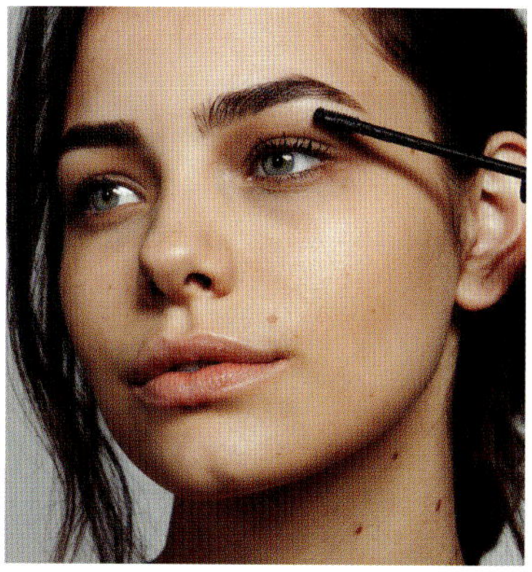

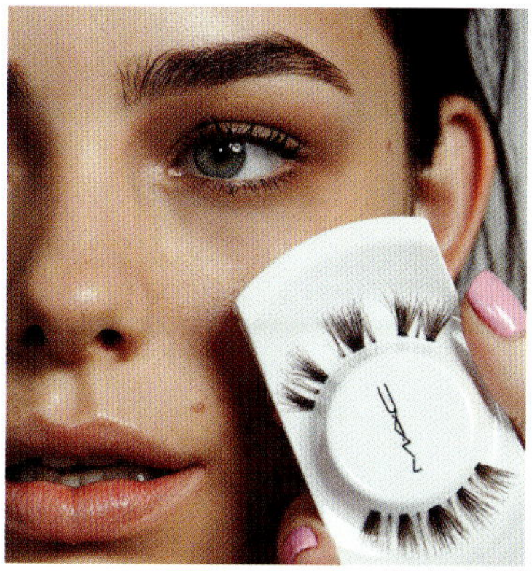

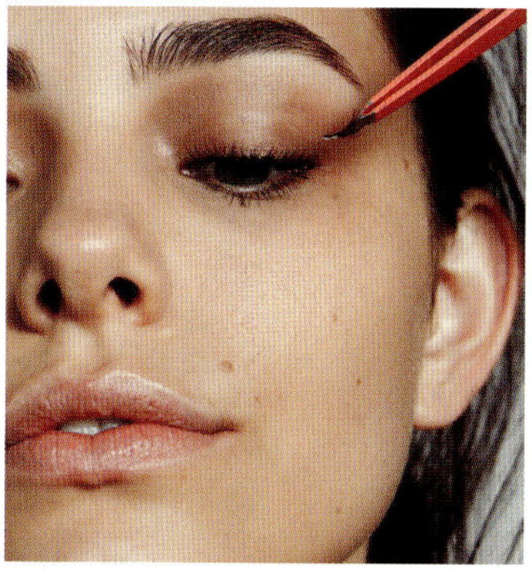

STEP 5

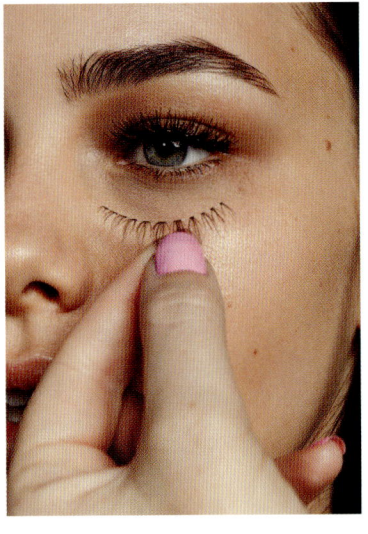

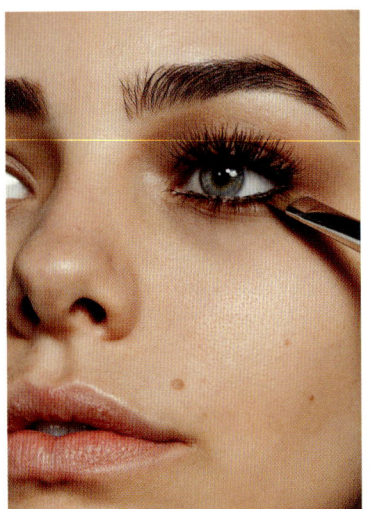

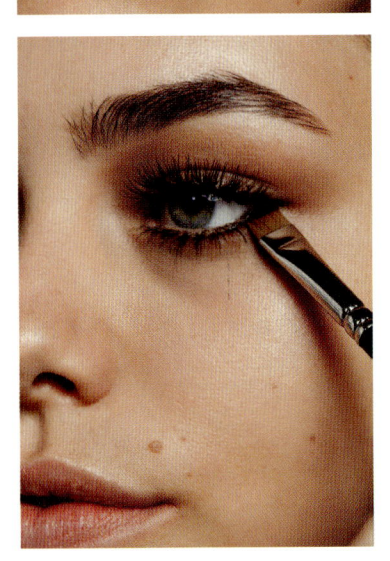

Wearing false lashes on the bottom lash line has for a long time been reserved for dress-up parties imitating Twiggy. This is no longer the case. Nowadays the lashes are so sheer and delicate, they are easily slotted into your lash line, both top and bottom, without anyone being the wiser!

If you are applying a full strip it is much easier to do so on the bottom lid. Lay a thin line of lash glue along the band of the lash, and place the lash beneath the bottom lashes, as close as you can possibly get them to the roots of your actual lashes.

> **TIP!** Lashes top and bottom will make your eyes look so much bigger! To enhance this look even further, add a soft wash of brown, slightly shimmery shadow for a natural look smoky eye that will bring the whole look together.

STEP 6

Use a flat eye shadow brush to really push the lash into place, wriggling and pushing it closer to the roots. Once again, you have a little less than a minute to secure the lash in the optimum position.

STEP 7

Use a dark matte eye shadow with the same flat brush to further disguise the clear strip of the lash. Creating a soft V shape, press the shadow to the outer bottom edge of the eye and the top outer edge together for a soft flick that can help mask the 'fakeys'.

> **TIP!** Eyelash glue! How much to add? Drag a cotton tip covered in glue along the lash base to draw a thin line. Then use the cotton tip to feather the glue out from the base on the underside of the lash about 1 cm. Spreading the glue out means the glue will adhere to more of the natural lash not just the roots so you will get a stronger hold for longer.

LASHES GET PASHES

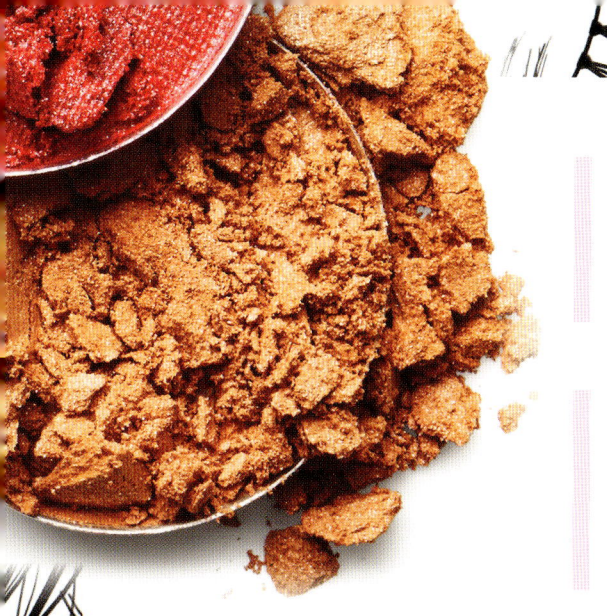

TIP! Applying a full strip of lashes takes a little practice. Peel the strip out gently from the pack and wrap it around your finger to give the strip a little bend and help it adhere to the curve of your eye. This is especially helpful if you have lashes that have a thick black base, as quite often they will lift on the eye.

TIP! Don't apply lashes with your eyes closed! I repeat. Do not apply lashes to closed eyes! You are more likely to get glue in your eye and make a mess if you attempt to do it with your eyes closed. Instead follow the guide here and open your eyes, looking down your nose while your chin is right up. The skin around the eye will be stretched out and you will find it much easier to apply!

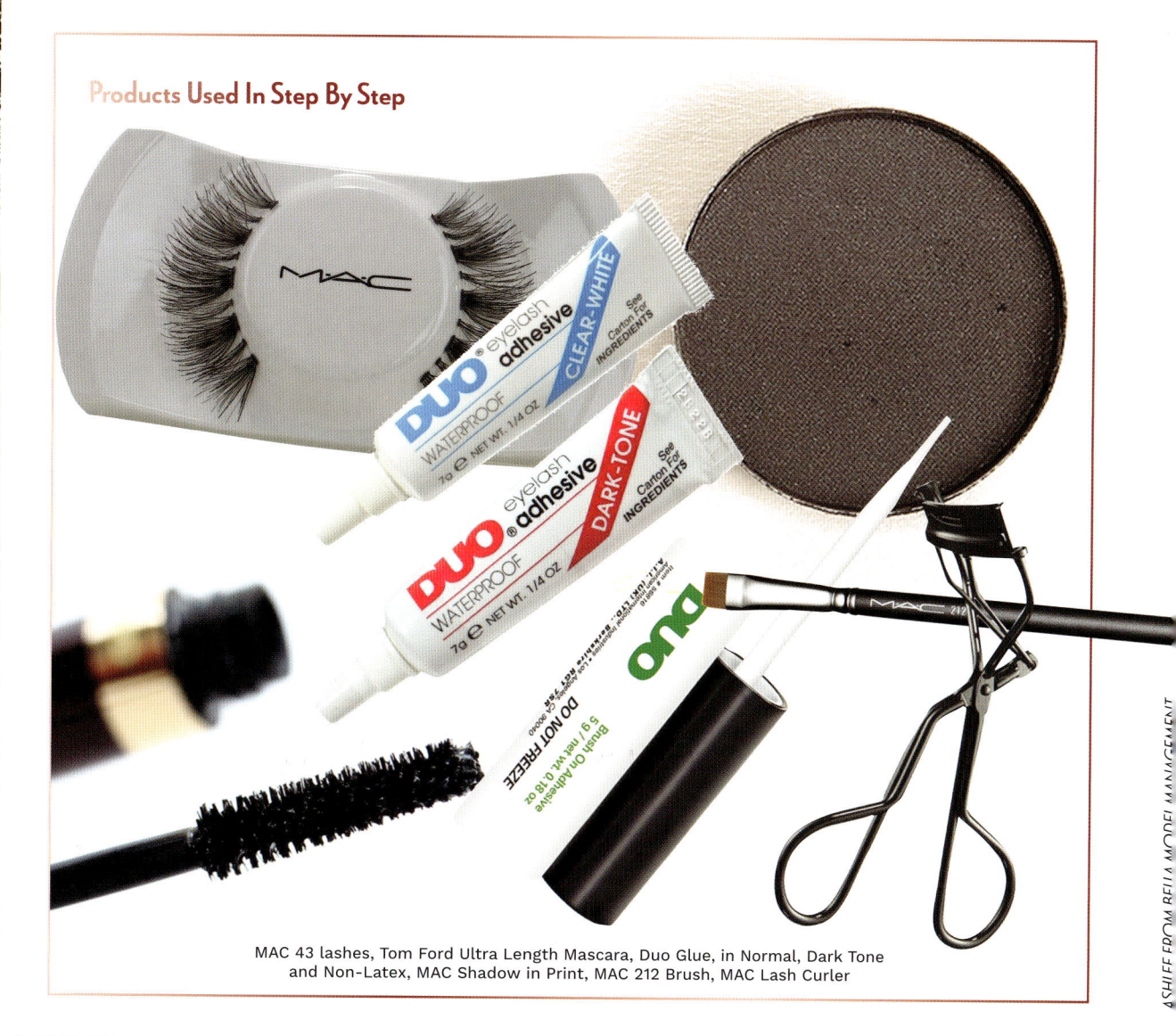

Products Used In Step By Step

MAC 43 lashes, Tom Ford Ultra Length Mascara, Duo Glue, in Normal, Dark Tone and Non-Latex, MAC Shadow in Print, MAC 212 Brush, MAC Lash Curler

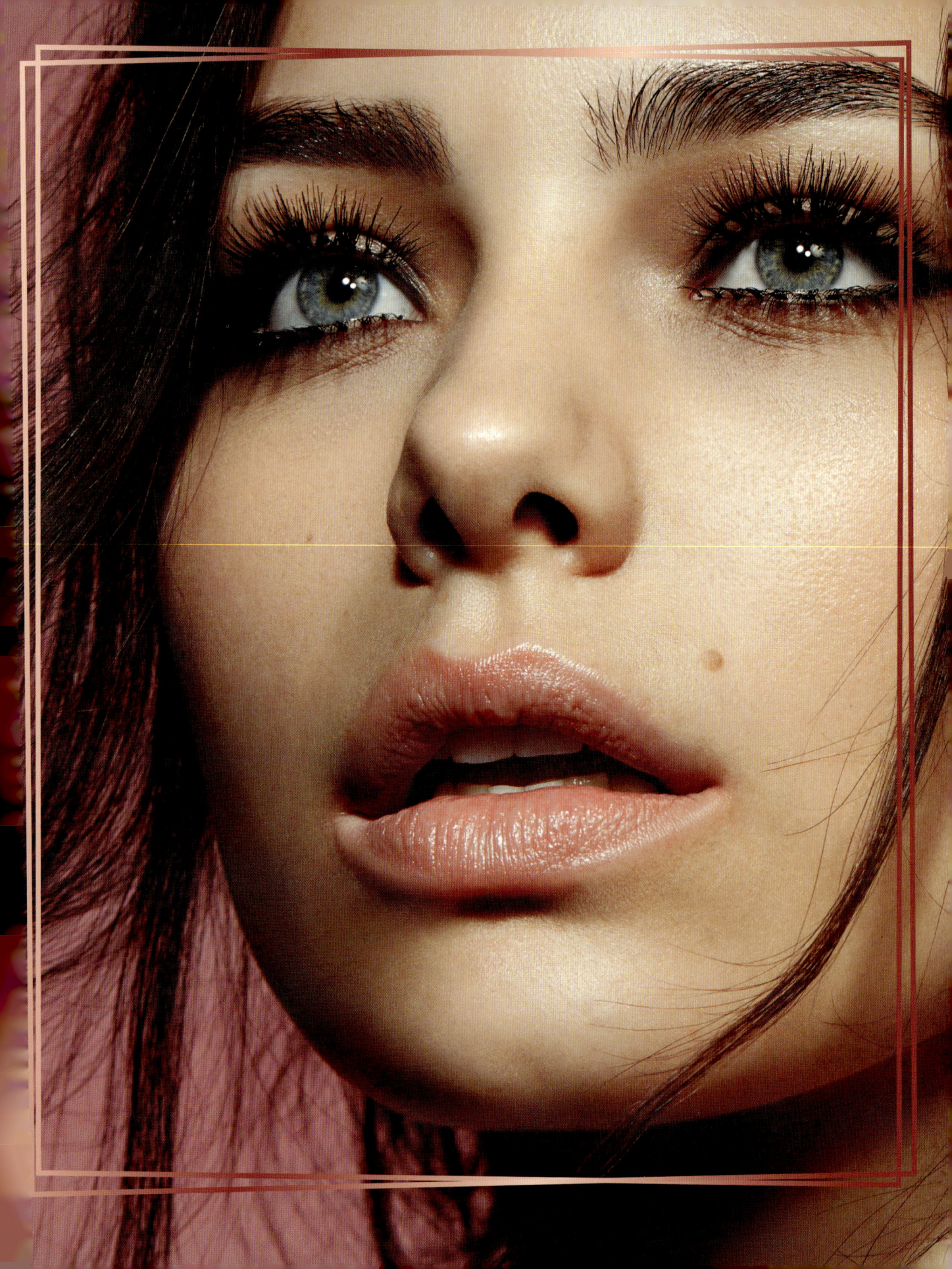

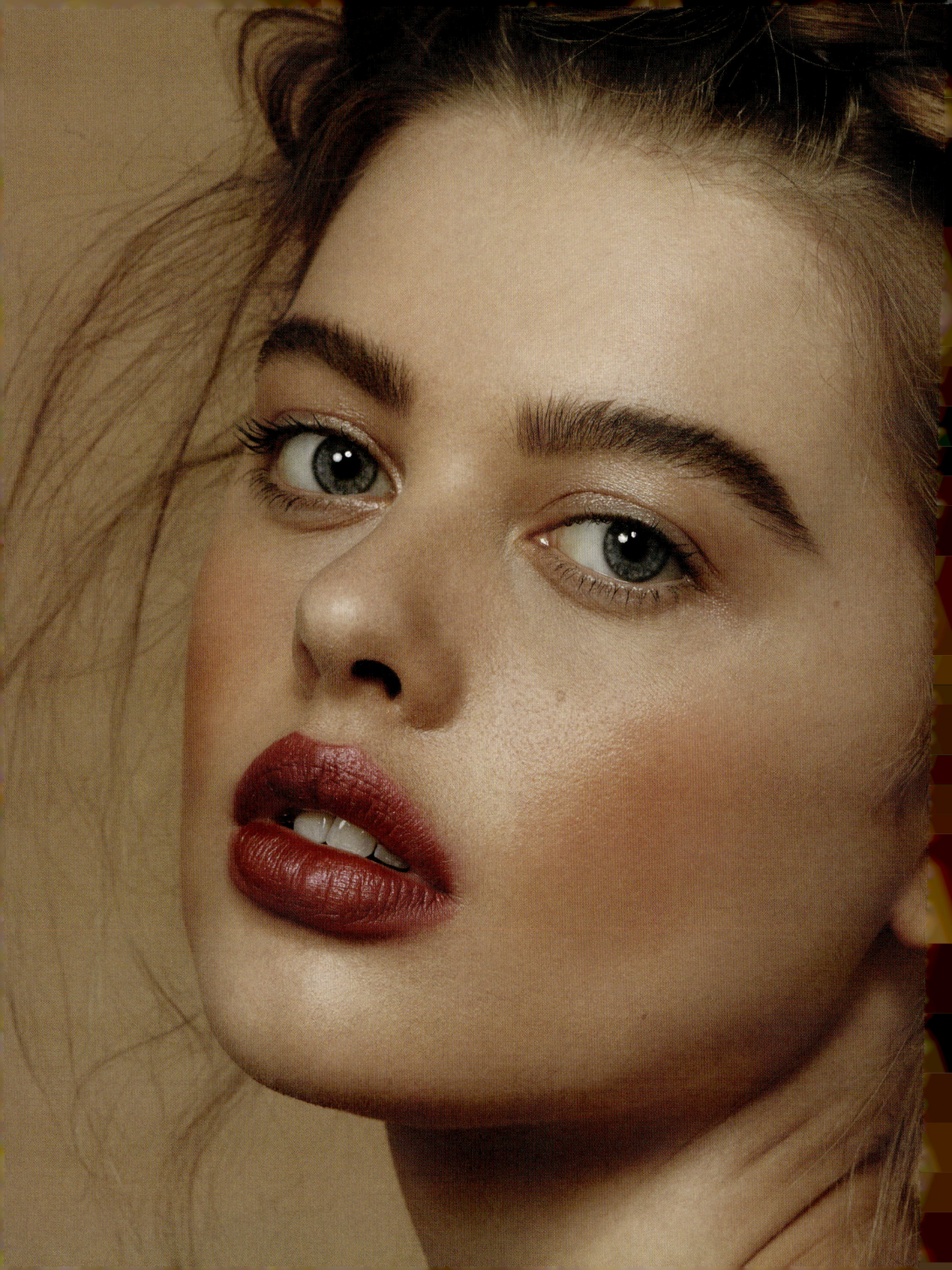

Power of the pout

We can never have enough lipsticks (am I right?!!). In the cosmetics industry, there is an incredible phenomenon called 'The Lipstick Effect'. Essentially what they find is that in times of economic downturn, lipsticks sales go up. Why you ask? Because putting on some lippy is a cheap and simple way to make yourself feel better. But you didn't need an economics lesson to know that.

My late grandmother was born in 1915 and lived a glorious 93 years. Whether it was for a fabulous function or a trip to the corner store, as far as I know she never left the house without her favorite rouge on. It was the one accessory she couldn't live without.

Lipstick holds serious power, and that power can be considerably enhanced depending on how you use it. Have you ever noticed that when you have found your soulmate of all lip colors applying it makes you instantaneously more fabulous and confident? Another question, has anyone else *cried* when their favorite lip color had been discontinued? Or is that just me again? However you feel about this makeup-bag staple, one thing is for sure, a good lip can make a statement or be the glue that brings your whole look together.

Before you get to the color, what's happening underneath? Just like under foundation, what happens underneath lip color will change it completely.

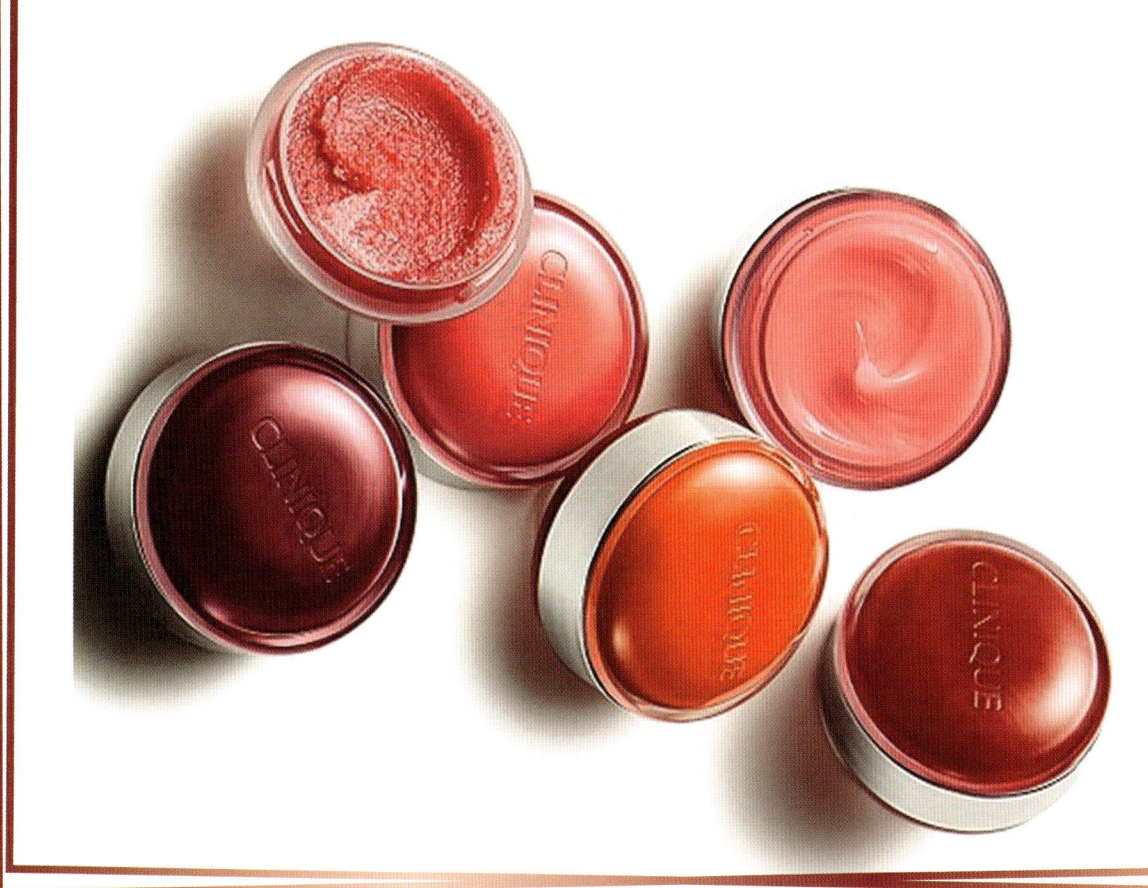

Exfoliation Is the Key

Take those lips one a one-way trip to supple town! There are a few different ways you can slough away the mortal enemy of the perfect lip – dry skin.

LIP SCRUB

Grab yourself a lip conditioner and scrub in one. They taste good and do great things!

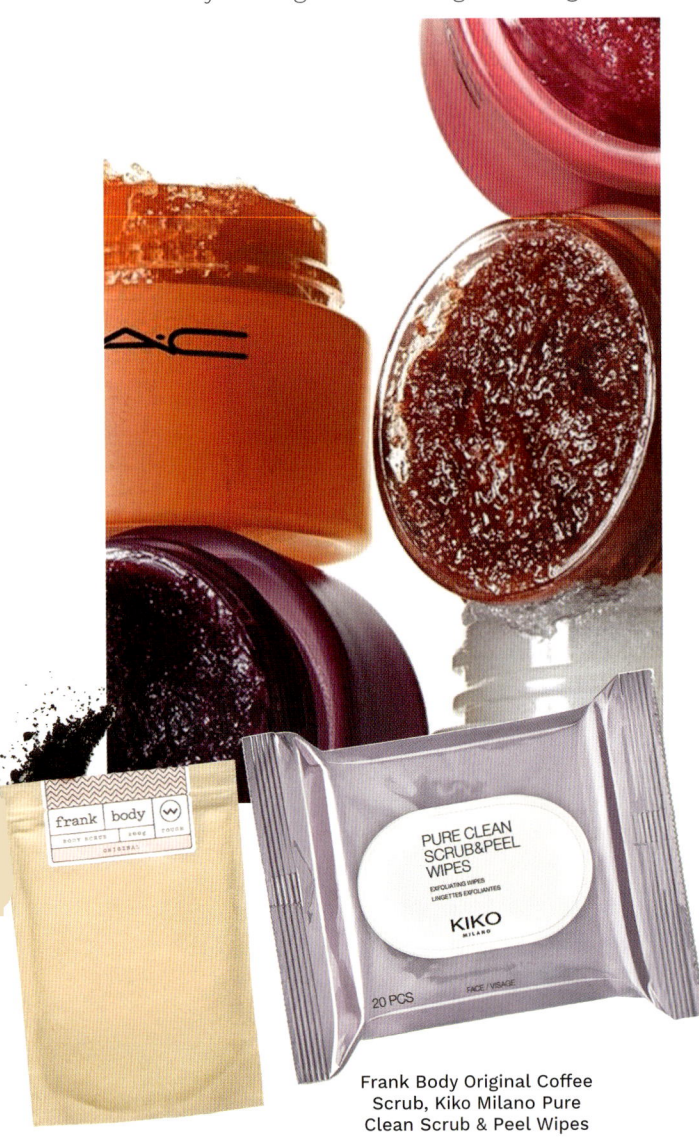

MAKE YOUR OWN SCRUB

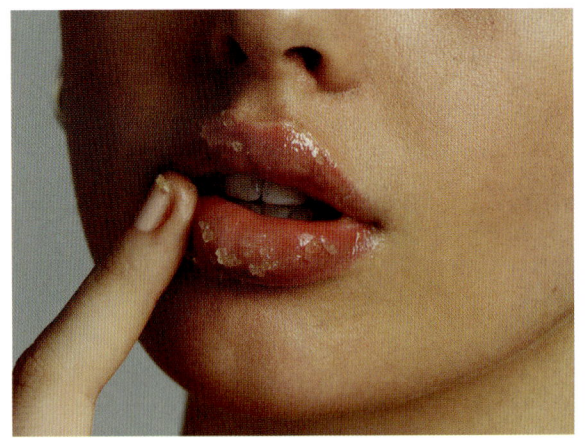

This is something that I have done many a time when I haven't had time to get to the shops. Mix sugar in with a lip balm you have at home and rub all over your lips. The mixture should be course and rough.

FACE EXFOLIATOR

Only have a face exfoliator? Have no fear, use it dry over the lips for a similar effect.

EXFOLIATING WIPES

I use these so much in my makeup kit for the ease and speed. There are heaps of options out there and they are inexpensive – supermarket to beauty store, the choice is yours!

TOOTHBRUSH

Cannot find any of the above? You gotta have a toothbrush! This is an oldie but a goodie, that actually works. Use a dry brush on wet lips and scrub vigorously to get rid of those dry bits. Bam!

Now you are ready to CREATE!

Frank Body Original Coffee Scrub, Kiko Milano Pure Clean Scrub & Peel Wipes

POWER OF THE POUT

NUDE FULL LIPS

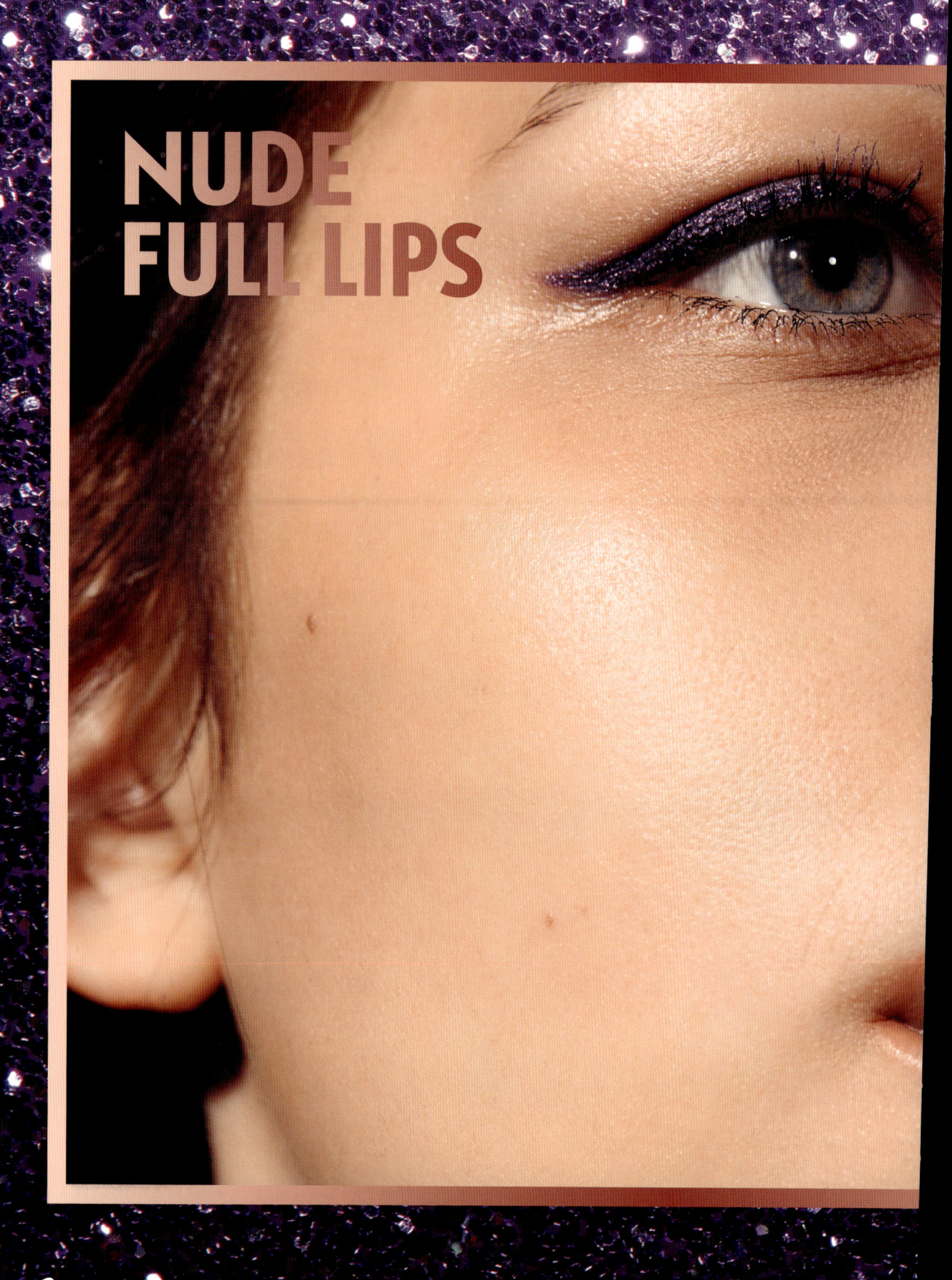

POWER OF THE POUT 183

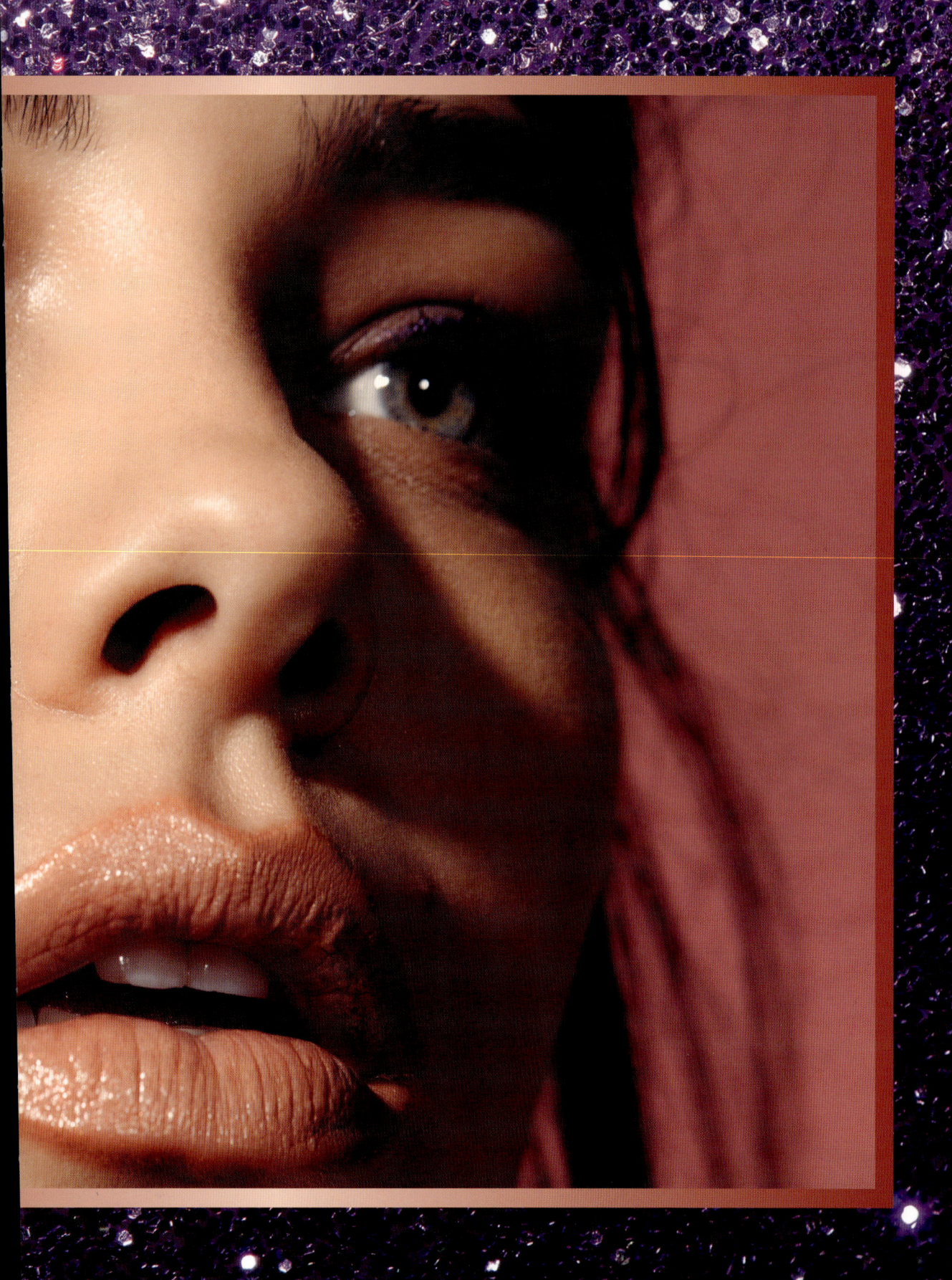

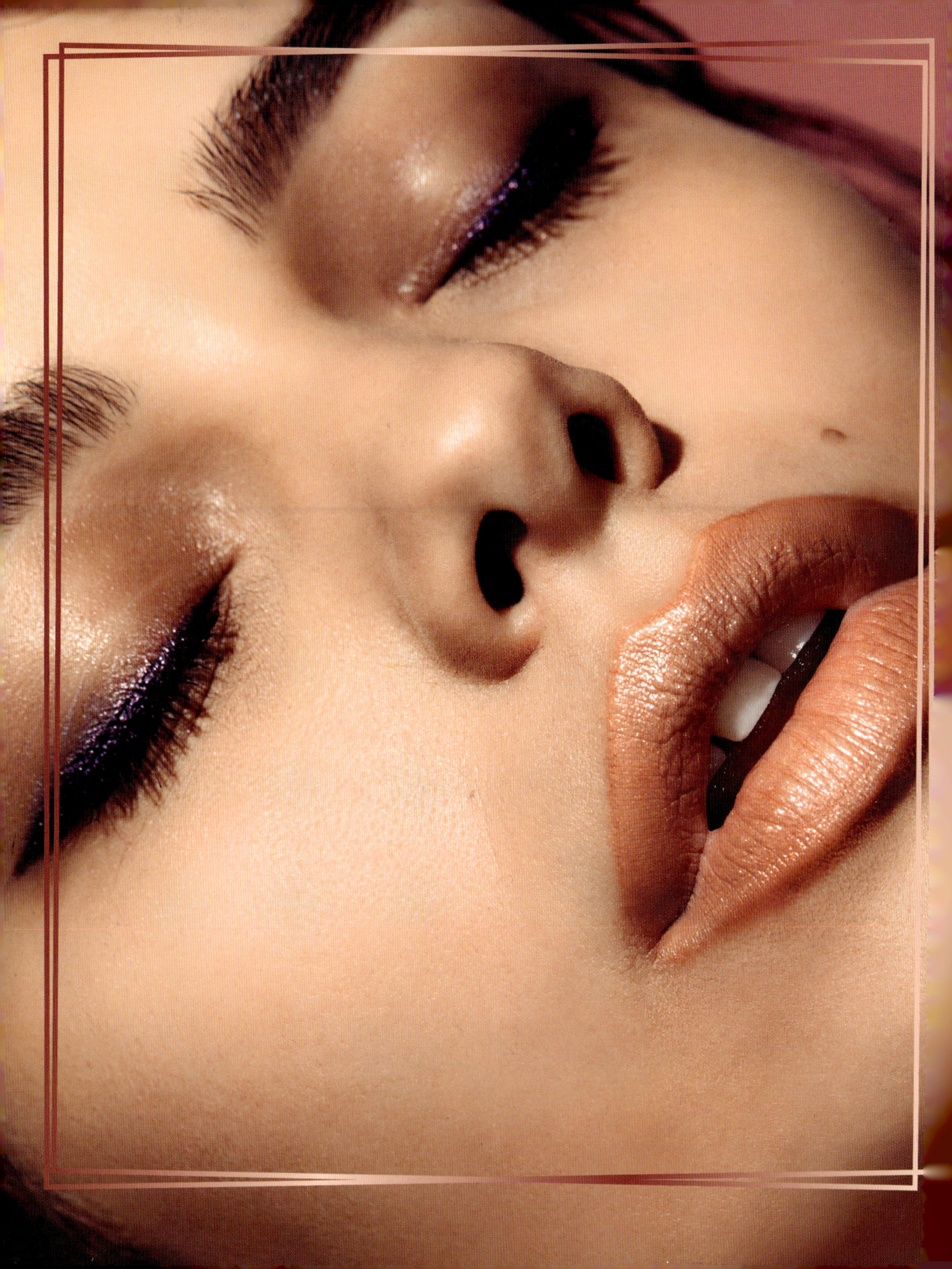

STEP 1

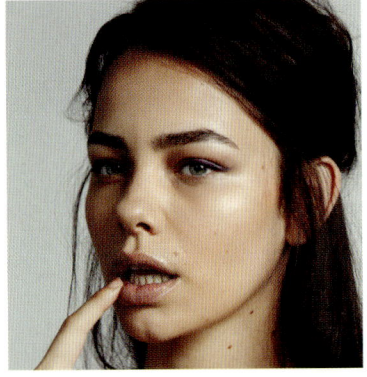

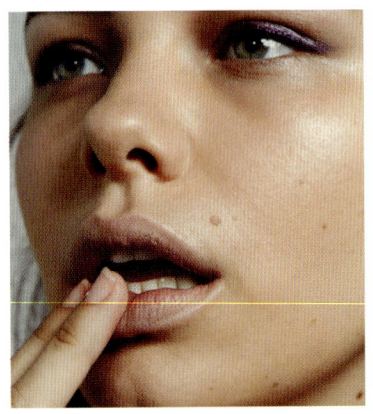

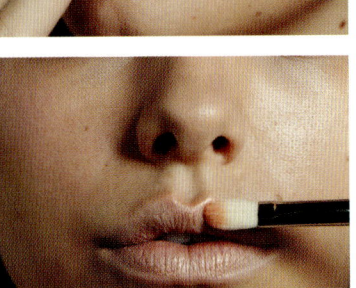

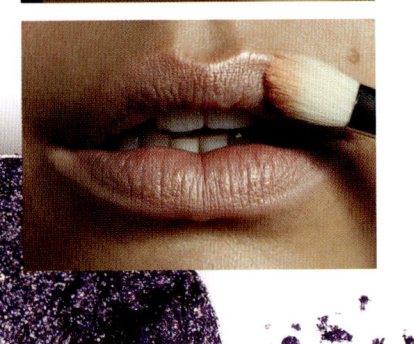

To get the best out of any lip look, the prep is important. Load on some lip conditioner to soften your lips; do this and complete the rest of your makeup then come back and they will be supple enough for product to glide on.

> **TIP!** Are you lips resembling the walking dead? A little dramatic, but you get my point. The *worst* thing you could do on top of dry flaky lips is a nude! Gah! Scrub away rough patches with a lip scrub, toothbrush or exfoliating wipes.

STEP 2

Tone down your tone. A nude lip won't be nude if your lips are naturally pink! Start with a blank canvas and pat on your foundation or concealer with your fingers over the lips and fading out across the lip line. If it is too thick it will only feel heavy. Just a little color from the edges softly blended inwards is perfect.

STEP 3

Ever attempted highlighting the Cupid's bow after you have painted on your lips and ended up with a nice pink lipstick mustache? Grand isn't it. Highlighting is so important to create the illusion of fullness to the lips – do it first!

I love using a powder highlighter with a fluffy brush as you can glaze the edges of the lips without the danger of producing a highlight that resembles a gathering of fine white hairs above your top lip. Be sure to apply the powder highlighter to your top and bottom lips, it will seal in the foundation you tapped on giving you a nice dry base to blend into.

> **TIP!** A purple flicked eyeliner (try MAC Pearlglide Intense Eyeliner in Designer Purple) is the perfect accessory to these perfect peach nude lips. Side note: it is literally one product! Swipe the pencil and blend with a small angle brush – easy as that!

POWER OF THE POUT

STEP 4

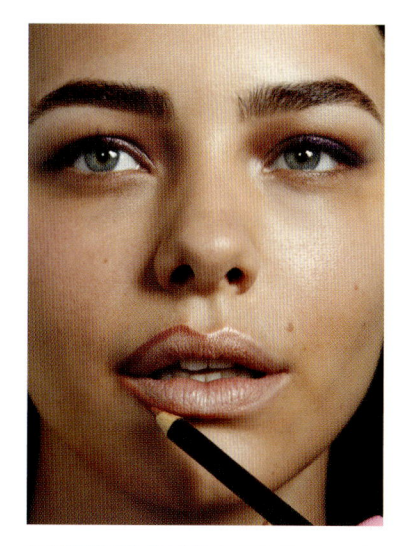

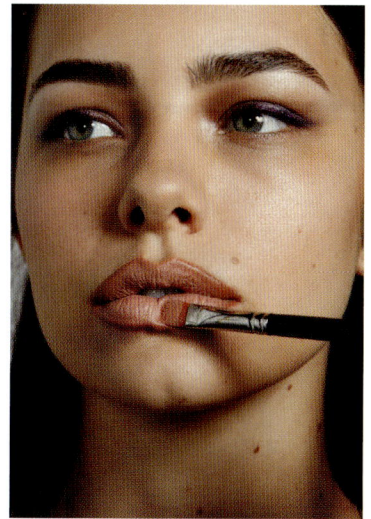

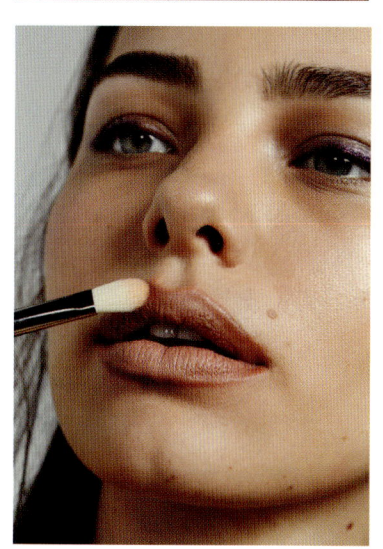

In we go with the pencil! Create the peak of your Cupid's bow first to ensure symmetry and feather the color out to the corners of the mouth. Feathering is the key here. A good nude lip pencil is often stronger in color pigment than you think; you shouldn't have to press too hard!

> **TIP!** Let's talk about the overdraw. I love to ignore my natural lip shape and give myself the lip shape I wish I was born with! Have you also wanted to do the same thing but weren't too keen on looking like a blow-up doll? You will want to start small and get bigger because I have seen it (both on my face and others) go horribly wrong when you jump straight into drawing a line too far from the natural edge of the lip. Instead, feather the color in from your natural lip shape, then once you have your shape reassess how big you want to go. Take the line further out, concentrating on the top lips and center of the bottom lips first. Keep checking as you go. Often when you adjust the line in these areas first it is enough!
>
> If you have a fuzzy upper lip, you have two choices. Stay away from overdrawing too high into the hairs, or get hair removing! Lipstick and pencil into the hairline will just highlight what you would rather disguise.

STEP 5

Paint on a nude lipstick that is slightly lighter than the pencil color; you want to craft a subtle ombré effect. You can use a brush here for a professional finish, or you can apply straight from the tube dabbing and blending with your fingers.

STEP 6

Use face powder to set and clean up the shape. This is especially important when you have gone beyond your natural lip shape. What you need to do is to blend the lip texture between skin and lip so it creates the impression that your lips are actually this size! Matting down the edges will do this, as creamy shiny things will just highlight the difference more.

You can use a soft fluffy brush for ease, and use a colored face powder or translucent setting powder. A gentle hand is a must.

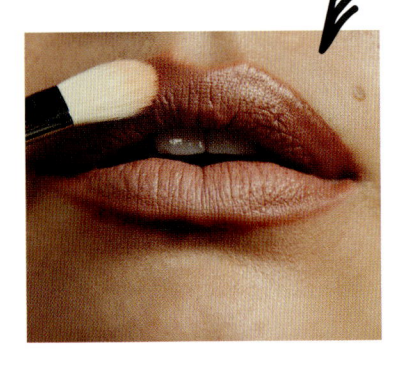

TIP! I love to take it that little step further and instead use a nude shadow over the edges to give dimension to the lip and increase that juicy lip look!

TIP! To ensure a seamless blend, tap your finger with a slight amount of the nude lipstick all over your finished lip.

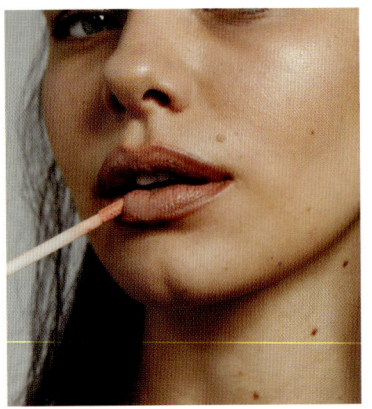

STEP 7

If you want max fullness finish with gloss! This part is not essential, especially if you prefer a matte, pressed-in nude. The more sticky the gloss the more shine you will get and the longer it will stay on your lips. If you have your hair out on a windy day avoid sticky gloss unless you want to eat your hair!. Go for a cream gloss with no stickiness or pop the lip conditioner you used at the beginning on to finish.

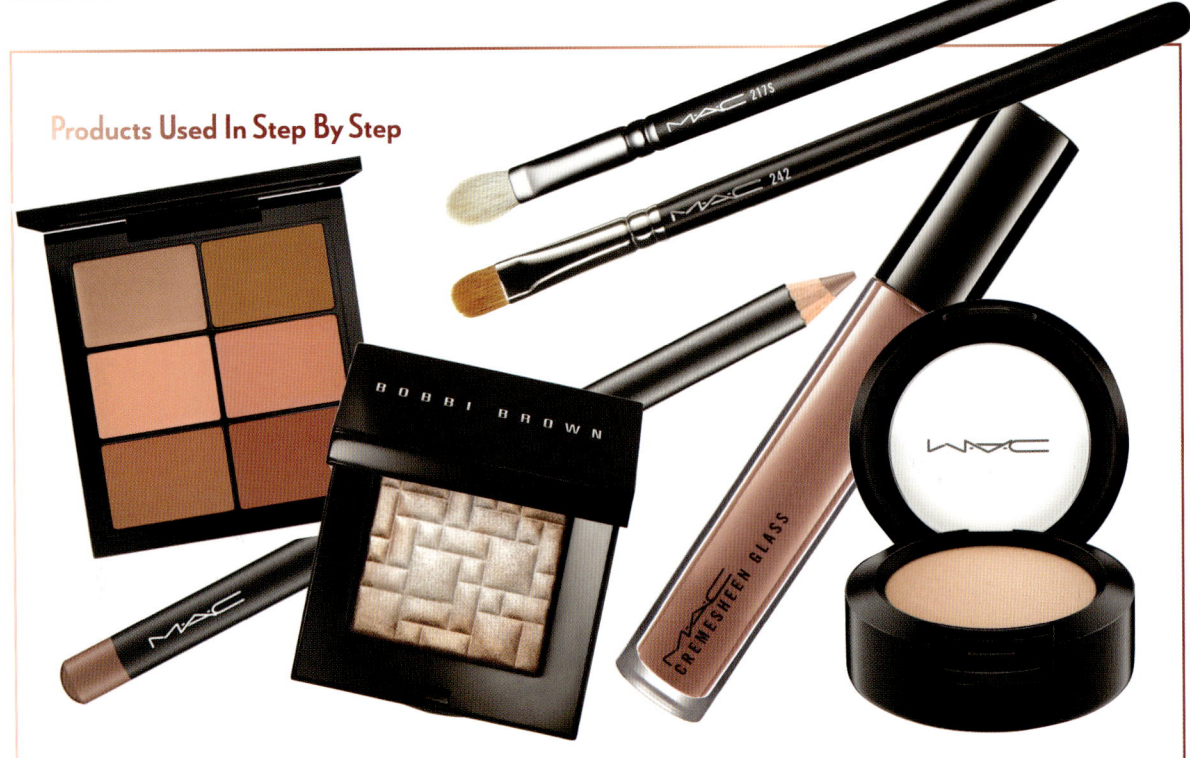

Products Used In Step By Step

MAC Lip Pencil in Stripdown, MAC Lip Palette in Necessary Nudes, Bobbi Brown Higlighting Powder in Pink Glow, MAC Cremesheen Glass in Boy Bait, MAC 217 and 242 brushes, MAC Eye Shadow in Arena over edges

ASHLEE FROM BELLA MODEL MANAGEMENT

POWER OF THE POUT

THE ART OF THE STAIN

POWER OF THE POUT

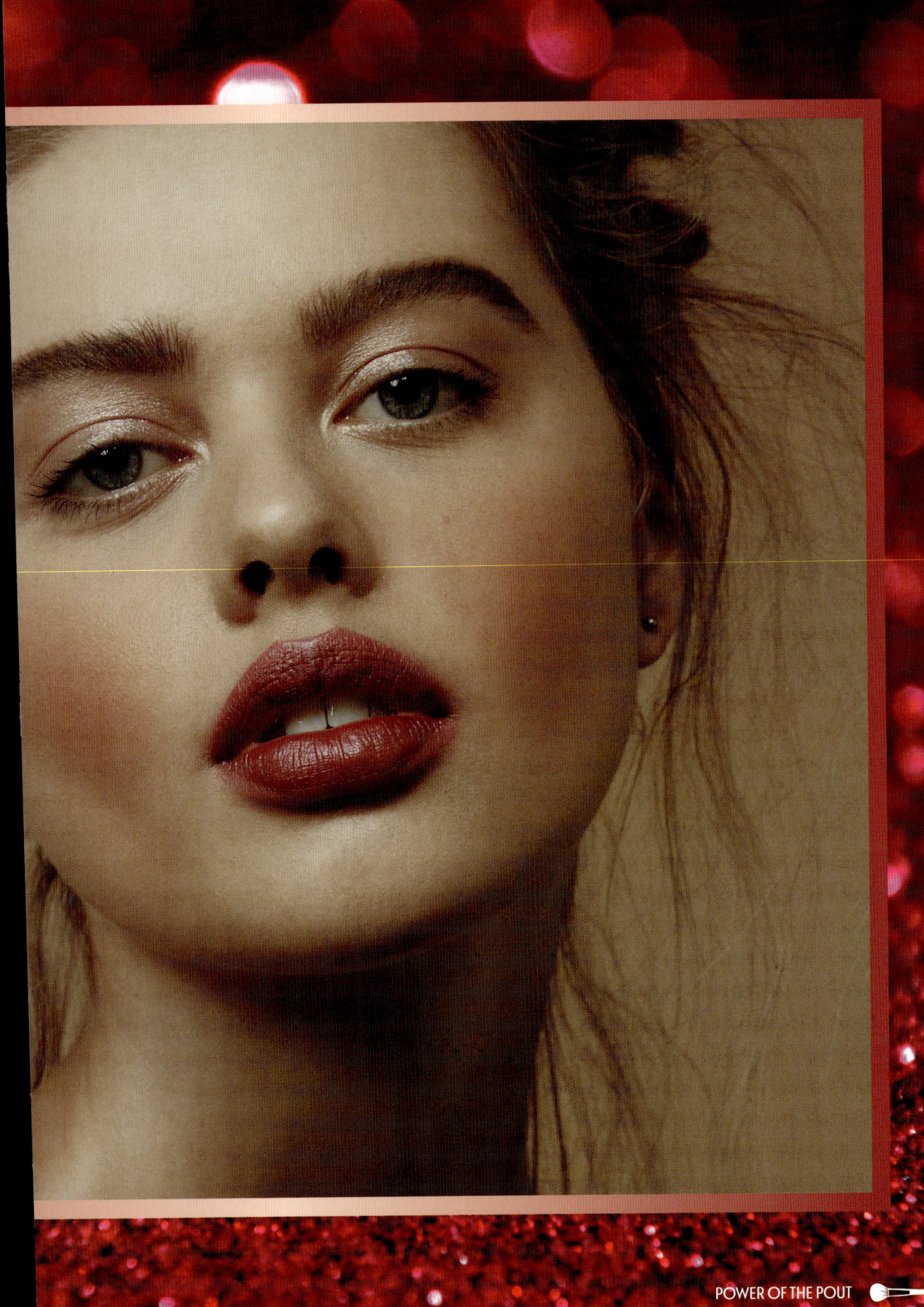

STEP 1

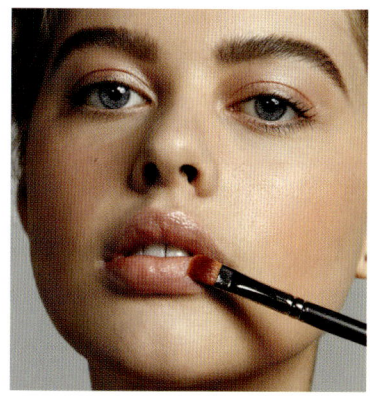

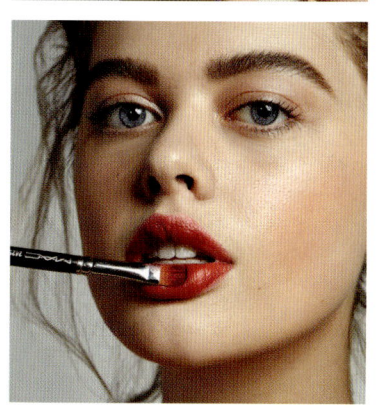

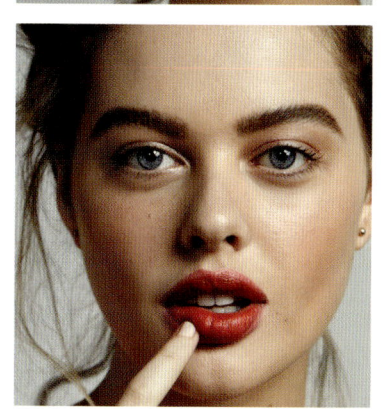

Dry, flaky areas have no place in this makeup look (do they ever have a place?) so it's time to whip out the lip conditioner. This glossy paste of goodness will instantly make the lips look and feel more supple. You will not require a primer for this lip.

STEP 2

Softly take your foundation or concealer over the lips, starting at the outer edge then blending inwards. This will stop the whole lip look from appearing messy and rushed at the end. Again, perfected surroundings are just as important as the feature!

> *TIP!* Don't go heavy with the 'foundie' as it will cause the lip color you layer over the top to change tone and appear heavy. Ideally use a sponge as it will absorb excess product.

STEP 3

Coat your lips with your choice of lipstick, working from the center outwards. Blend the color up to just before the edge without worrying about how perfect that edge is – we will get to that!

You may find it easier to go straight from the tube of lipstick and that is okay. Just make sure to apply it lightly so it doesn't become a smeared mess later!

STEP 4

Using your fingertips, blend the recently applied lipstick into your conditioned lips. If you forgot that step in the beginning, this is where you will notice the lip color becomes difficult to blend or patchy. The idea is not to rub all the color away! It you do feel the color is too heavy, soften it by continuing to work into your lips. Alternatively, if you think the color needs a bit more punch, add more lipstick and blend from the center, working outwards until you reach your desired depth of color.

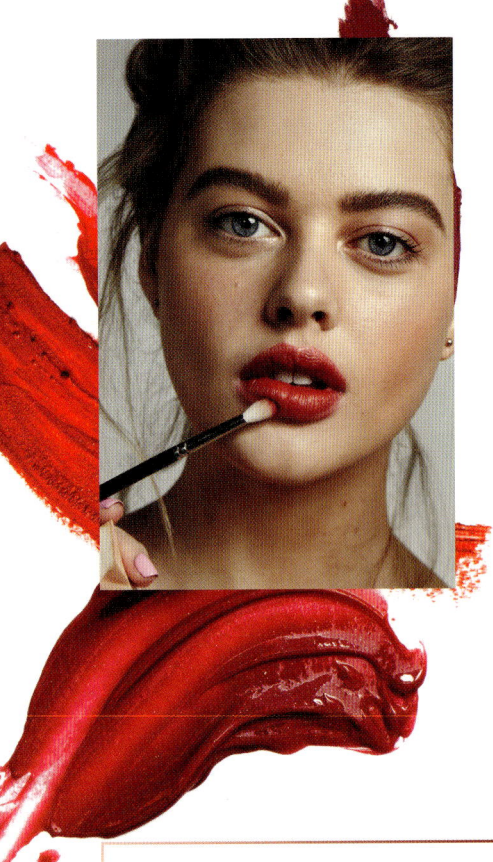

When you get to the outer edges, simply drag your finger tip along the perimeter of the lip line, subtly moving outwards. This will soften and spread the color, creating that lip tint effect.

STEP 5

With a soft yet small brush take some powder color, like a blush or an eye shadow, over the top to set the lipstick in place and amplify the lip look. A powder is super easy to glide over the whole lip and bring the look together while smoothing any uneven areas in your blending.

A slightly sheeny or metallic finish blush works a treat! A blush has less color pigment than an eye shadow so will blend easily over the top and not grab onto dry areas

Use a matte shadow with the same brush for a deeper look or a more bold finish!

TIP! Keep your foundation sponge or brush, with the left over foundation still on it, on hand to act like a little eraser and clean up any overzealous blending that has moved towards your chin to keep your look polished!

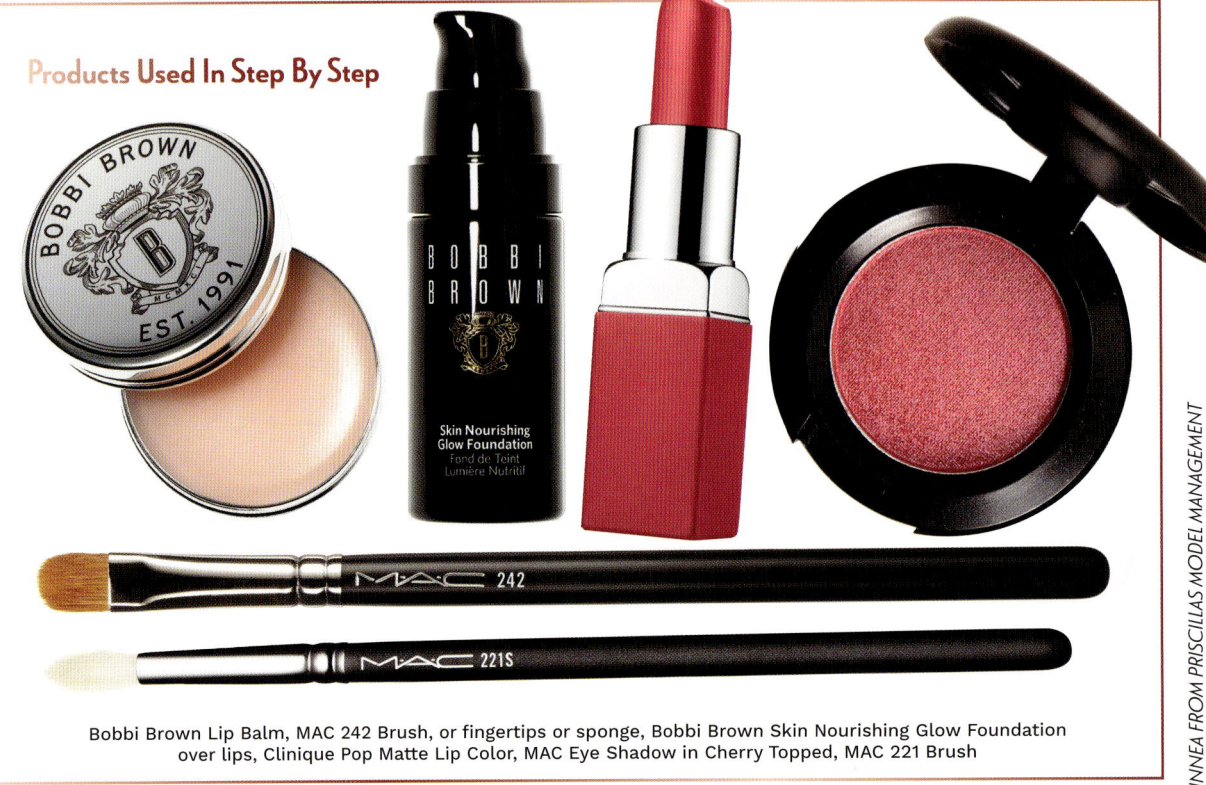

Products Used In Step By Step

Bobbi Brown Lip Balm, MAC 242 Brush, or fingertips or sponge, Bobbi Brown Skin Nourishing Glow Foundation over lips, Clinique Pop Matte Lip Color, MAC Eye Shadow in Cherry Topped, MAC 221 Brush

INNEA FROM PRISCILLAS MODEL MANAGEMENT

BOLD MATTE LIP

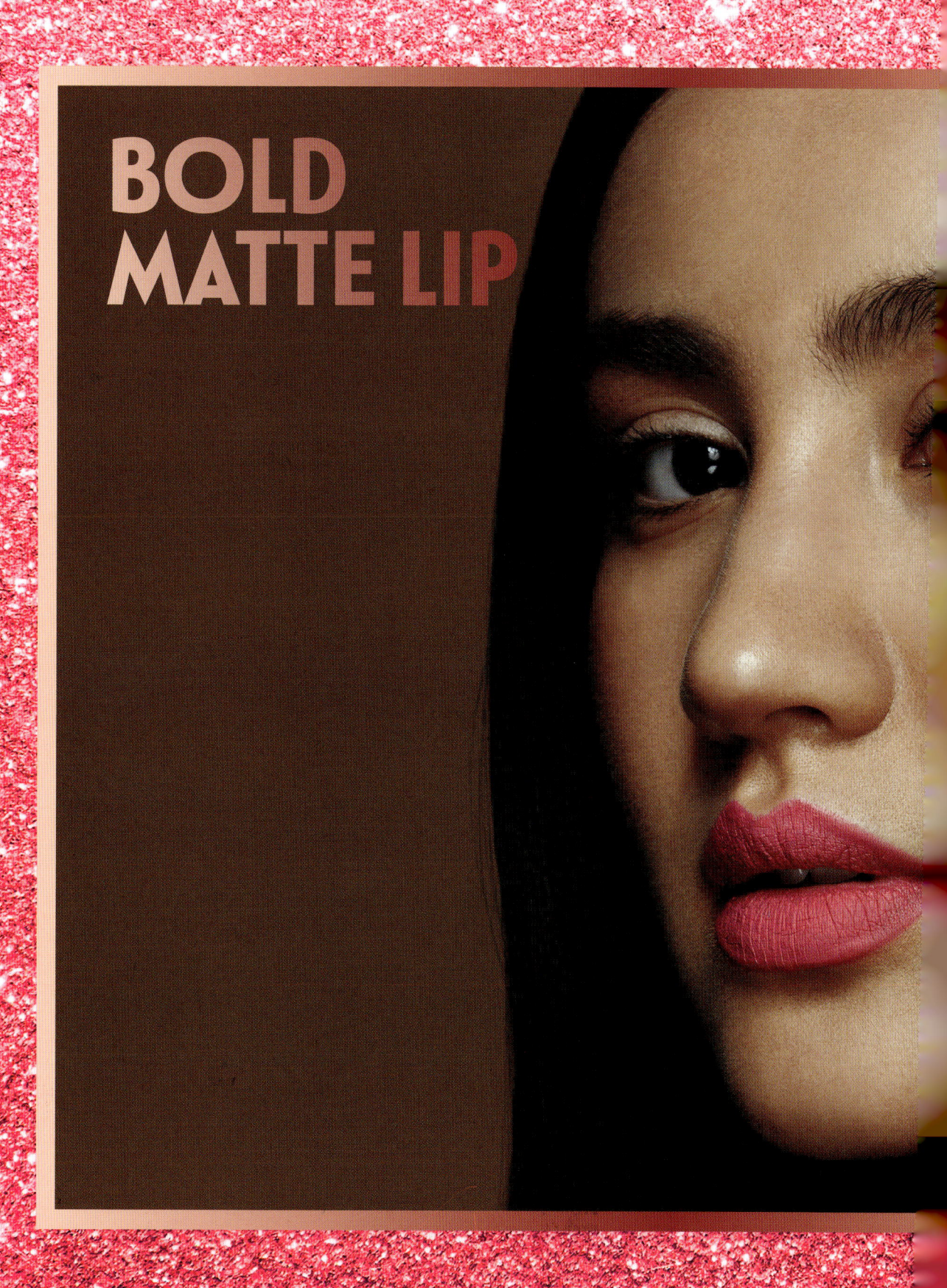

POWER OF THE POUT 193

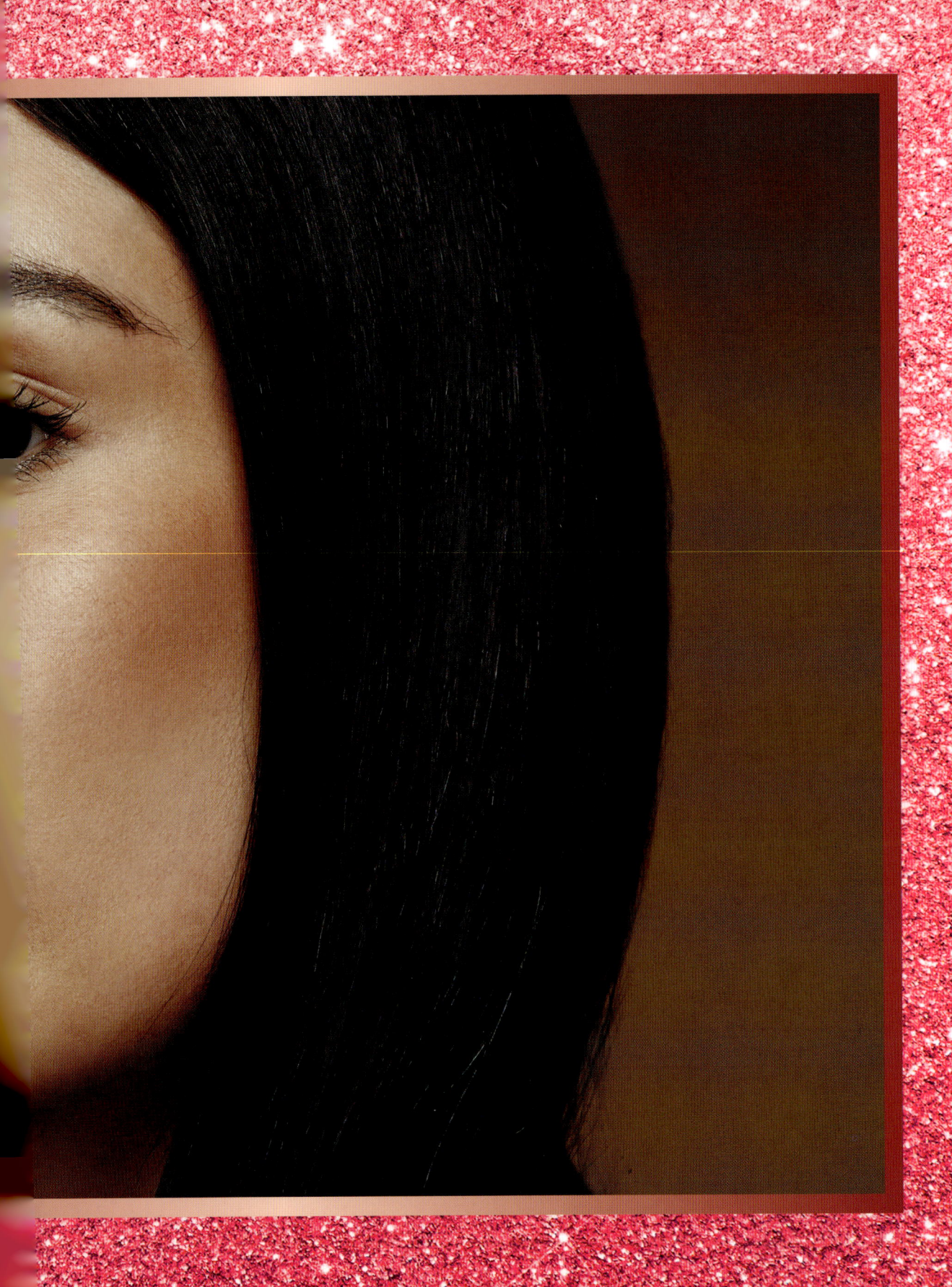

STEP 1

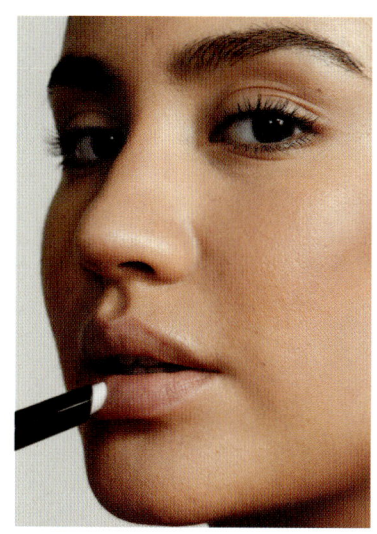

You do the applying, your lip primer does the holding! We have primers for all over the face now, and thank *you* makeup gods for coming up with this one! I *never* thought I would bother with a lip primer! But never say never, right? This guy has become a staple in my personal and professional kit. I mean, if you are going to put all this effort into the application, you want to see it on longer that your first coffee sip.

Take the moisturizing primer over your lips and also over the outer edges of your lips to stop the bleeding of the color.

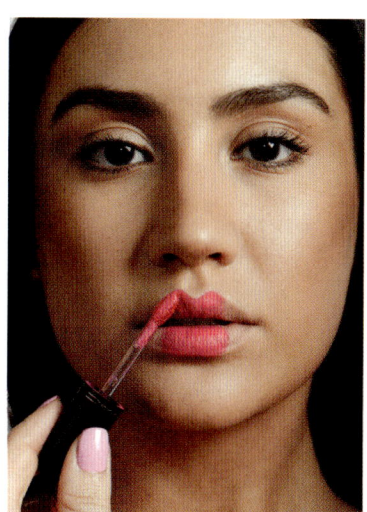

STEP 2

Once your lips are all evened out with your foundie and highlighter, go straight in with the lip product. Liner or lipstick first? If only we all did the same things in life! This is completely personal.

When I am using a super matte liquid lip product that sets, I don't mess with them, I get them on first! Often they are so opaque in color and set for so many hours you may not need a lip liner at all – gasp!

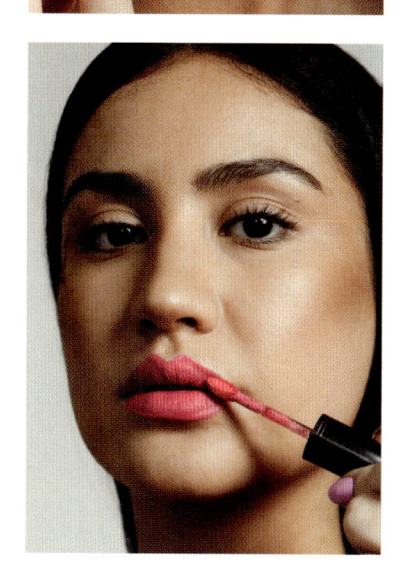

STEP 3

Start the color in the center. High impact lip colors will show up any unsymmetrical shape so it is best to start in the center. Create the bow of the lip, get that perfect, then drag the color down towards the outer corners.

On the bottom lip, start in the center and then paint upwards toward the corners. Work quickly with that color and open your mouth wide to make sure you completely fill your lips in, no edges or gaps.

STEP 4

Now with your matching pencil (or slightly darker to give dimension) use it as a corrector. You have more control than with

a brush and cream. It is so much easier to tidy edges and not add any more product and make a mess.

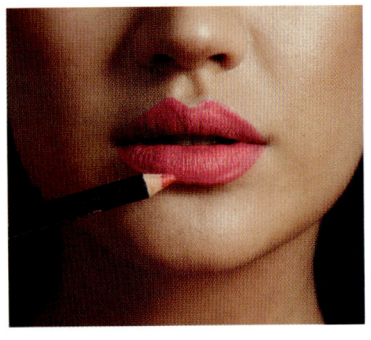

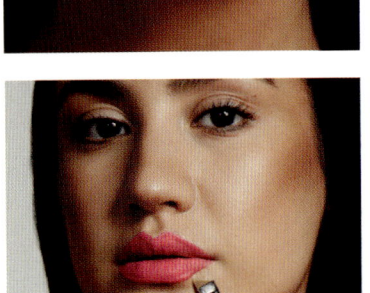

STEP 5

Clean up any soft smudges with a flat brush and colored face powder. Make sure the color is not too light or it will look like a white halo around your lips.

> *TIP!* If you make a big mistake or smear, have no fear! Stop crying, and do *not* wipe off your entire lip color! Instead, use the flat brush, this time with waterproof makeup remover, and swipe the brush through the smear, backward into the lip. You should have created a hole in the lip color. This hole is way faster to paint in than to do the whole lip again!

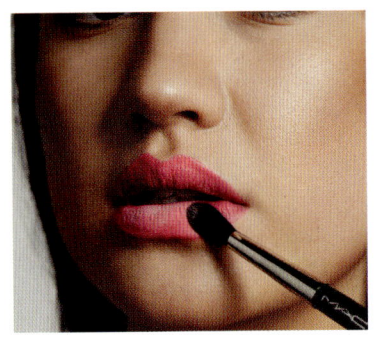

STEP 6

Powder with very sheer, invisible loose powder to set and smooth the lip.

> *TIP!* Don't have time for all these steps? Your favorite lip liner can be a fast and controlled alternative matte lip color. Draw over primed lips so the color won't be patchy and color your whole lip in.

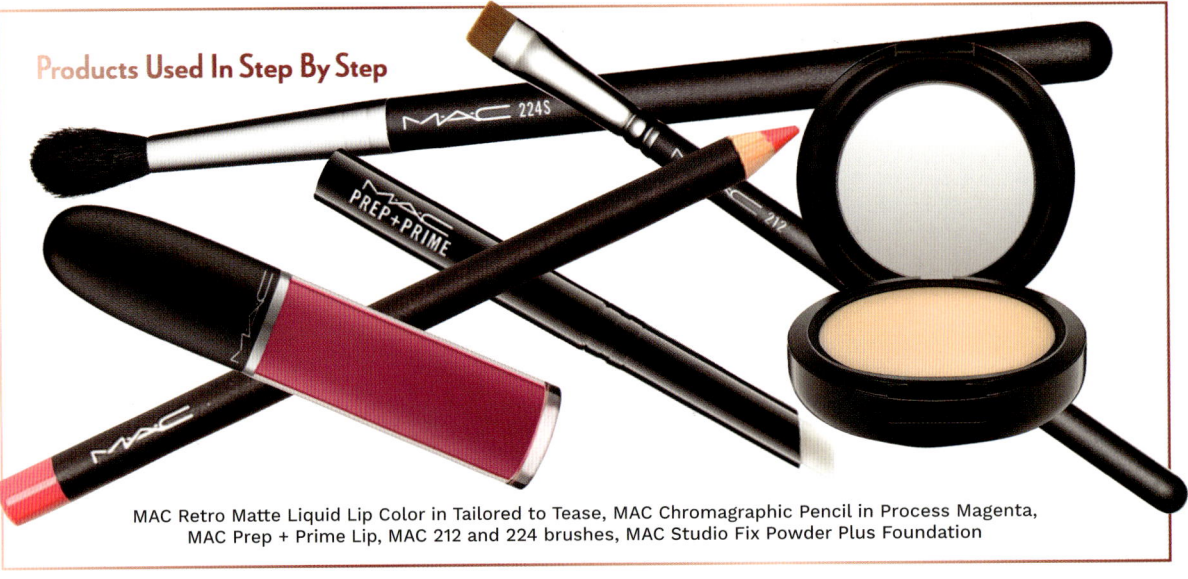

Products Used In Step By Step

MAC Retro Matte Liquid Lip Color in Tailored to Tease, MAC Chromagraphic Pencil in Process Magenta, MAC Prep + Prime Lip, MAC 212 and 224 brushes, MAC Studio Fix Powder Plus Foundation

TIARE FROM BELLA MODEL MANAGEMENT

POWER OF THE POUT   195

DARK LIP

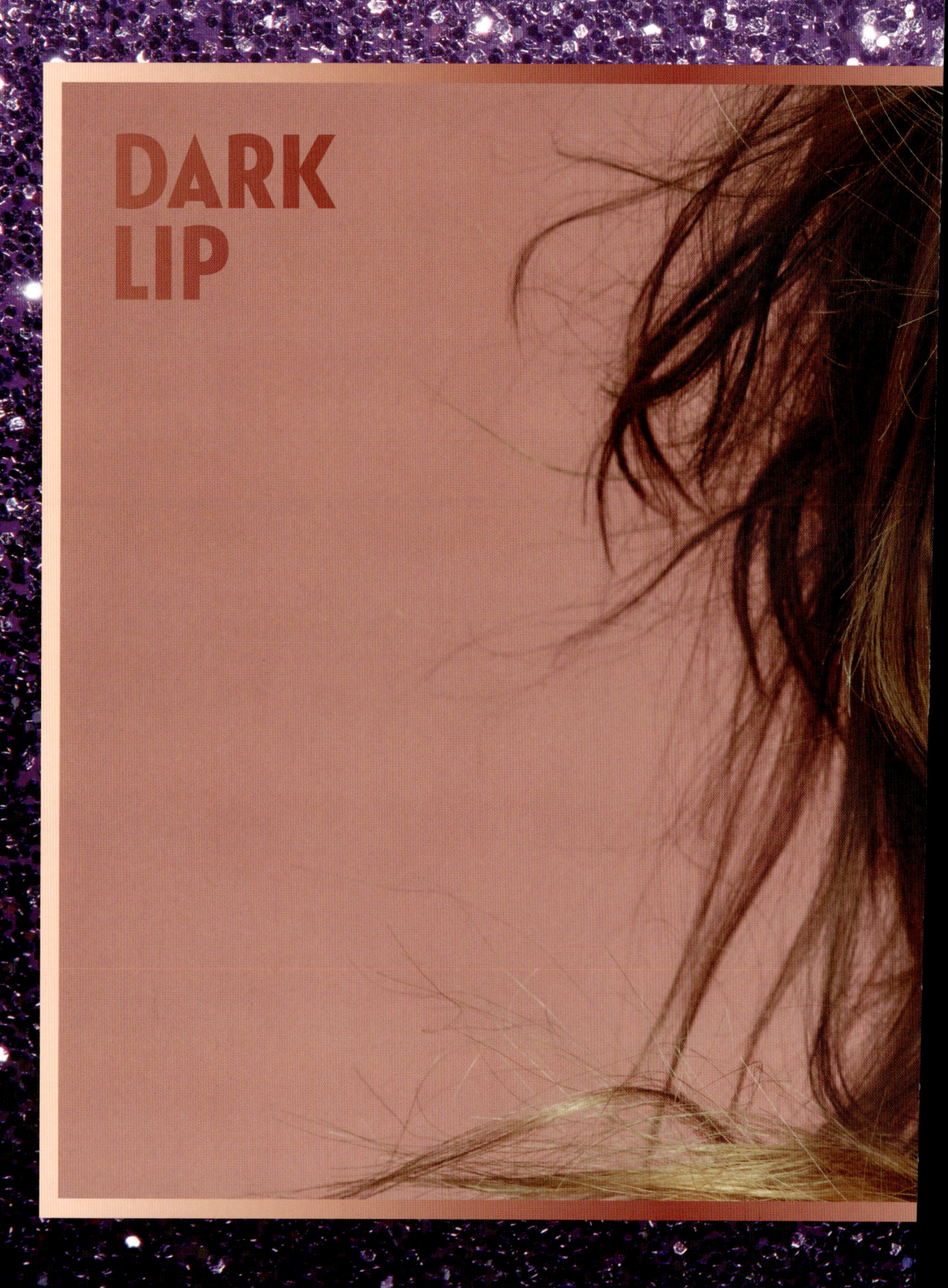

POWER OF THE POUT   197

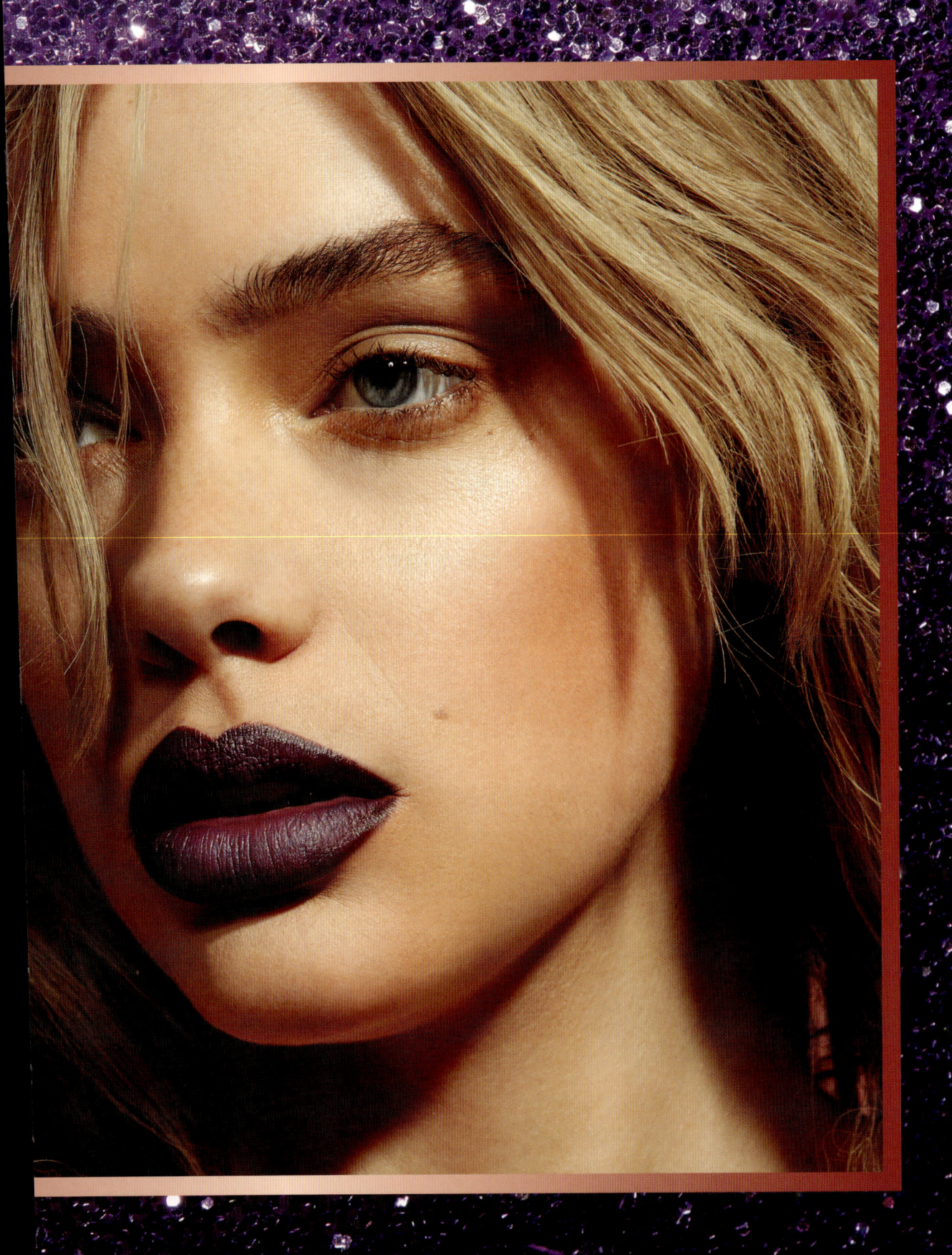

STEP 1

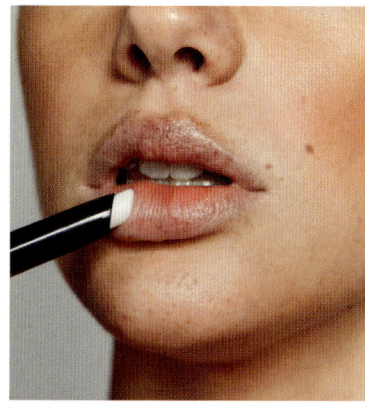

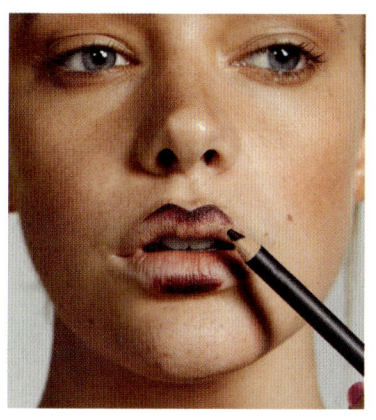

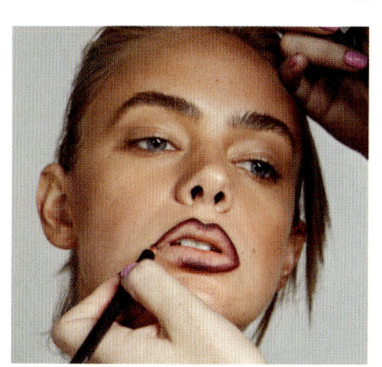

Primer ahoy! Smooth all over the lips and tap in with your fingers to start – standard lip operating procedure.

STEP 2

See a theme here? Take your foundation lightly over the lips and up over the edges, creating a flawless base on the skin around the lips. Whether you are doing a dark lip, brown lip or red lip, redness or discoloration next to the lips will ruin your entire look!

STEP 3

Start your lip-shape engines! With your pencil, starting in the center with the bow of the lip has never been more important. Draw the curve of the Cupid's bow and the center of the bottom lip line. It doesn't need to be perfect so take a deep breath. We can always tidy and correct later.

> **TIP!** Warm up your pencil! If the pencil is too sharp it can make our hands shaky. I like to soften the point in a tissue so you get a slightly softer line.

STEP 4

Tilt your head to complete the liner. I wish I could explain this more but trust me, tilting your head while you go from side to side has helped me when I am strapped for time! Feather the liner, working inwards from the edges. This will make for a more seamless lipstick color application on top.

STEP 5

Liner and feather that color into every nook and cranny of your lips. Get right up in there! There is nothing worse than when you are doing your best candid yet planned wide laughter shot on Instagram and the lipstick is all messy in the corner, like you are

recreating Heath Ledger's Joker. Or worse still, you haven't even reached the corners. Oh the horror of it all.

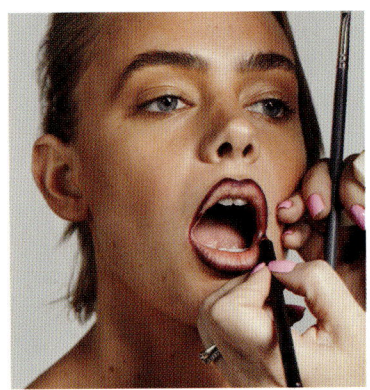

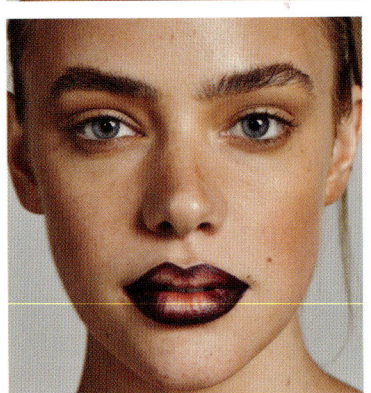

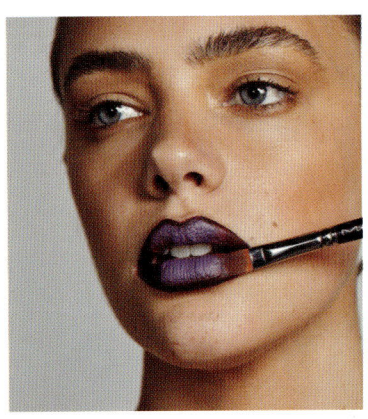

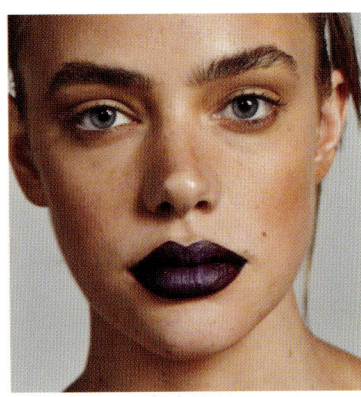

STEP 6

Now we color in! A dark lip as on its own can tend to look super thin so for this look we want to create shape and dimension. This is achieved by using two lipsticks, the first is the actual dark shade, and the other is a few shades lighter – in this example a pastel version of this deep plum.

Paint the dark lip around the outside first and blend inwards with your brush or your fingertip.

STEP 7

Swipe the lighter color through center and blend for that 3D effect!

TIP! Customize your own lip plumping shade combo. Use a light nude lipstick and wear through the center of any high-impact lip color to pastelize and give fullness. Try it!

STEP 8

Keep the rest of your makeup simple. I will not say wear *nothing* with a dark lip – that goes against my religion. We all need a little love on our skin and eyes to look and feel good, but keep your look simple and chic.

Skin should be as flawless as possible; a little glow in the skin will take the gothic edge off a dark lip. Golden, ocher-toned bronzes look incredible with a deep plum lip – take the same shadow over the eyes and to warm up your cheeks. A lashing of mascara with brushed up brows and woolah!

POWER OF THE POUT

STEP 9

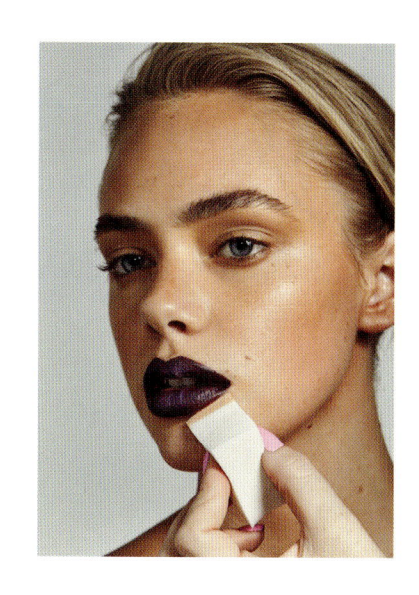

Use the flat edges of the pencil to softly trace over the edge of the lip. This will make the lips appear larger and it will stop the dark lipstick from wearing you! You can also use that flat sponge to clean up the skin around the lip with a skin-toned powder.

TIP! Don't forget to check your teeth! Why oh why are we punished by the universe with lipstick on our teeth, only when we are talking to someone new or important? Gah!

Bend your index finger, and pop your knuckle in between your lips to catch any excess lip product that would have been devastating later on!

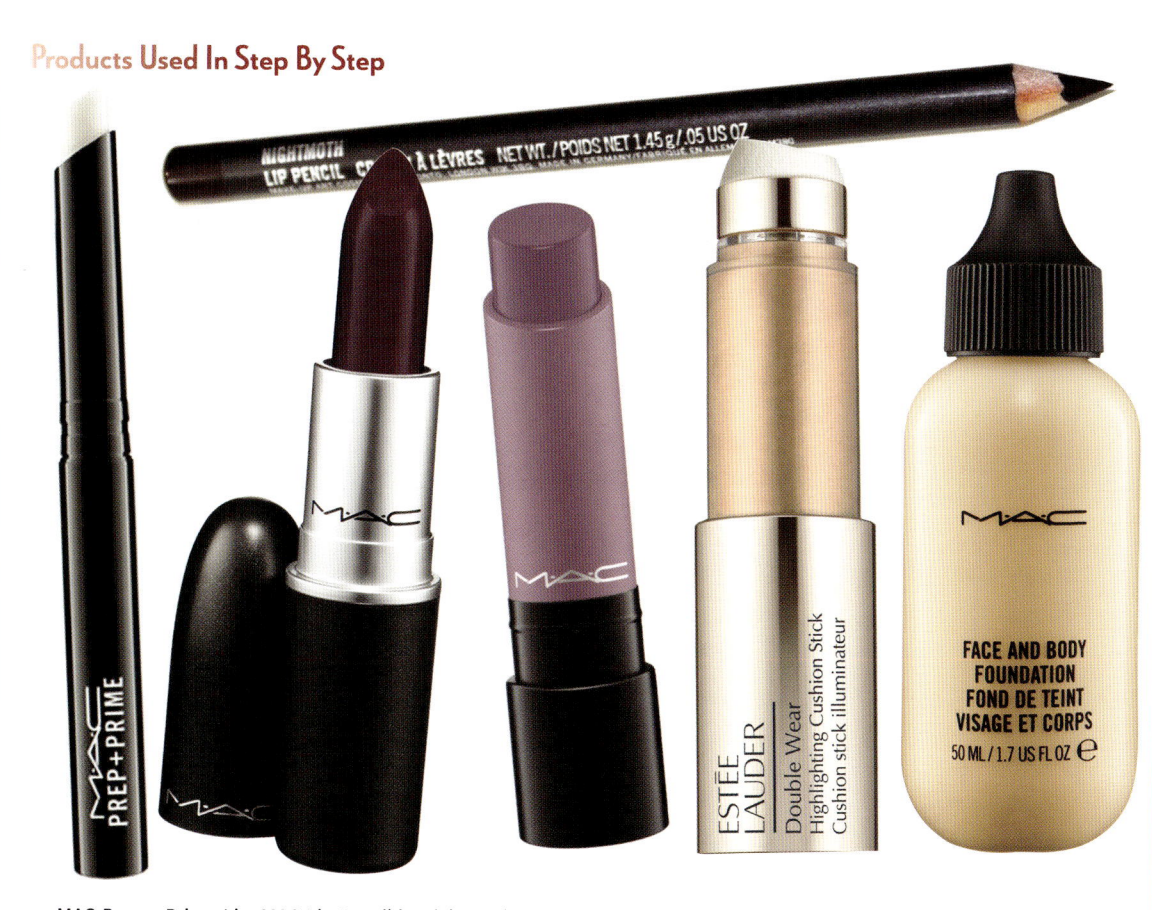

Products Used In Step By Step

MAC Prep + Prime Lip, MAC Lip Pencil in Nightmoth, MAC Lipstick in Cyber (dark lipstick), MAC Liptensity Lipstick in Galaxy Grey (lighter lipstick), Estée Lauder Highlighting Cushion Stick in Bronze Glow, MAC Face and Body Foundation

PHOEBE O FROM CHADWICK MODELS

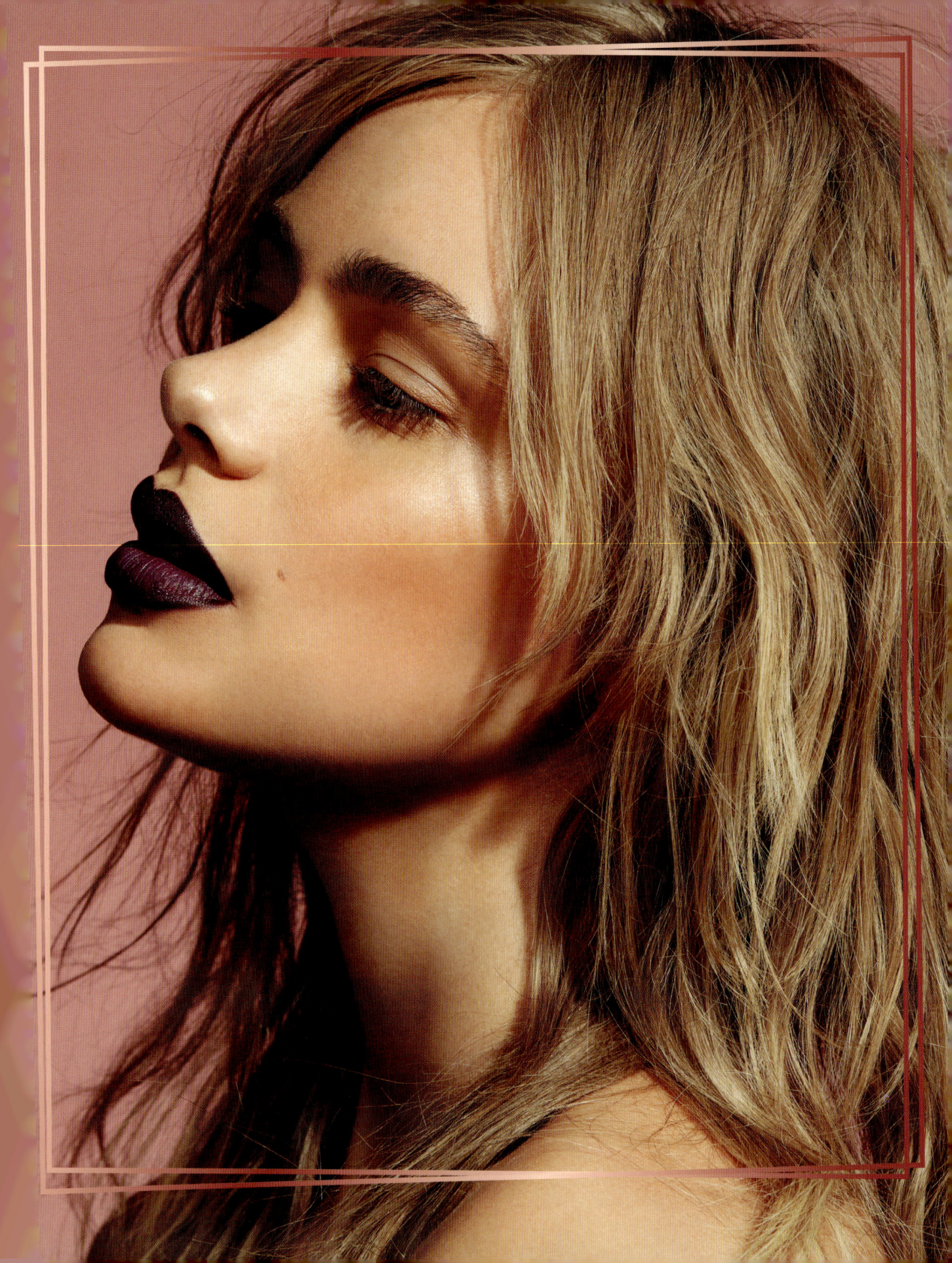

METALLIC LIPS

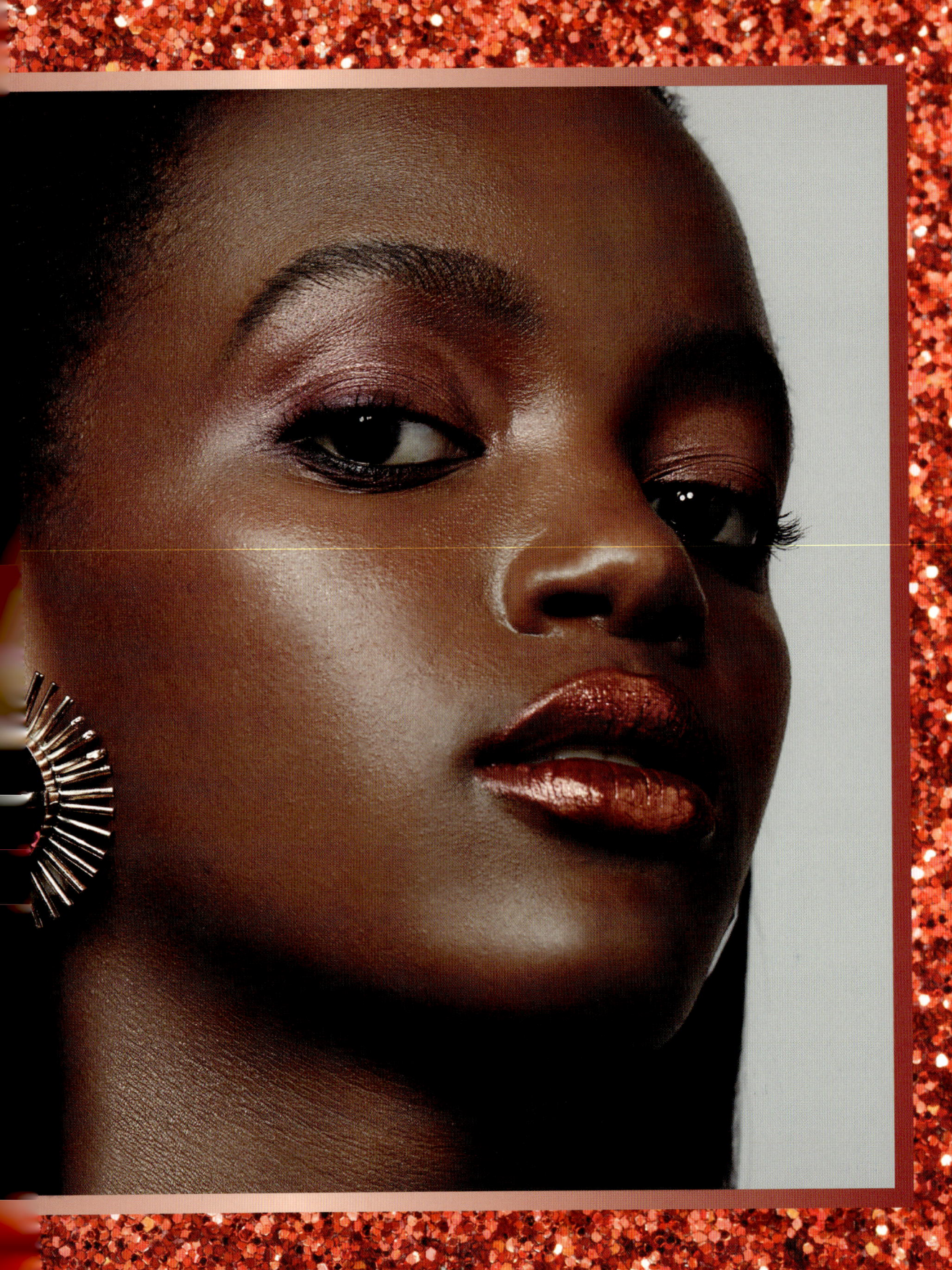

POWER OF THE POUT

STEP 1

Hello our old mate lip primer! You know what to do by now!

STEP 2

Let's lay down the base. I've chosen a super long wearing matte liquid lip as I want max hold for my metallic finish! Use the applicator that comes with these lip colors instead of a brush. It will mean you can get the perfect shape faster and without the edges.

> *TIP!* You can use your favorite lipstick as the base, regardless of whether it is cream, matte or glossy.

STEP 3

Draw a matching lip liner, or even one shade darker, around the edges of the lip. Pencils are far easier to use than a brush when defining the edges of your lip. It will provide you with so much more control over the product.

STEP 4

Blend your chosen metallic shadow/s over the lips with a flat brush, starting from the center. Spritz your brush with Fix+ to amp up that metallic vibe.

Nailing a good metallic look comes down to balance. If less is more for you, try a pressed metallic shadow to reduce the fallout of color. If this part gets your engine going, try a loose powder metallic pigment, they tend to give a richer, bolder color payoff!

> *TIP!* Flat brush I say! This guy will make your life easer; it will give your lips clean edges and denser color!

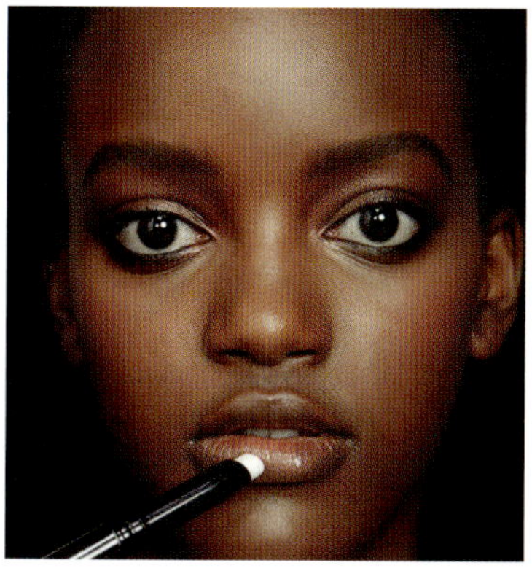

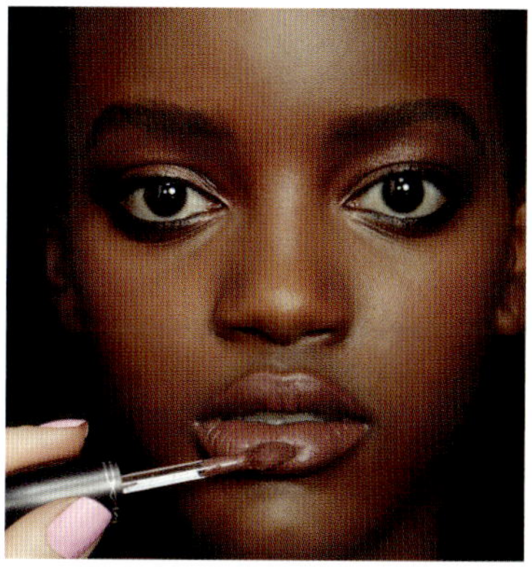

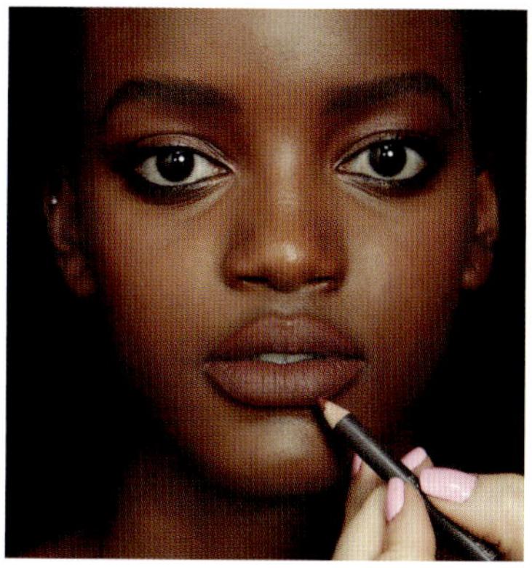

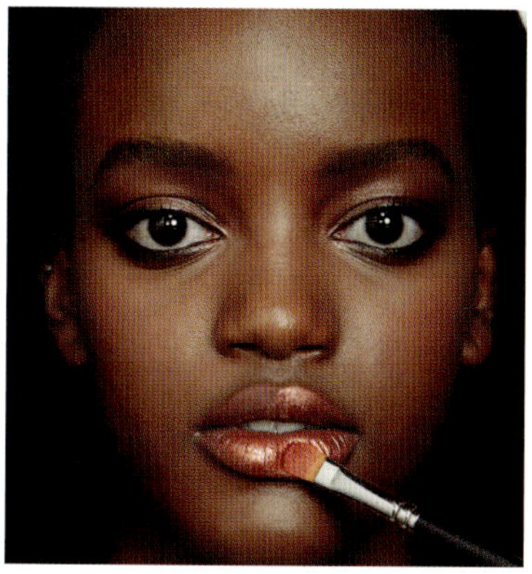

STEP 5

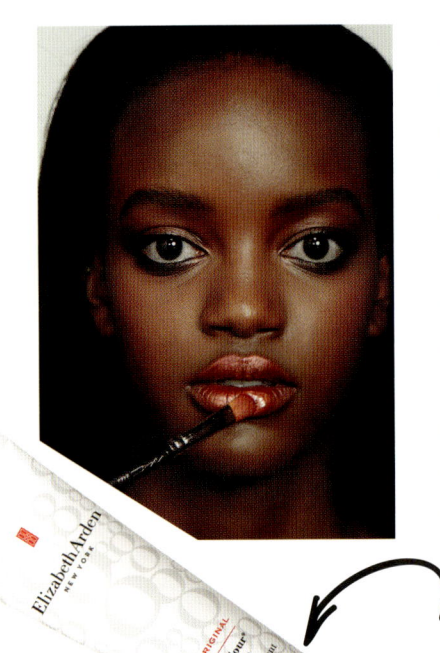

For next level reflection, apply a gloss over the lips. Paint it on through the center of the lips and spread outwards. You don't need to pile it on at the edges unless you want to have it moving down to your chin within the hour! For supreme shine, you cannot go past MAC Clear Lip Glass – serious shine that won't move.

Let this metallic lip stand out by taking the rest of your makeup down a notch. Try subtle hints of a similar shade on the eyes and cheeks, with defined features to enhance the pout, not compete with it.

TIP! For those of you with long hair that you would prefer didn't get tangled up in this metallic moment, try a non-sticky gloss or clear shiny lip conditioner to finish it off!

Elizabeth Arden Eight Hour Cream Skin Protectant

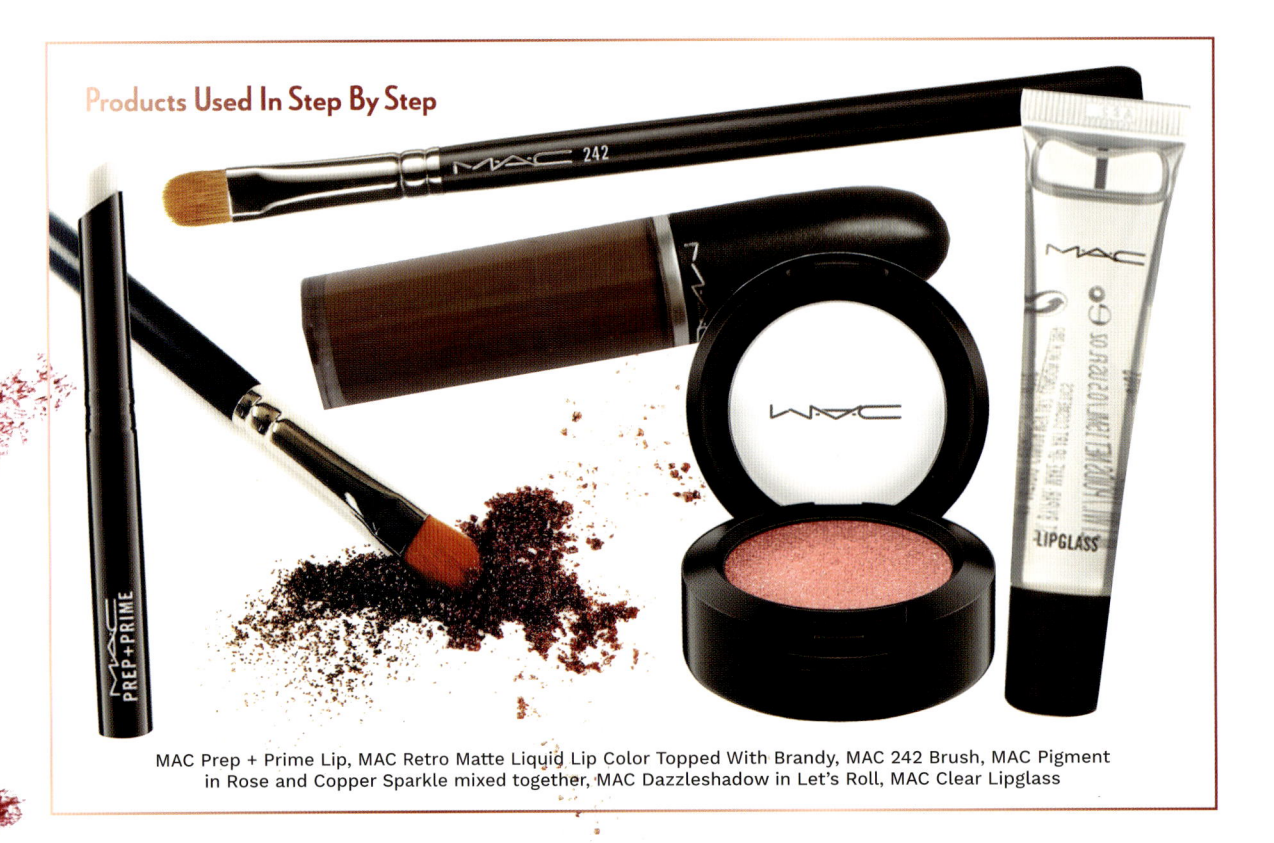

Products Used In Step By Step

MAC Prep + Prime Lip, MAC Retro Matte Liquid Lip Color Topped With Brandy, MAC 242 Brush, MAC Pigment in Rose and Copper Sparkle mixed together, MAC Dazzleshadow in Let's Roll, MAC Clear Lipglass

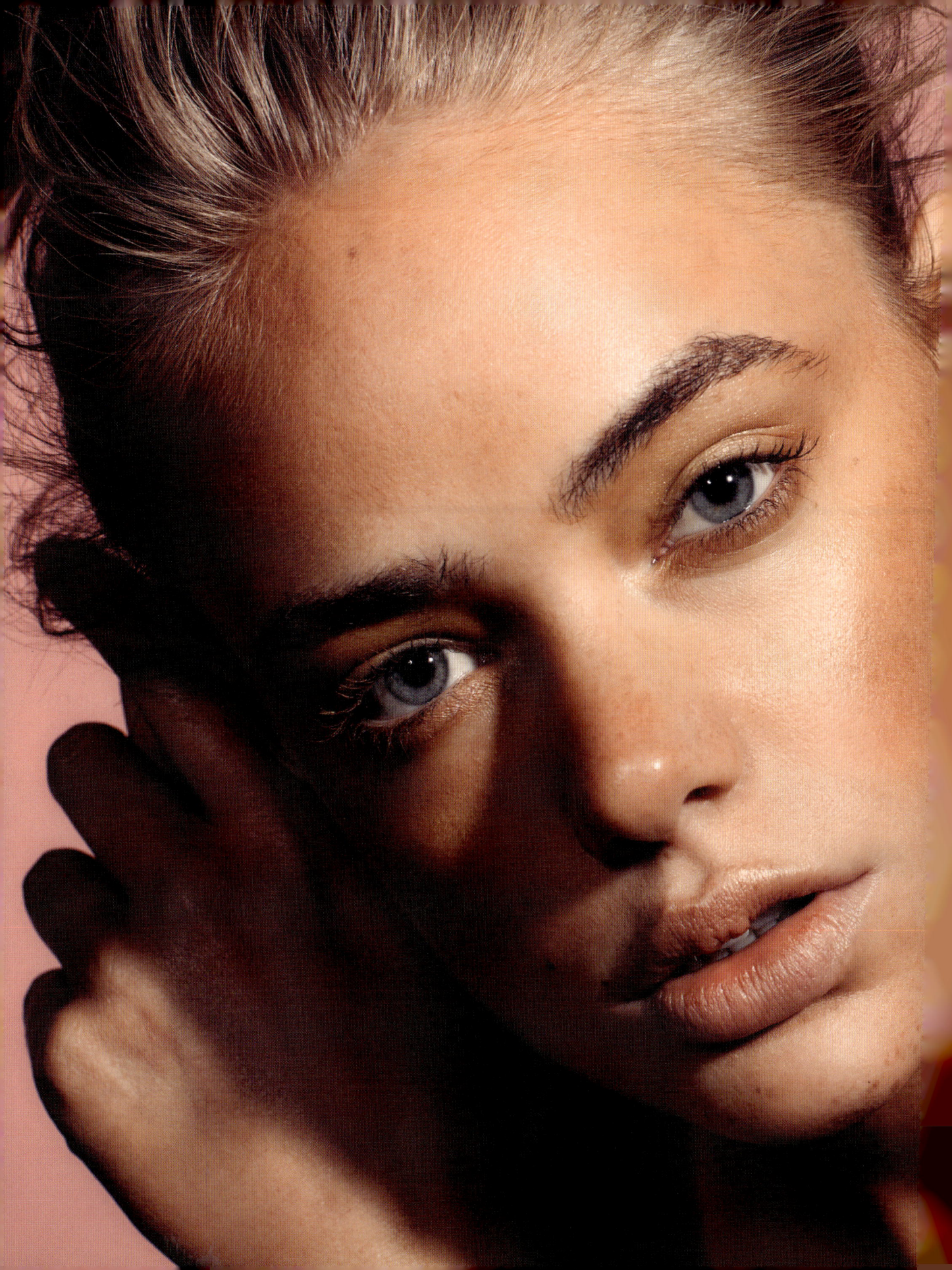

Cheeks on fleek

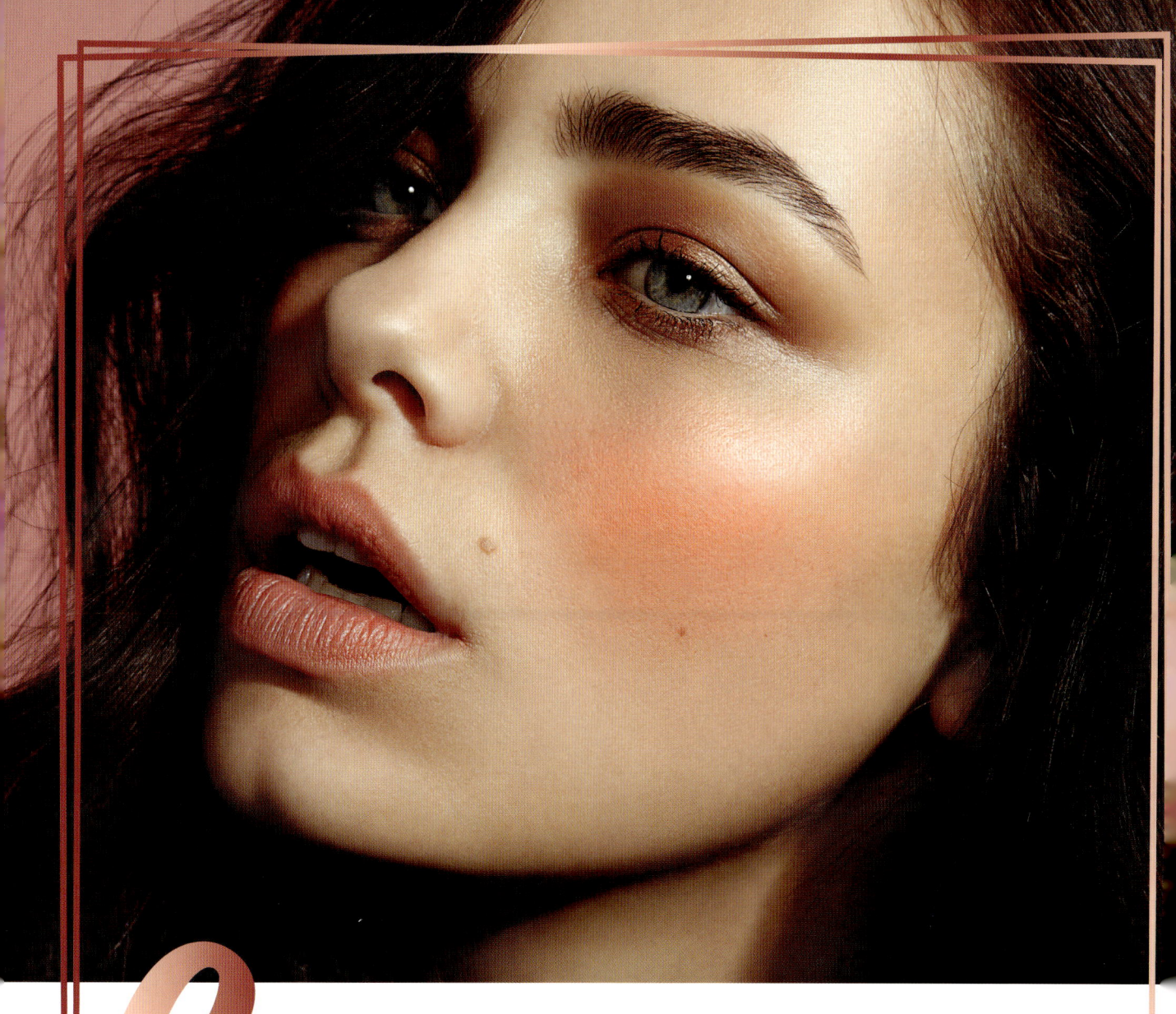

Cheeks take up the most real estate on your face, so getting them on point should be a priority. When most people think of makeup on cheeks, they conjure up images of the Renaissance or Shirley Temple looking flushed with blush. I like to imagine Native American peoples, warriors both men and women, their face paint a part of their armor, a deep red smeared across their cheeks, the color of war.

Makeup for me isn't about covering up, it is a piece of my armor and lets me and the rest of the world know I am ready for whatever the day wants to throw at me. What I wear on my cheeks will sum up whatever side of my personality I want to bring out to play. The differences between bronzing and wearing blush go far beyond the product you use. As they say, it's not just about what you've got, it's what you do with it that counts. So let's get into cheeks, like a grandma to a baby at Christmas!

Bronzing

Bronzer is a great staple in anyone's makeup bag, from novice to pro. Applying a bronzer to the face is all about shaping the face through enhancing a healthy skin tone. Cream or powder bronzing techniques can give you the color without the sun exposure or awaken tired or pale wintery skin to create a fabulous healthy illusion.

While bronzer can be the magic wand of your makeup bag, if used incorrectly you can end up looking orange and dirty and perhaps resembling an Oompa Loompa from *Charlie and the Chocolate Factory*.

Here are my favorite techniques to master the tanned glow.

Blush

Ah, blush – the 'easy' part of your makeup routine. **Insert laughter here**

Ever rushed through your makeup, loved what you created while at home in your mirror, then you have looked at yourself later in much more natural and unforgiving light and thought, why do I look like the evil guy from the movie *Saw*? No? Just me? Well I can bet that not everyone out there gets it right every time!

People talk about the dark lip or flicked liner being the trickiest parts of makeup, but sometimes the makeup moments that seem the simplest can be the toughest to master. Your blush can be a beautiful subtle complement to the rest of your makeup or alternatively a full-blown statement, it will just come down to your color choice and how much product you chose to apply. But one thing I know for sure is that once you get it right, blush is far easier to apply in the back of a taxi than a red lip!

Blush has gone far beyond that tinted powder that was thrown on just before you headed out. Good cheeks are sleek and stand on their own, looking matte or looking creamy, through a range of techniques, using powders, creams and even one of my favorites – lipstick!

CREAM BLUSH

Cream does not have to be scary! No way! It is actually my preferred product of choice when I am doing makeup on my clients as I can blend it smoothly into the skin in a natural way or I can build it up to make it pop. Like a good coffee bean, it's all in the blend.

POWDER BLUSH

I love the look of blush high on the cheekbones for an instant face lift. If you don't love a blush up high, these simple techniques can be used for any color and any positioning, so move the color around your face until you find that sweet spot to flush!

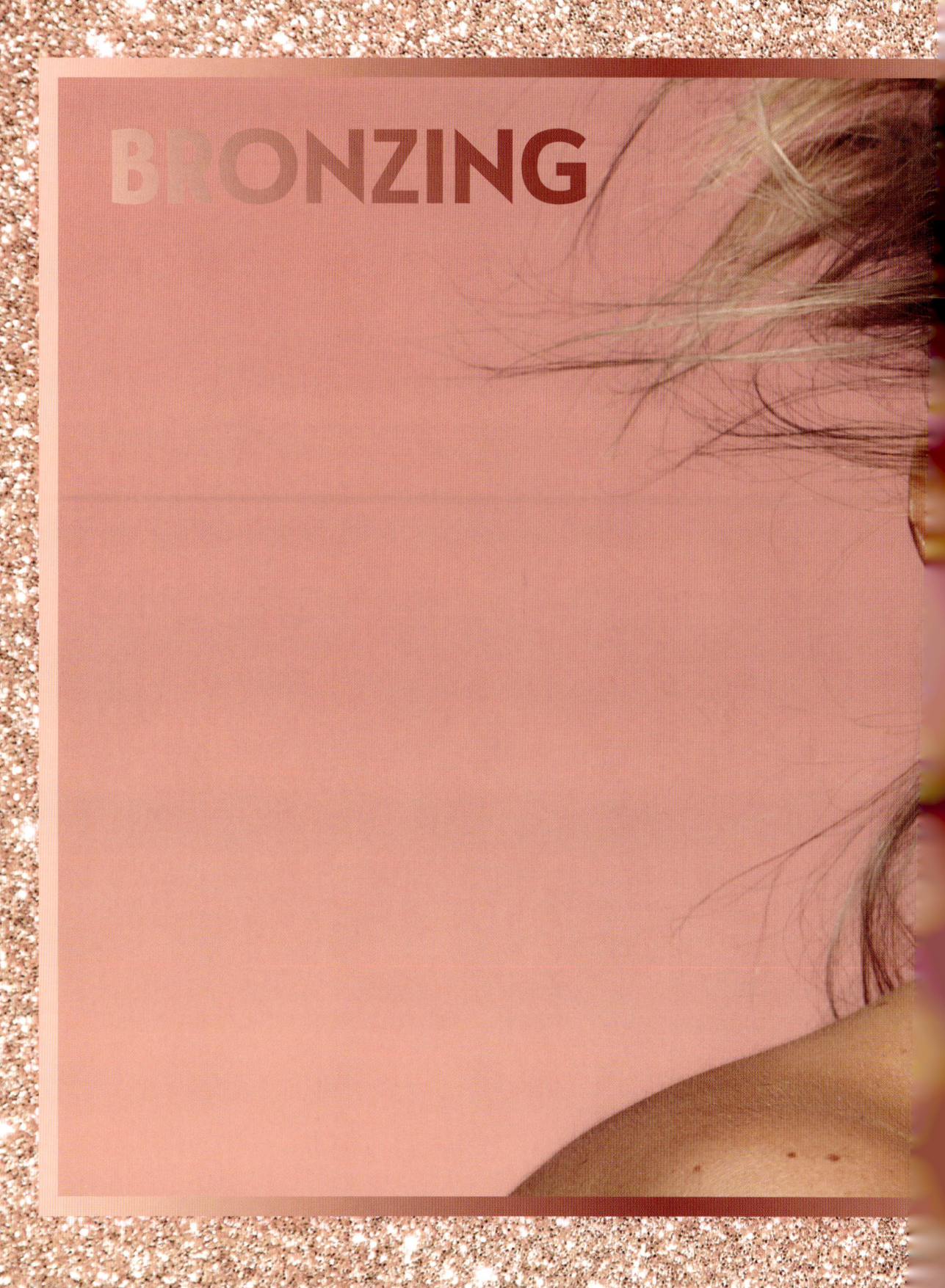

BRONZING

CHEEKS ON FLEEK

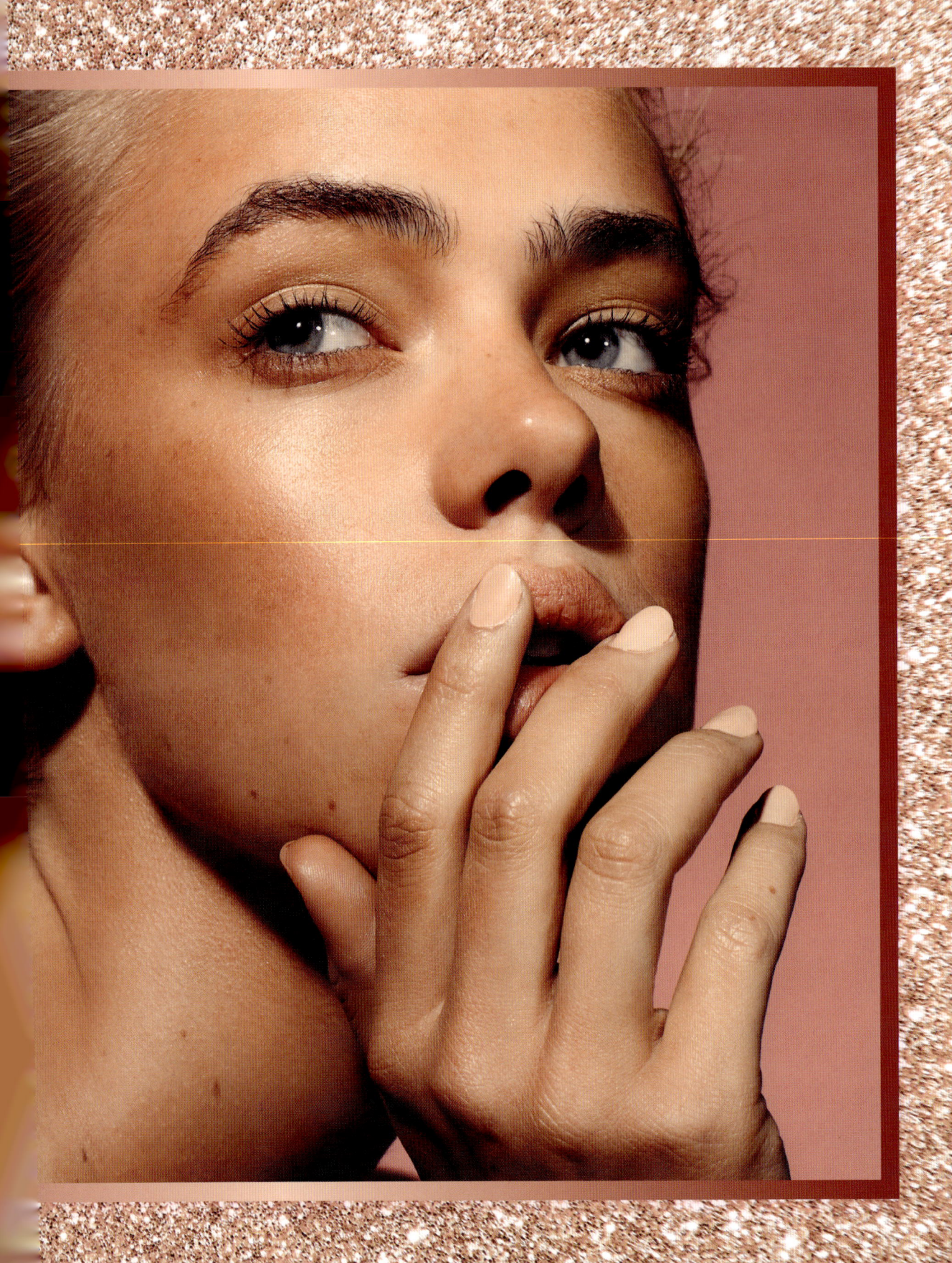

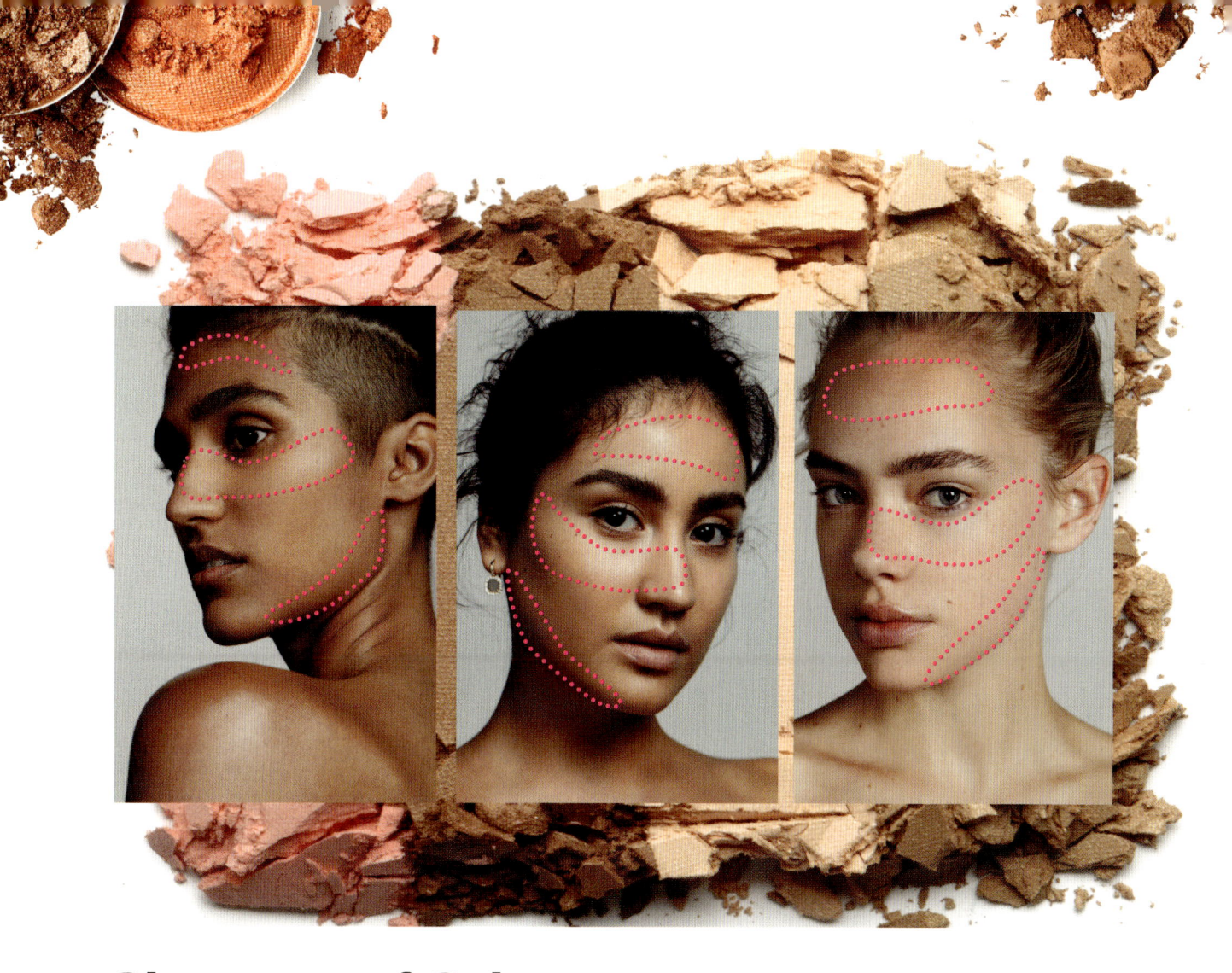

Placement of Color

Whether you are using a cream or a powder bronzer, or adding a little or a lot of color to your skin, the placement of product will stay the same. First think about *why* you are applying bronzer. The aim is to warm up the skin and fake that sun-drenched holiday glow – no matter what time of year it is.

You want to add the color your skin would naturally tan if you were out in the sun, where the sun would hit your skin. As opposed to contouring, which is designed to carve the face with shadows by sitting underneath the bone structure, bronzer should tint the tops of your facial structure, décolletage, and across the front of the face.

You want to glaze the skin with color starting with a giant '3' shape across the forehead, along the tops of the cheekbones and following the jawline. Then blend excess across the bridge of the nose, down the neck. Don't forget the collarbones and shoulders for a unified, flawless look. Hit that bone structure!

Color Choice

You want to choose a color that is one or two shades deeper or richer than your skin color or foundation color – a shade that will mimic the look of a natural tan on your skin. This color will change from person to person that is for sure!

Dark isn't always better. Too many times have I seen someone go for the 'I just got back from Mykonos tan', but come out looking like they have been looking through a trash can. A good starting point for color tones is that for fair skin tones warm, nude camel tones, with a hint of peach or rose, are great. For medium skin tones golden toffee tans work beautifully. Rusty, brick-toned brown shades mimic the suntan well on deeper skin.

> **TIP!**
> Before buying anything try the product on your skin and check it out under natural light to make sure it is the one for you. I do suggest looking in a full-length mirror with your shoulders exposed to check the color. Pop a shoulder like you would for a selfie and assess if the color on your face matches!

Tools

Soft and fluffy are the names of the game. The more dense or small the brush the more product you will add, resulting in uneven skin. A soft brush will ensure you have a seamless edge to your blending.

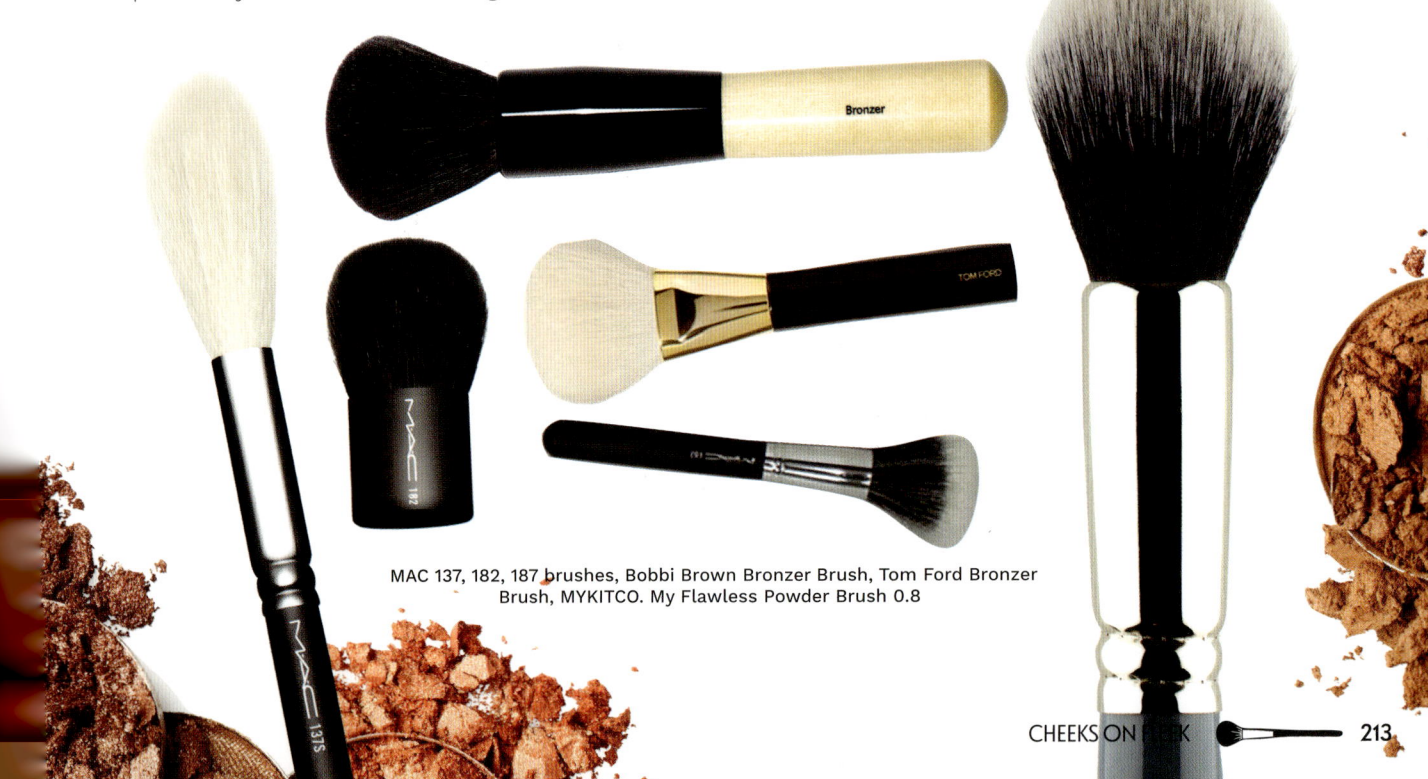

MAC 137, 182, 187 brushes, Bobbi Brown Bronzer Brush, Tom Ford Bronzer Brush, MYKITCO. My Flawless Powder Brush 0.8

Blend

This deserves its own moment, because... patchy face. Take a moment to check all angles of your application in good light and blend. Then when you have finished, blend again. Trust me.

Which Texture Is the One for You?

Choose a *cream bronzer* if you have dull or dry skin and want to give it life. Also for if you wish to go hard with the color and want zero danger of powder fallout mess.

Choose a *shimmer cream bronzer* if you want beaming skin. Sheeny, shiny and easy to blend – go! Reconsider if you have overly textured or blemished skin as shimmer will just enhance this.

Choose a *matte bronze powder* if you have oily or problem skin. Matte powder will set and stay!

Choose a *shimmer bronze powder* if you want all that the glow without the slip; perfect for oily skin shimmer lovers and people (like me!) who have a fear of creams on their skin.

Choose a *bronzer stick* if you want the color and the control. There is something so familiar about holding a bronzing stick like a texta as a child – just don't draw on your face like you drew on your parents' walls!

Choose a *tanning gel or cream* if you want to complete the most accurate tanning little white lie. Sheer in color and virtually no coverage, the gel won't mask your skin so you will not look like you are wearing anything at all yet magically you look fresh, healthy and fabulous. Oh, and lasting a few days through washing faces and showers is also a bonus.

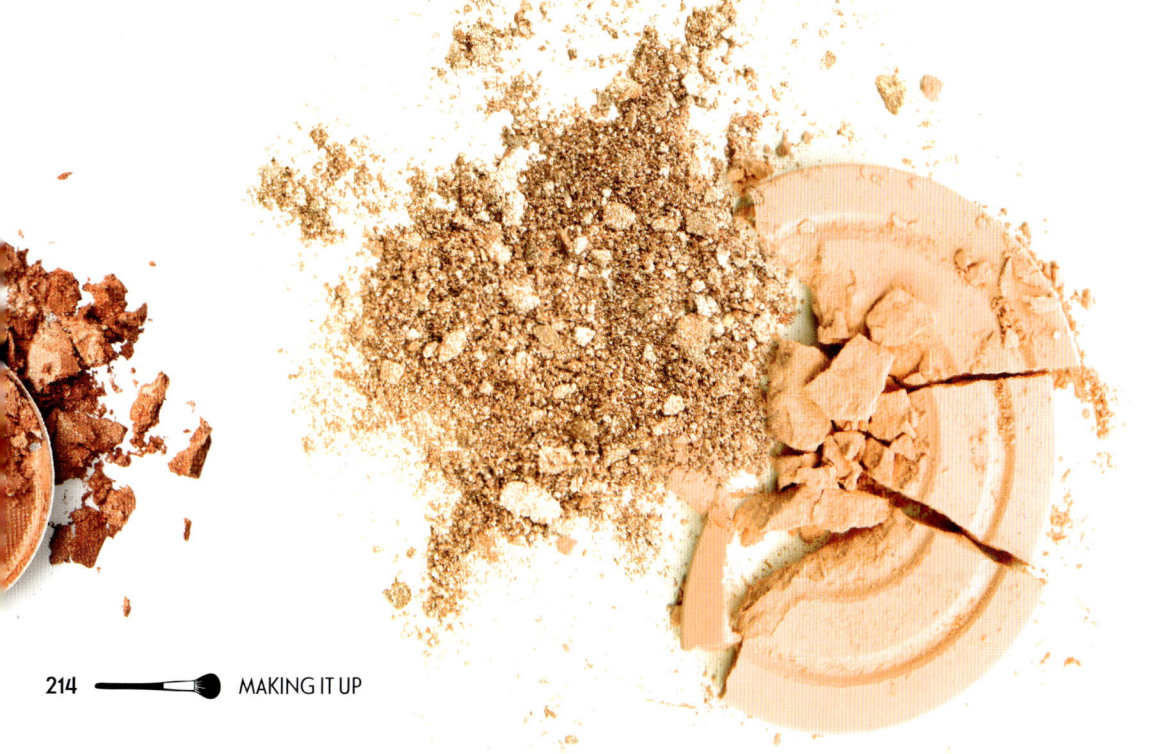

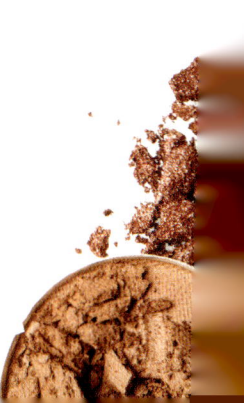

CHEEKS ON FLEEK   215

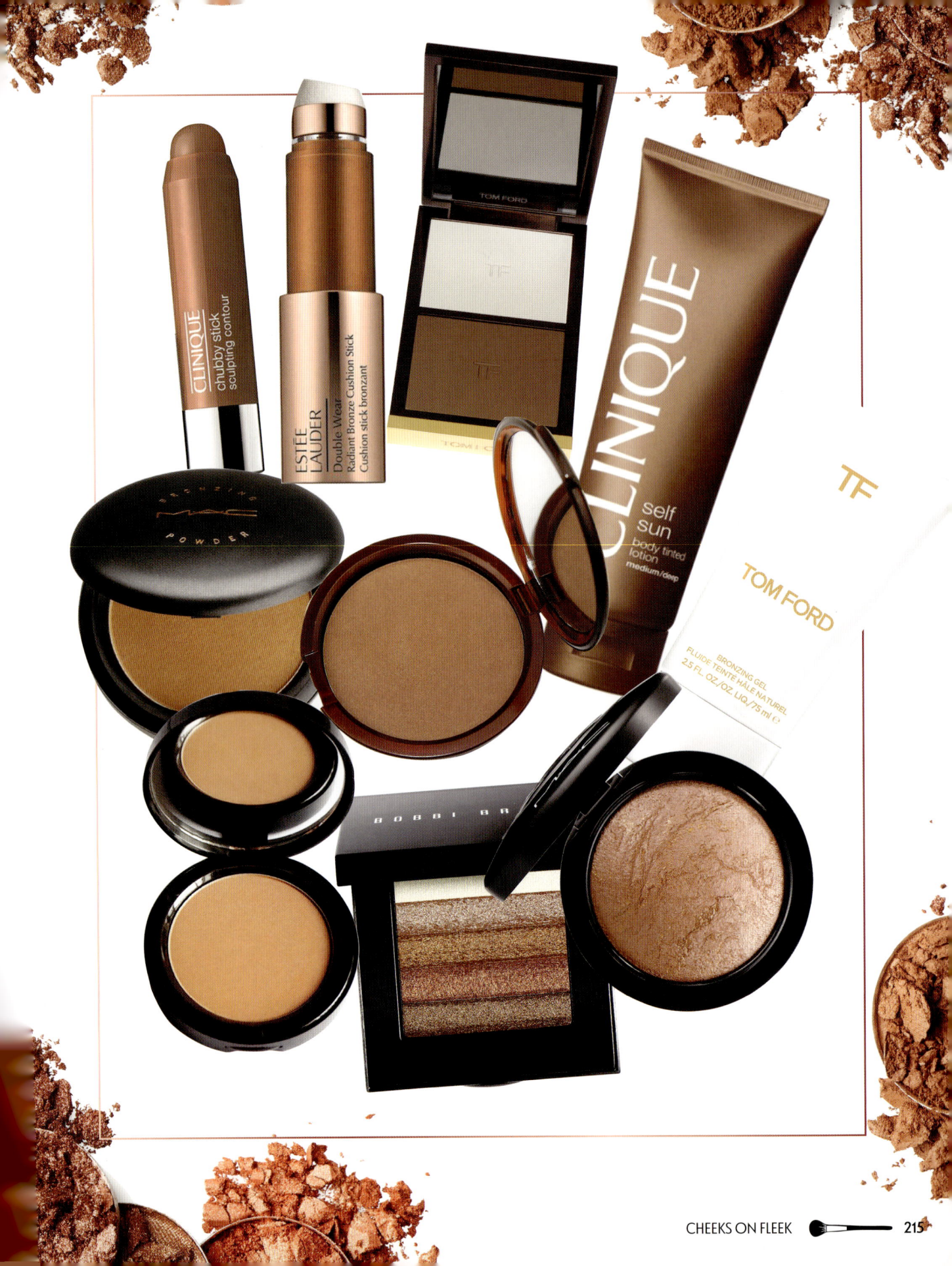

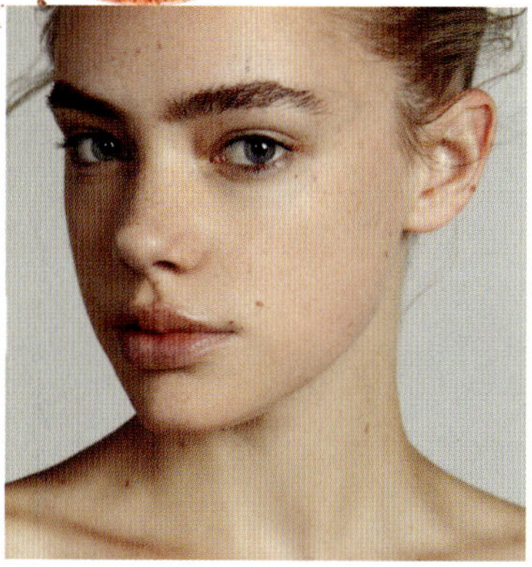

STEP 1

Start with a finished and powdered foundation base as you are taking bronzer everywhere and if the skin is wet the color will grab! This is especially important for cream bronzer. The light coat of powder underneath will help hold the cream bronzer in place once blended.

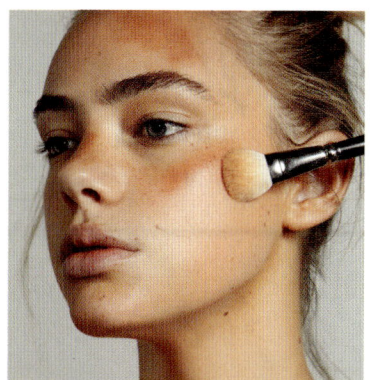

STEP 2

Tap the cream color onto the tops of cheekbones, forehead, across the nose, along the jawline and blend away.

Remember when you are blending the color, you are *not* contouring! Tint the skin where the sun would hit: on the tops of the cheekbones, brow bone, bridge of the nose and décolletage. Take the color down the neck and across the collarbones. The underside of the neck is always paler than your face so you may need some extra product here. Hitting the shoulders and décolletage will ensure your next selfie is flawless. Thank me later!

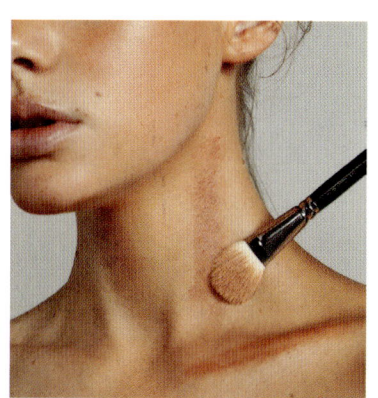

STEP 3

Finish with highlighter to polish. Use a subtle shiny powder or cream that will bring your whole look together and amplify that glow.

> *TIP!* Want a cream bronzer multitasker? The answer may already be lying in your makeup bag. Try a warm brown, or dark nude lipstick! Super easy to swipe and blend, a lipstick also generally has good strong color pigment, so work quickly and it will stay in place once applied.

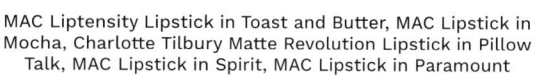

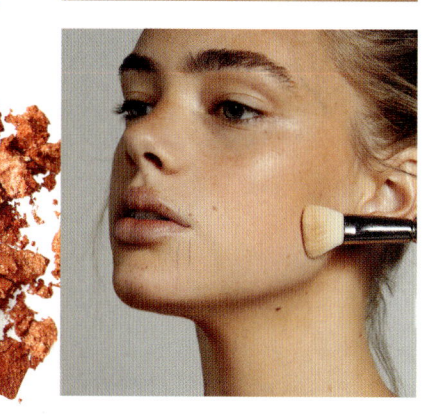

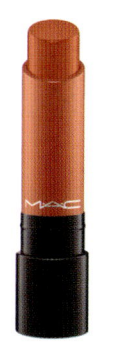

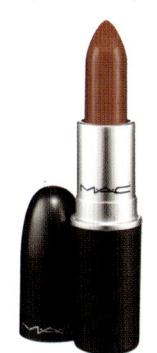

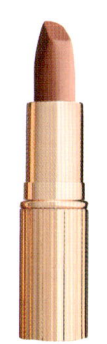

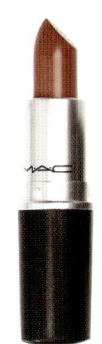

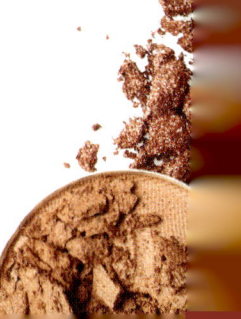

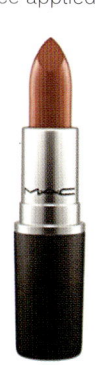

MAC Liptensity Lipstick in Toast and Butter, MAC Lipstick in Mocha, Charlotte Tilbury Matte Revolution Lipstick in Pillow Talk, MAC Lipstick in Spirit, MAC Lipstick in Paramount

MAKING IT UP

STEP 4

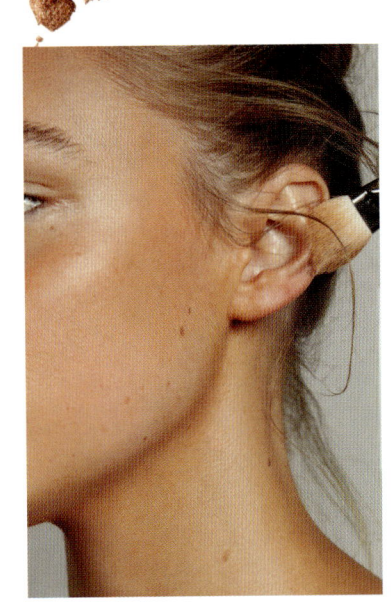

Don't forget the ears! Bronze and highlight those bad boys to finish off your look so your red ears don't jump out in photos.

TIP! I hardly ever say less is more, except for bronzing! Build the color slowly rather than going too hard too quick. It is always easier to add more than it is to take it away.

TIP! Layer a powder bronzer over your cream bronzer for maximum tan with that extra hold. The different textures will set together and last the distance. Be sure to go in with a giant fluffy brush for the powder application to stop it becoming too dark or heavy.

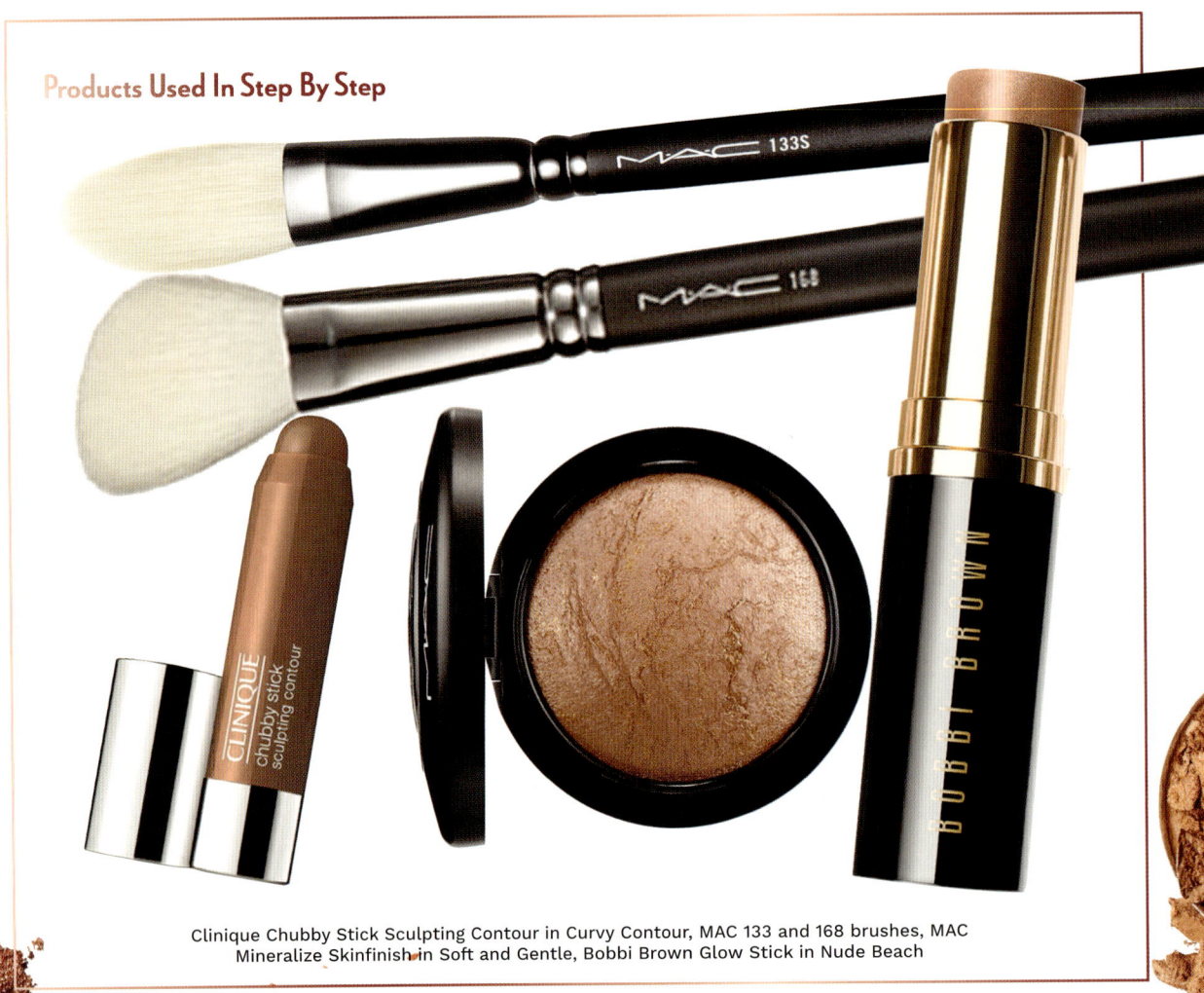

Products Used In Step By Step

Clinique Chubby Stick Sculpting Contour in Curvy Contour, MAC 133 and 168 brushes, MAC Mineralize Skinfinish in Soft and Gentle, Bobbi Brown Glow Stick in Nude Beach

PHOEBE O FROM CHADWICK MODELS

CHEEKS ON FLEEK

CREAM BLUSH

CHEEKS ON FLEEK   219

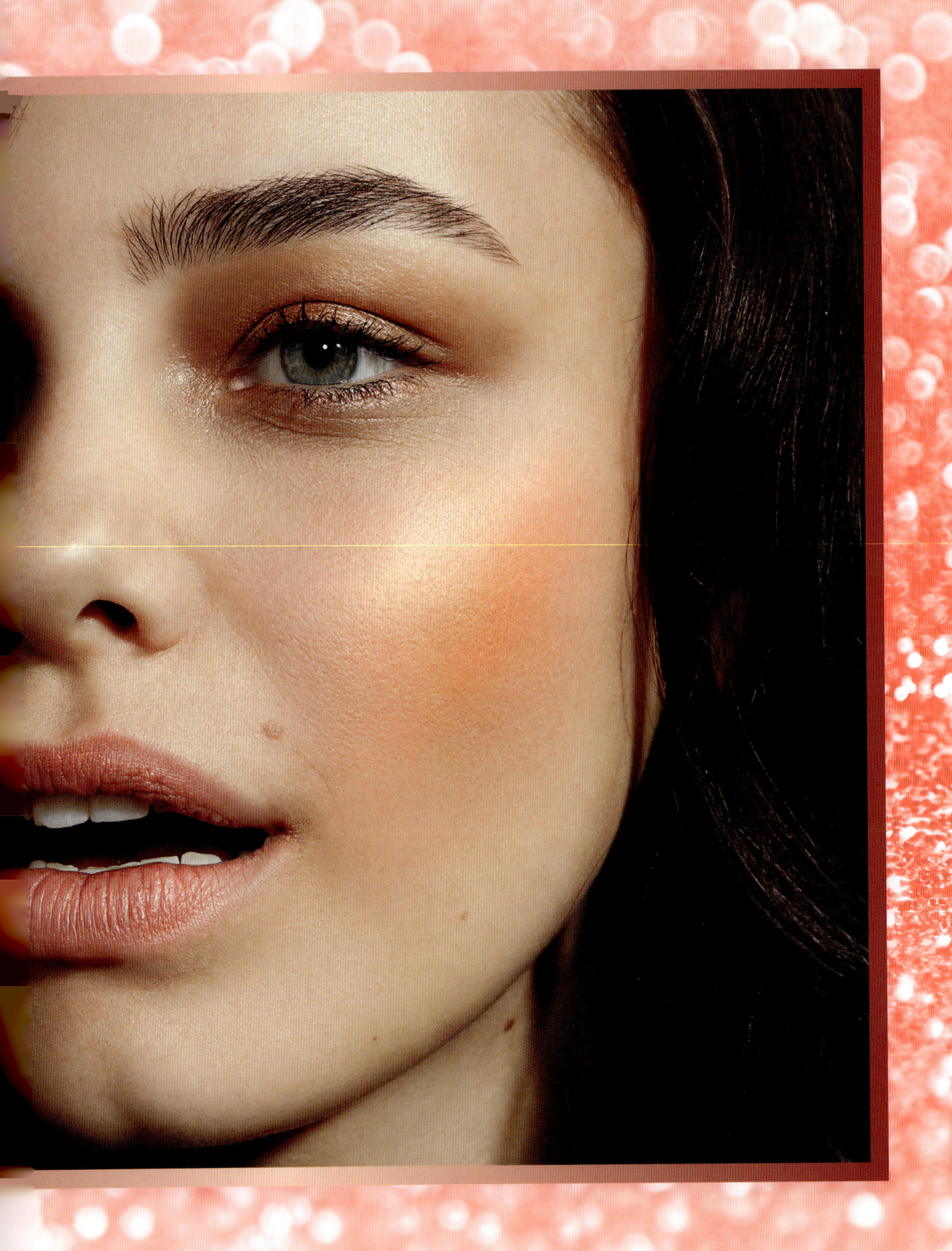

STEP 1

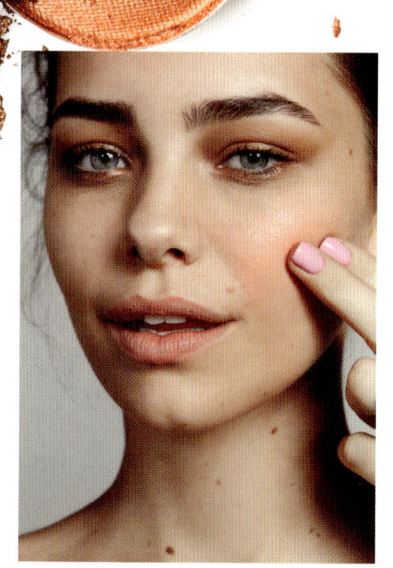

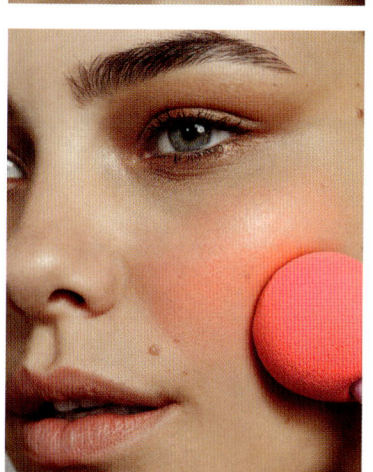

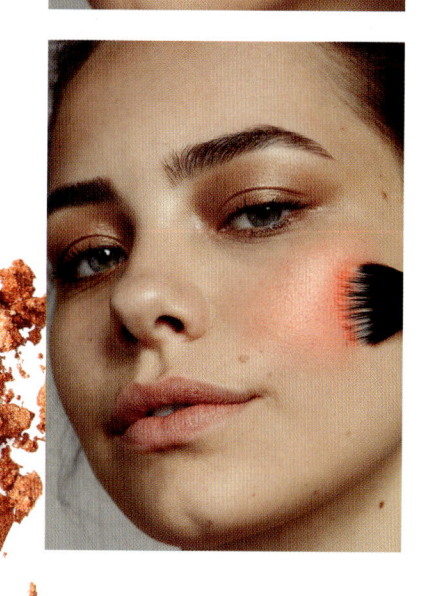

On finished and softly powdered skin, dab the cream color onto the apples of the cheeks. Now while I like to swipe it directly from the lipstick tube, you may prefer to dab the color on with your fingertips. Either way, don't worry about perfection yet – we are going to blend!

> **TIP!** If you are using a matte or highly pigmented lipstick, dab and blend swiftly! Otherwise the lipstick may set quickly, get patchy and have you looking like a rodeo clown.

STEP 2

Blend and layer the color using a round sponge to avoid streaks or edges. If you prefer to blend with your fingertips, make sure to look in the mirror with your face at different angles while applying. Different light sources will show the unblended color and moving your face around will help you escape fingerprints of color!

STEP 3

Once you have built up to the color you are happy with, feel free to stop right there for a fresh flush on your cheeks. If you want a slightly bolder look and stronger hold apply a powder blush over the top. Use a small fluffy brush for an easy blend. Remember you are doubling the formulas not doubling the color. Use each product sparingly to start with and remember you can always add more but it is hard to take it away!

> **TIP!** Customize your blush color by switching up the cream and powder combinations. Try a candy pink cream with a coral powder, or a rosy cream with a mauve powder – mix and match!

> **TIP!** I love using the same lipstick I am wearing on my lips as the base for my cream blush look. Not only is it fewer products you need to carry with you but it can really unify your overall beauty look.

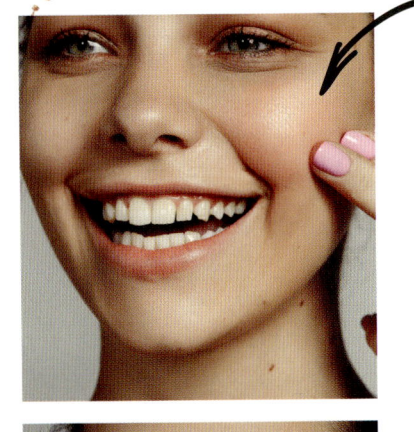

TIP! Give yourself a little smile in the mirror to show you where to dab your color on. Make sure to hit the top of your cheekbones with color rather than the underside when you are doing this so the color does not end up on your jawline when you relax your face!

STEP 4

For extra staying power layer a powder and cream and then repeat a few times. The layering of the textures will hold everything where you want it for longer. Please don't use a colored powder for this unless you are going for an embarrassed circus performer look. Try a translucent or sheer skin tone powder instead.

Finally don't forget to set. Spritz your Fix+ spray on top lightly and pat on with the palms of your hands to set.

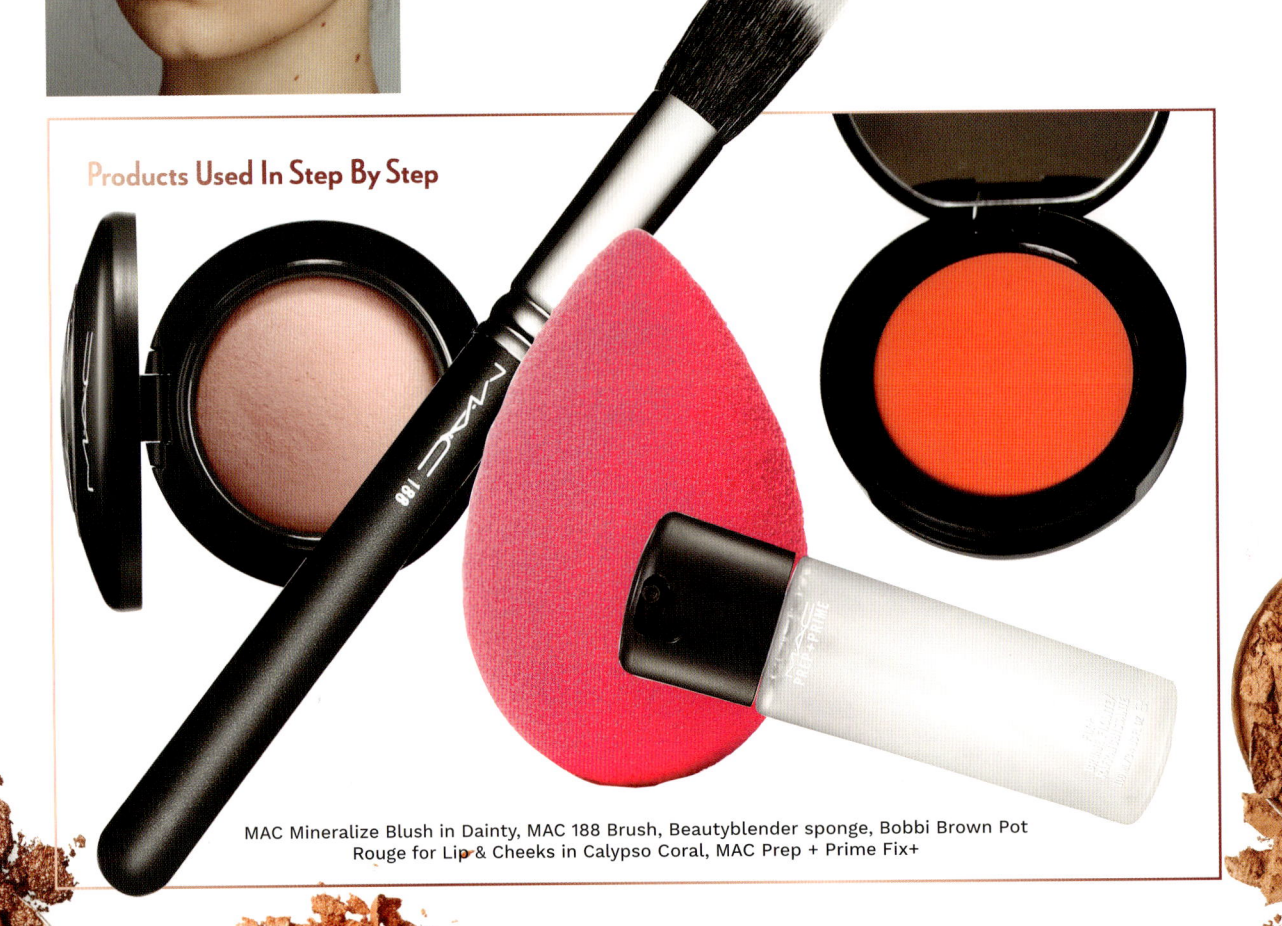

Products Used In Step By Step

MAC Mineralize Blush in Dainty, MAC 188 Brush, Beautyblender sponge, Bobbi Brown Pot Rouge for Lip & Cheeks in Calypso Coral, MAC Prep + Prime Fix+

ASHLEE FROM BELLA MODEL MANAGEMENT

CHEEKS ON FLEEK

POWDER BLUSH

CHEEKS ON FLEEK

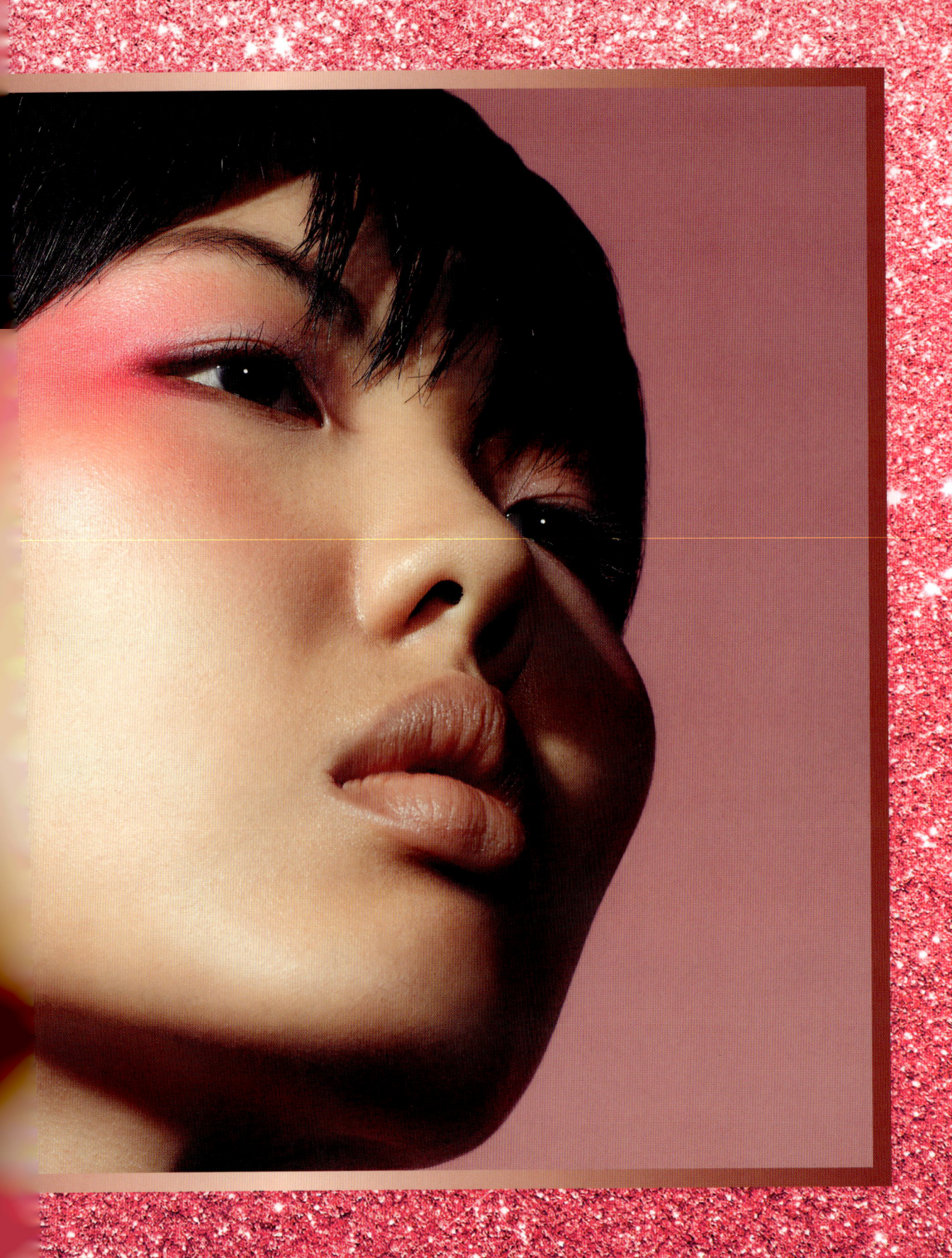

STEP 1

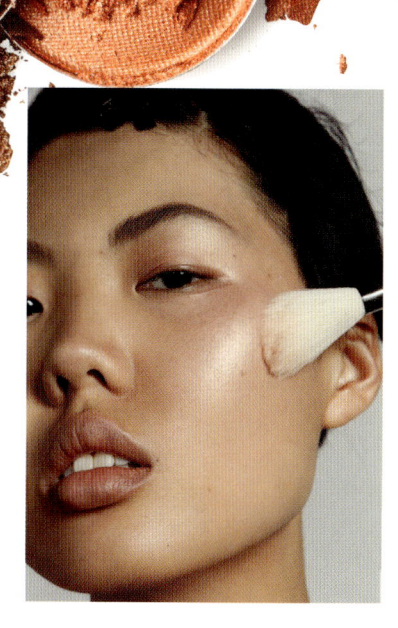

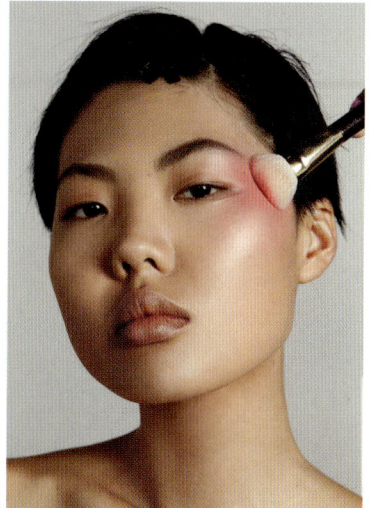

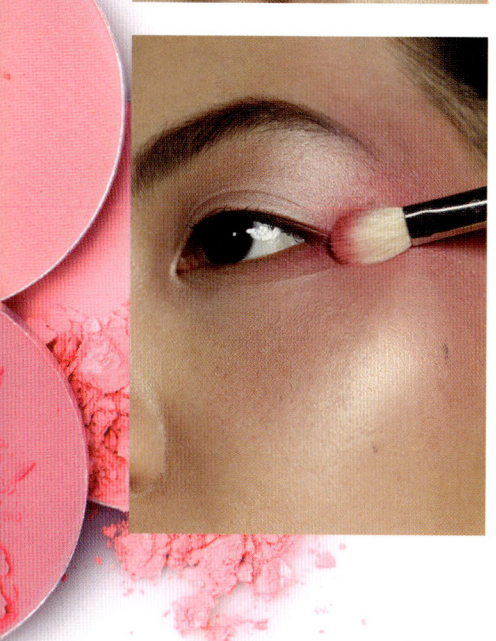

Start with polished skin and highlighting. Super important! Rosy will enhance rosy. You really need to have evened out skin tone underneath your blush application to have something for it to blend into so it looks flawless and not patchy.

If you have textured skin due to wrinkles, pimples and other fun imperfections, steer clear of using a shimmer blush as it will just highlight it, unfortunately. Stick to matte blushes applied in the same way for a more flattering look.

> **TIP!** Don't get *too* excited with your powder highlighter! Too much powder underneath will make it hard for you to build up colored powder blush on top. Just a subtle amount of highlighting is good to start.

STEP 2

Just like foundation and bronzer, blending blush is made easier with a fluffy brush. Work in circular motions from the outer corner of the eye onto the tops of the cheekbones.

Don't blend the blush too far onto the cheekbone and have it appear as though you are contouring with it – we have contour products for that

> **TIP!** I love makeup multitaskers! Blush is one of those products you can use in many ways: from cheeks, to eye shadow to lip shading. When you are in a time crunch blush can be used all over in a jiffy.

STEP 3

If you kept blending with the same brush, the color would get stronger, and also bigger. To give you more control use a smaller brush to build up the color intensity without spreading it everywhere. Tapping the powder blush color on with your fingers to enhance the color is also a great cheap option.

> **TIP!** Highlighter has the magic ability to bring your makeup pieces together in a photo. As light jumps out, it can help to disguise any edges improve the appearance of your blending. With a big soft brush, take your powder or cream highlighter over the top to refine your look.

Products Used In Step By Step

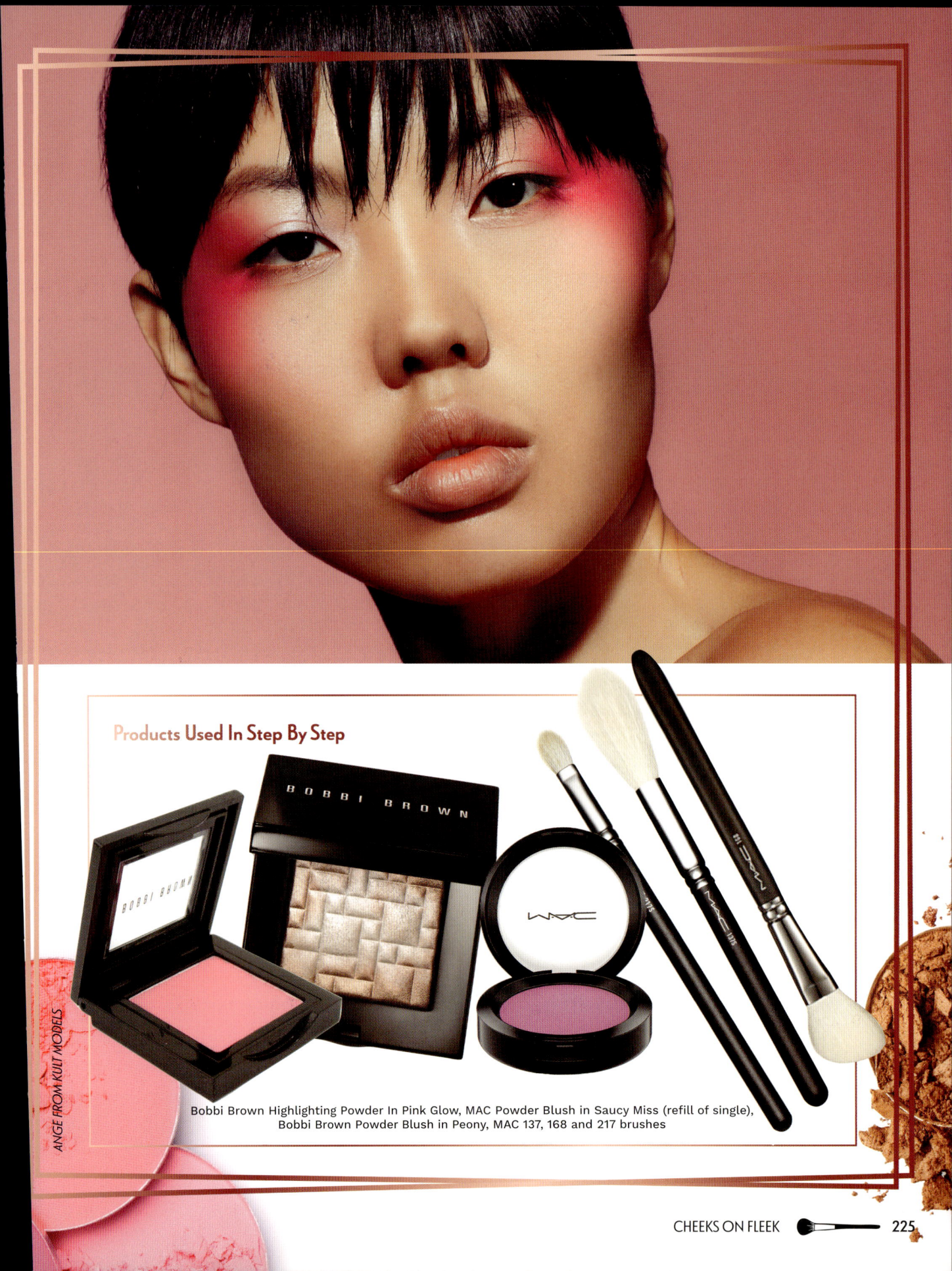

Bobbi Brown Highlighting Powder In Pink Glow, MAC Powder Blush in Saucy Miss (refill of single), Bobbi Brown Powder Blush in Peony, MAC 137, 168 and 217 brushes

ANGE FROM KULT MODELS

CHEEKS ON FLEEK

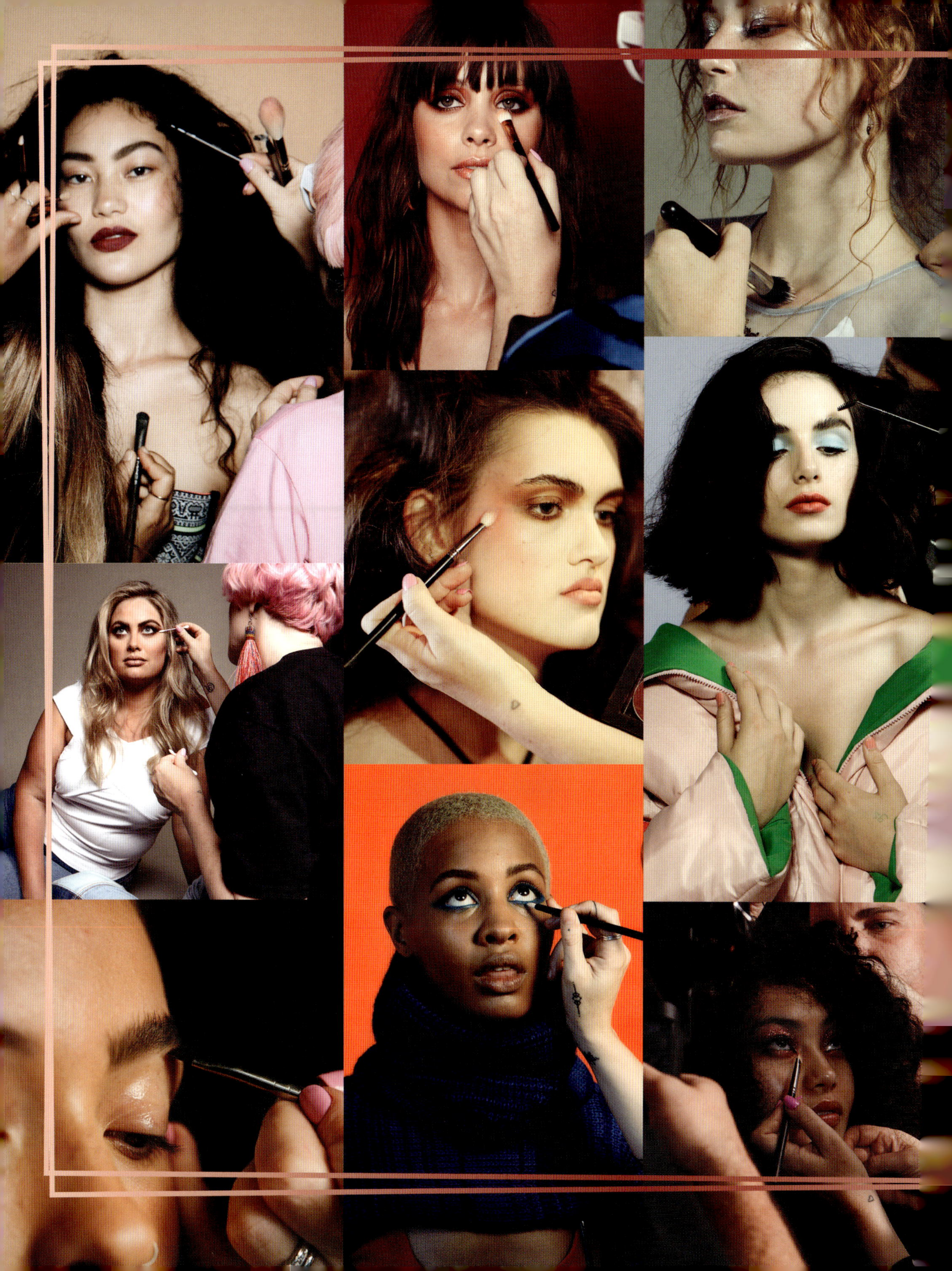

Mama didn't raise no tool

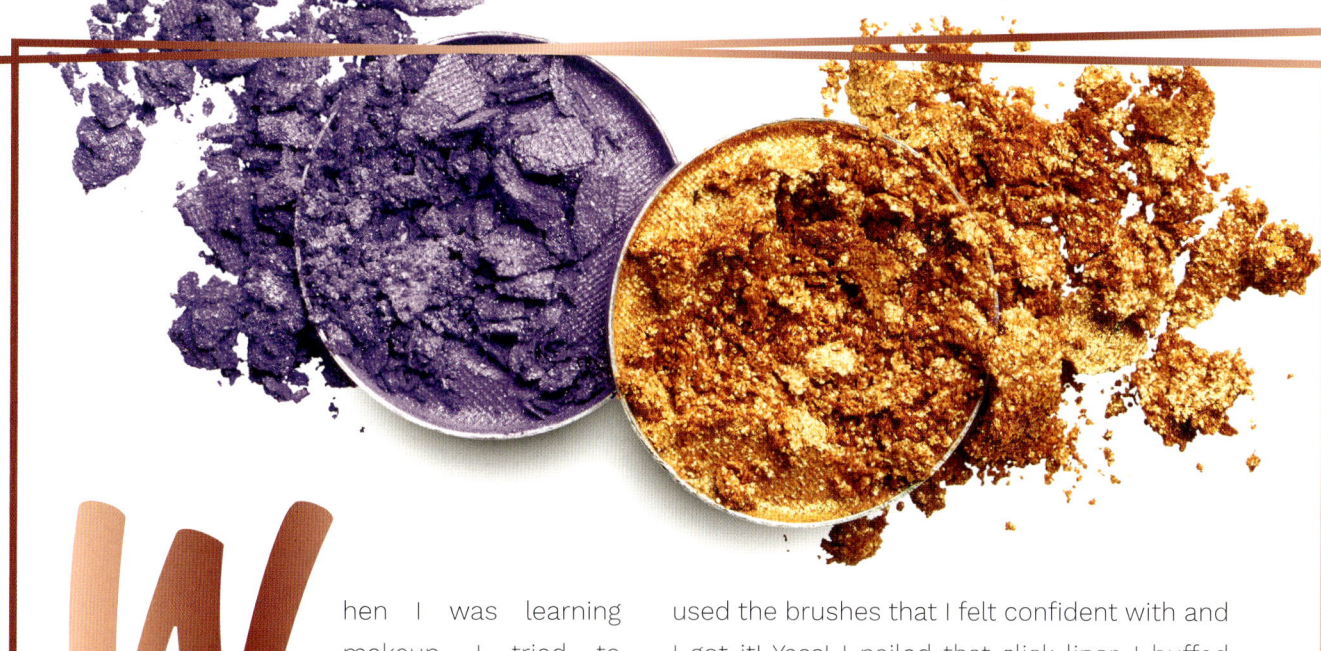

When I was learning makeup, I tried to copy everything my teacher told me to do, including the brushes I chose. Halfway through my course I wanted to give up; I just could not get the effect I wanted in my head from the exact brush she was using. I thought I sucked. Nope, I just needed to listen to my instincts. When I finally did I used the brushes that I felt confident with and I got it! Yass! I nailed that slick liner, I buffed the hell out of that skin – I never looked back! Sometimes we are weird, and that is great. If you want to apply foundation with a small angle brush you go gurl!

One thing I do know is you simply can't get the results you seek by just using fingers and a few cotton tips. At some point you must treat yourself and get some toys!

Brushes

Now before you think I am going to send you into credit card debt, I believe the shape and the density of the brush is way more important than the brand. There are brushes to infinity and beyond these days and once you understand what the style of brush is going to do, you can confidently decide what brushes you need to add it!

No matter what part of the face you are talking about, when it comes to brushes, it's always simpler than you think: the smaller the denser the brush, the more product you are delivering to the skin instantly; the larger and fluffier the brush the less product you are applying to the skin and the softer the finish. Simple as that.

The brush you choose comes down to the effect you are trying to achieve and the confidence you have with it in your hand. Some brushes just feel good to us. This is a choose your own adventure situation.

As much as I love to play with new tools, I know as a makeup artist, if disaster struck I could survive with a few simple brushes.

BUFF THAT BASE

Boy do I love a fluffy brush when it comes to perfecting that foundie! When first applying the product to the skin I prefer a smaller brush to help me control this full coverage situation. I then whip out the big momma to soften any edges and take it further across the skin to blend out.

When loading up the skin with a fuller coverage foundation try a small, stumpy foundation brush, I really like the round ones as they don't give you streaks like a paint brush often does.

To get that seamless airbrushed effect on the skin what you need is a larger soft brush. Soft being the operative word. This is your buffing buddy. You can use this type of brush to buff into the skin what you applied with your other brush and make sure there are no edges. Don't worry if the brush says 'powder' on it, those large fluffy bad boys sometimes make the best liquid blenders. You can build your foundation into a more natural full coverage by buffing in layers to build to perfection.

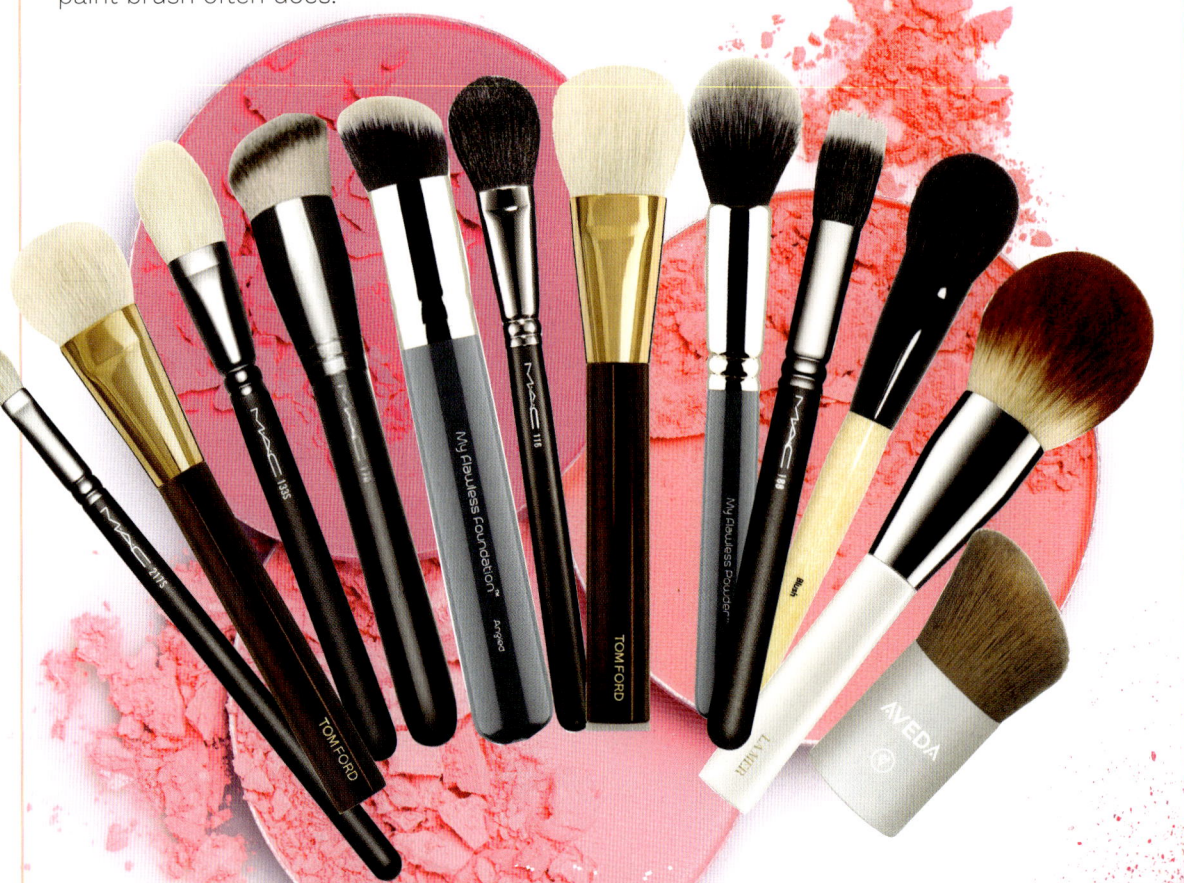

MAC 217 Brush, Tom Ford Cream Foundation Brush, MAC 133 Brush, MAC 170 Brush, MYKITCO. My Flawless Foundation Brush, MAC 116 Brush, Tom Ford Cheek Brush, MYKITCO. My Flawless Powder Brush, MAC 188 Brush, Bobbi Brown Blush Brush, La Mer The Powder Brush, Aveda Inner Light Brush

CONCEAL IT

For serious coverage on trouble spots like under eyes, blemishes and pigmentation, paint into those specific areas.

If you need softer cover and no edges go for the fluff and buff technique.

A new favorite of mine is using a combination of the two – a small and soft pencil brush to conceal blemishes perfectly with cream or powder!

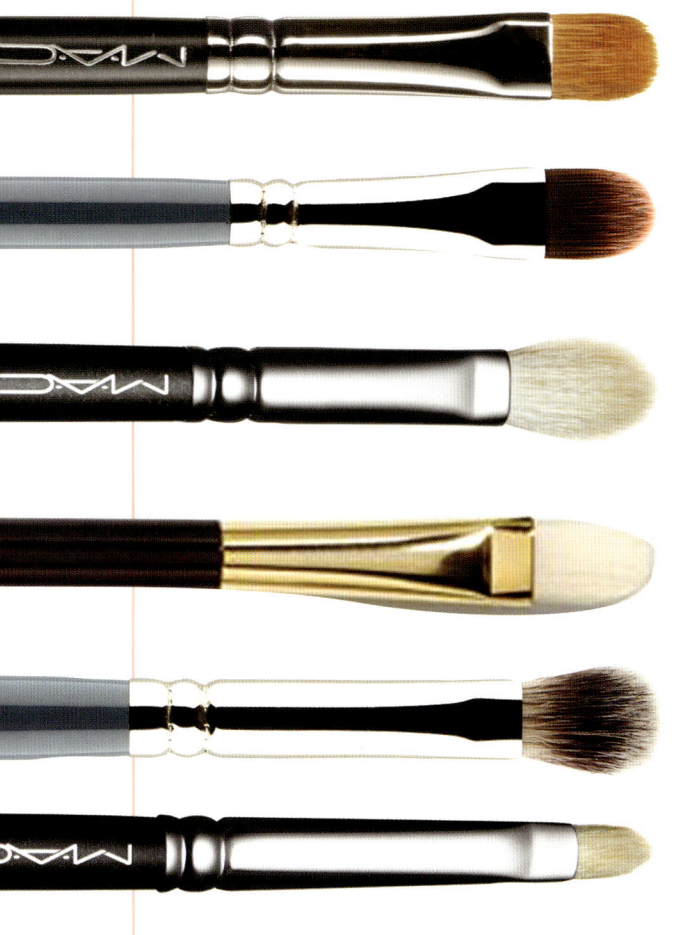

MAC 242 Brush, MYKITCO. My Precision Concealer Brush, MAC 217 Brush, Tom Ford Concealer Brush, MYKITCO. My Fluffy Concealer Brush, MAC 219 Brush

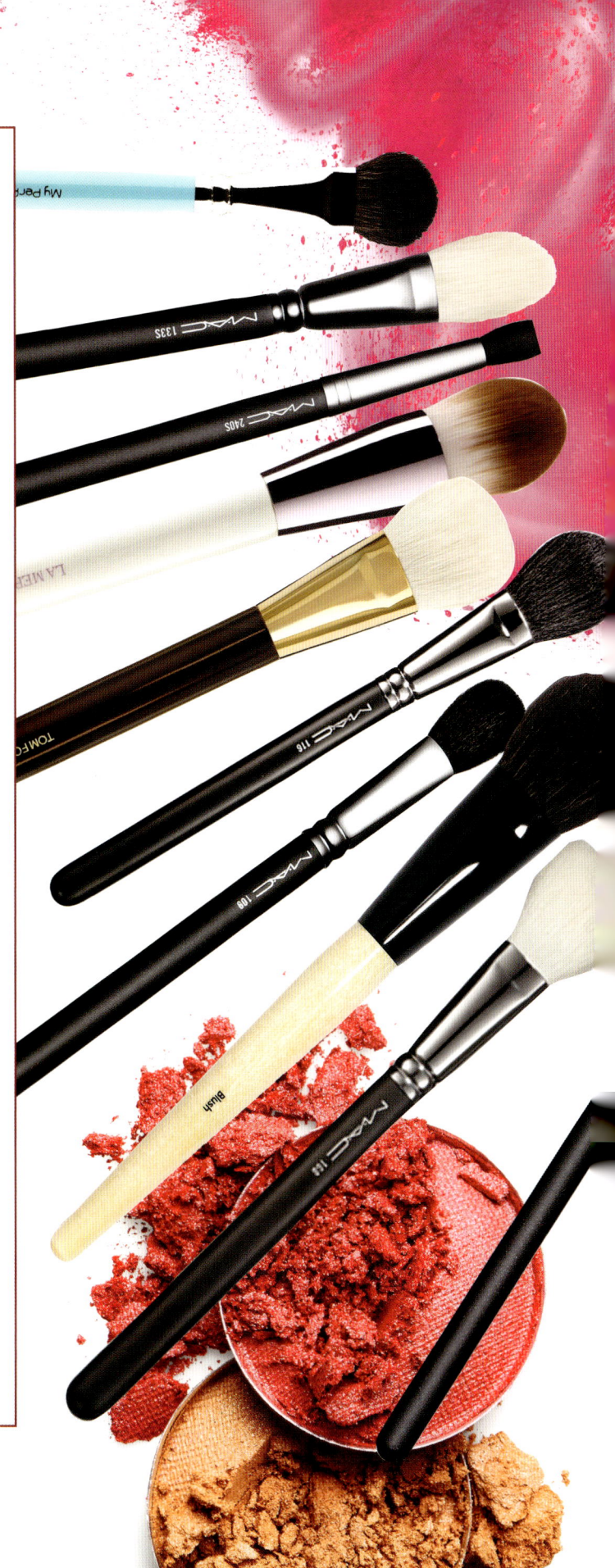

SET, SHAPE AND ENHANCE IT

So you are looking for precise powder application to eliminate that shine right where you need it. Don't be shy, press a smaller powder brush through all the shiny spots on your face for specific hold and set power.

Angled brushes are great for perfecting your contouring and shading so that it sits right on the bone structure.

HIGHLIGHTING SUPERSTARS!

Your smaller brush will get the shine popping and the soft fan brush will glaze the skin for effortless sheen.

When you are applying bronzer or a sheer color on face and body, these are the tools for you. They also work extremely well for all over setting powder.

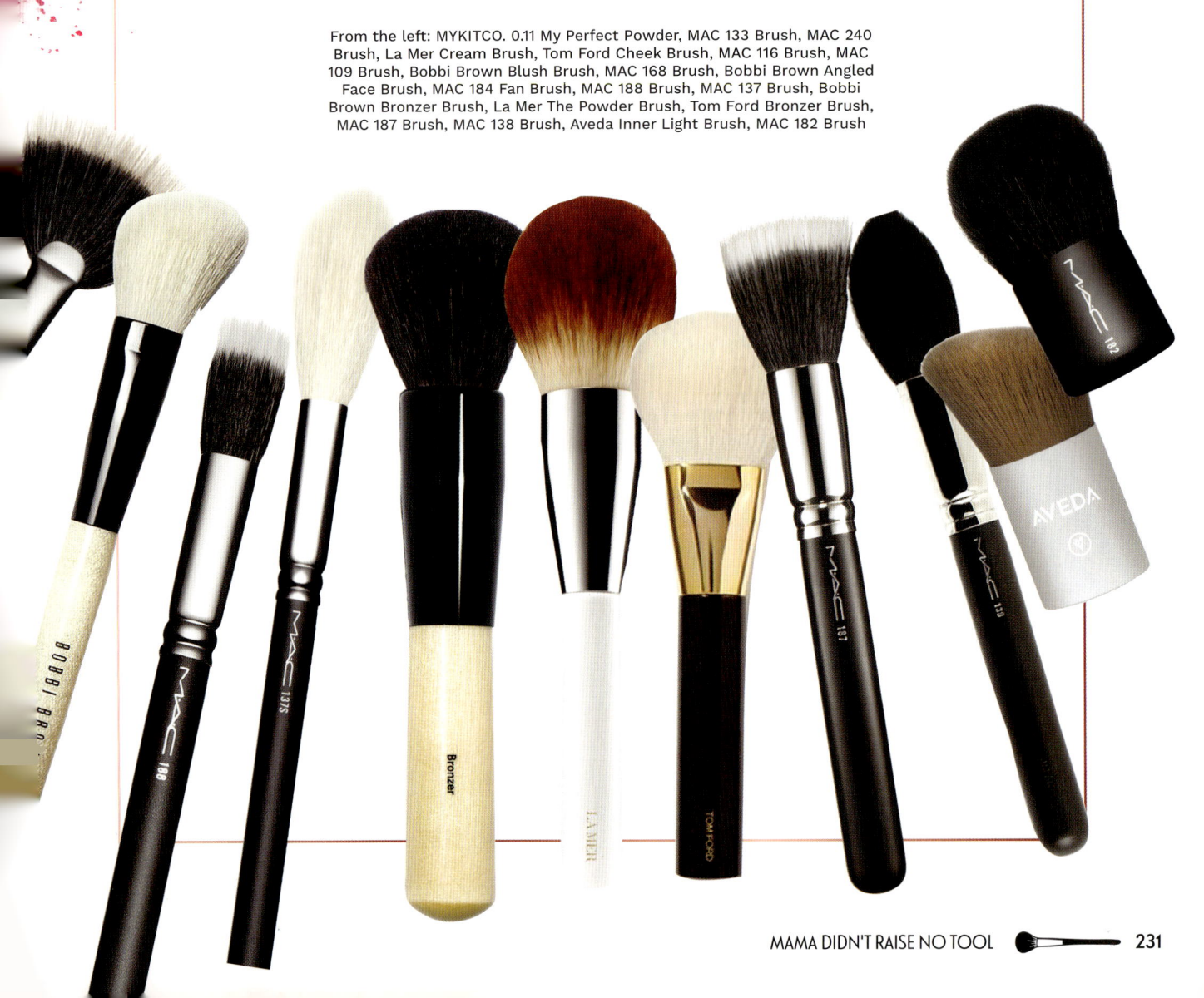

From the left: MYKITCO. 0.11 My Perfect Powder, MAC 133 Brush, MAC 240 Brush, La Mer Cream Brush, Tom Ford Cheek Brush, MAC 116 Brush, MAC 109 Brush, Bobbi Brown Blush Brush, MAC 168 Brush, Bobbi Brown Angled Face Brush, MAC 184 Fan Brush, MAC 188 Brush, MAC 137 Brush, Bobbi Brown Bronzer Brush, La Mer The Powder Brush, Tom Ford Bronzer Brush, MAC 187 Brush, MAC 138 Brush, Aveda Inner Light Brush, MAC 182 Brush

ALL ABOUT EYES

Smaller pencil brushes are great to smudge pencils and intense colors first or pump up density of color later. The flatter soft brushes work perfectly to pat on intense color and shimmer and sharpen up that cut crease.

The larger ones here are your blenders, once you've got your color laid down on the eyes these will take away your edges.

When you need a more definitive blend in that crease.

The small fan brush is the silent magician for fine or fat lashes.

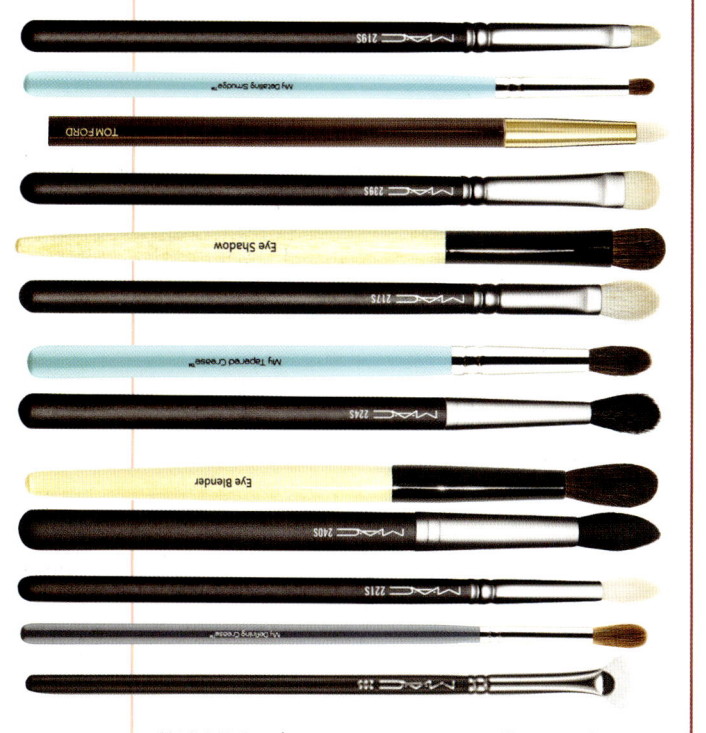

MAC 219 Brush, MYKITCO. 1.13 My Detailing Smudge, Tom Ford Smokey Eye Brush, MAC 239 Brush, Bobbi Brown Eye Shadow Brush, MAC 217 Brush, MYKITCO. My Tapered Crease Brush, MAC 224 Brush, Bobbi Brown Eye Blender Brush, MAC 240 Brush, MAC 221 Brush, MYKITCO. 1.3 My Defining Crease, MAC 205 Mascara Fan Brush

SHARP LINES

Thin, synthetic angle brushes are all about razor sharp eye lines and creating believable hair strokes, For perfect stamped definition the flat thin brush is the one for you.

We use pointed brushes for fine detail work. Use the longer haired pointed brush when looking to accentuate an elongated stroke.

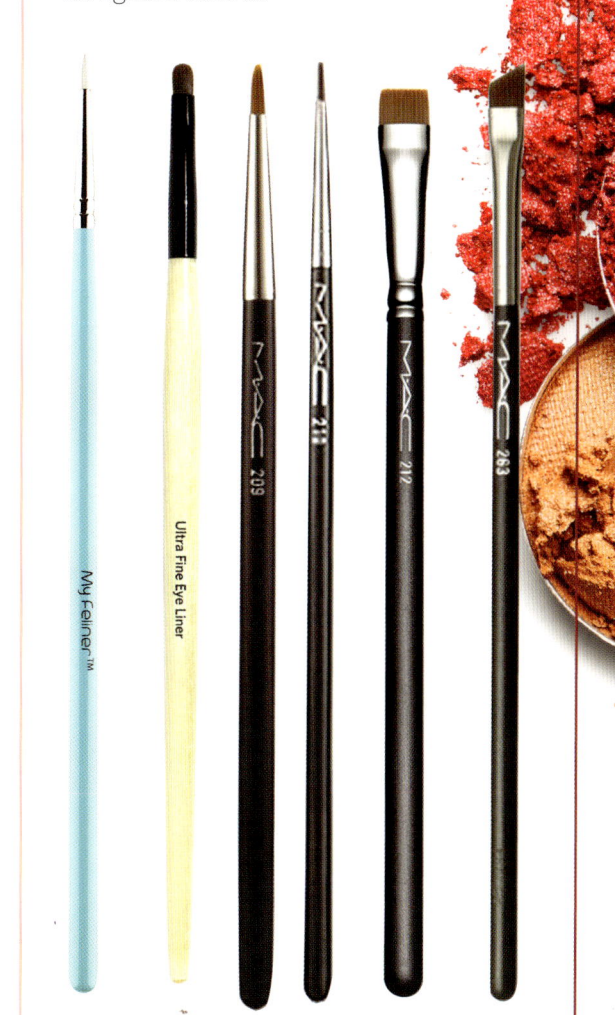

MAC 263 Angle Brush, MAC 212 Flat Definer Brush, MAC 210 Fine Liner Brush, MAC 209 Pointed Liner Brush, Bobbi Brown Ultra Fine Liner Brush, MYKITCO. My Feliner

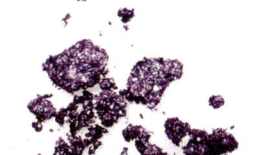

BROWS

The bigger the brush the bigger the brow. A larger angle brush is perfect for fuller, more bold brows, and a thinner angle brush used wet will give you hair-like strokes. My secret weapon for brows is the spoolie brush, as it gets your hairs moving the same direction and evens out any color.

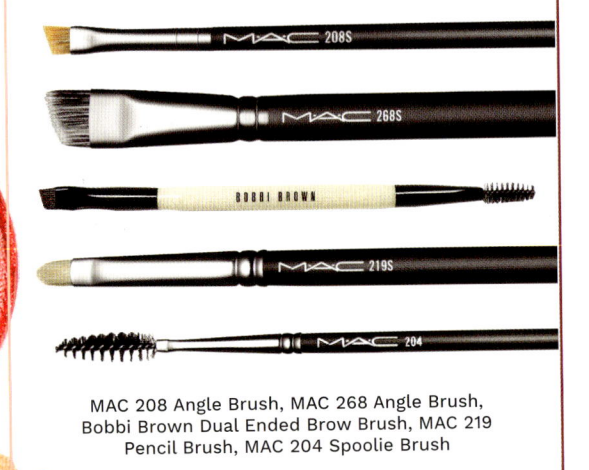

MAC 208 Angle Brush, MAC 268 Angle Brush, Bobbi Brown Dual Ended Brow Brush, MAC 219 Pencil Brush, MAC 204 Spoolie Brush

LIPS

Slightly rounded brushes make application easy by mimicking the shape of the bow of the lip and loading on lip product. The small, soft smudger is great for softening hard edges and to ramp up the fullness.

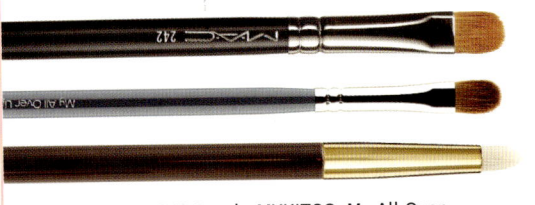

MAC 242 Brush, MYKITCO. My All Over Lip, Tom Ford Smokey Eye Brush

MY TOP SIX MUST-HAVE BRUSH SHAPES FOR ALL-OVER APPLICATION

1. MAC 170 Foundation Brush (Stipple that foundation, pat on that cheek color and highlighter!)
2. Tom Ford Bronzer Brush (Buff that skin, and brush bronzer on face and body)
3. MYKITCO. My Perfect Powder Brush (Precise powder blotting and contouring)
4. MAC 263 Angle Brush (Perfect eyeliner and brow defining)
5. Tom Ford Smokey Eye Brush (Smudge your pencil liner, apply the color and pump it up!)
6. MAC 221 Brush (Blend, blend, blend your concealer and your eye shadow)

Sponges and Puffs

Sponges are the pusher – the foundation pusher. I bring out my sponge when I want that crazy flawless coverage and a little face massager in one. Are sponges or puffs better than brushes? Better, no, but they do serve their own specific purpose. I will never head to a makeup job without these three items.

BEAUTY BLENDER

This is the name of the brand, but so effective have they become I am putting them in a category of their own. Look after these as they aren't cheap. They have a pointed end for the application of product and then rounded side for blending. A super versatile piece of kit!

WEDGE SPONGE

An oldie but a goodie. The wedge sponge is multipurpose, working well for blending while the straight sides makes them handy to fix up edges or lines. These are disposable, so if they no longer look white, they are definitely *not* alright.

POWDER PUFFS

A brush can only hold so much powder, so when you need to lay it on heavy turn to the trusty puff.

TIP!

Sponges will absorb creams; that is the nature of the sponge. There is no real way to avoid it, in fact, that is the magic of them! When you are wanting to create a super-duper flawless coverage, by using a sponge you are building up the coverage while sucking up the excess product that is sitting on top of the skin, so essentially you are not going to look cakey!

Stipple don't wipe! Stippling is the action of patting on the skin. Wiping a sponge across your skin will give you nothing in terms of coverage. Stippling will push the makeup onto the skin and more pressure will give you more product – stipple away!

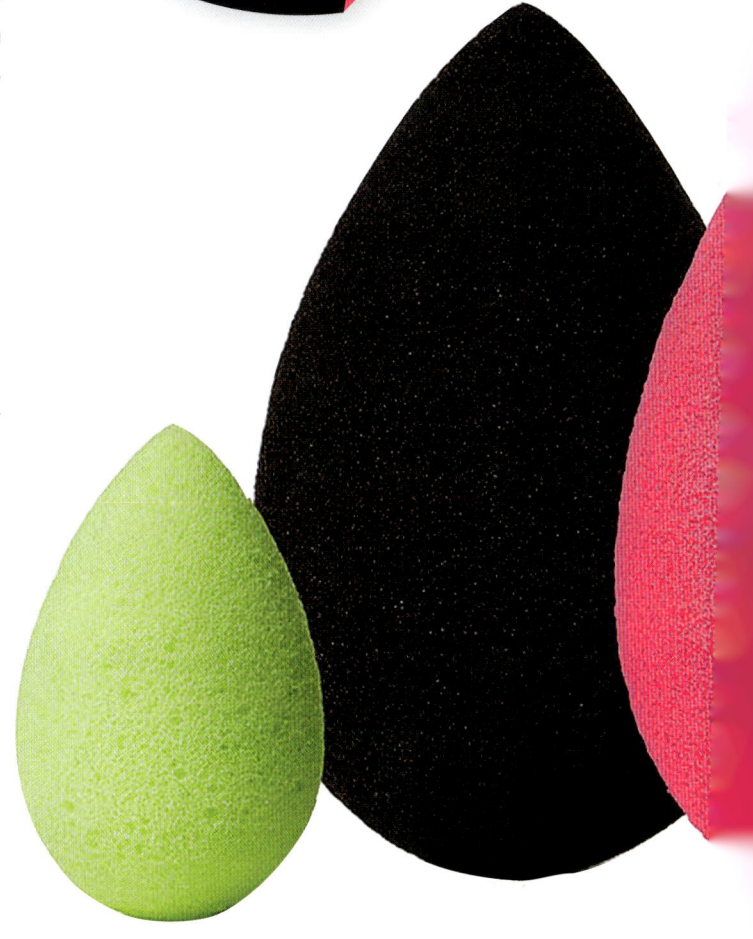

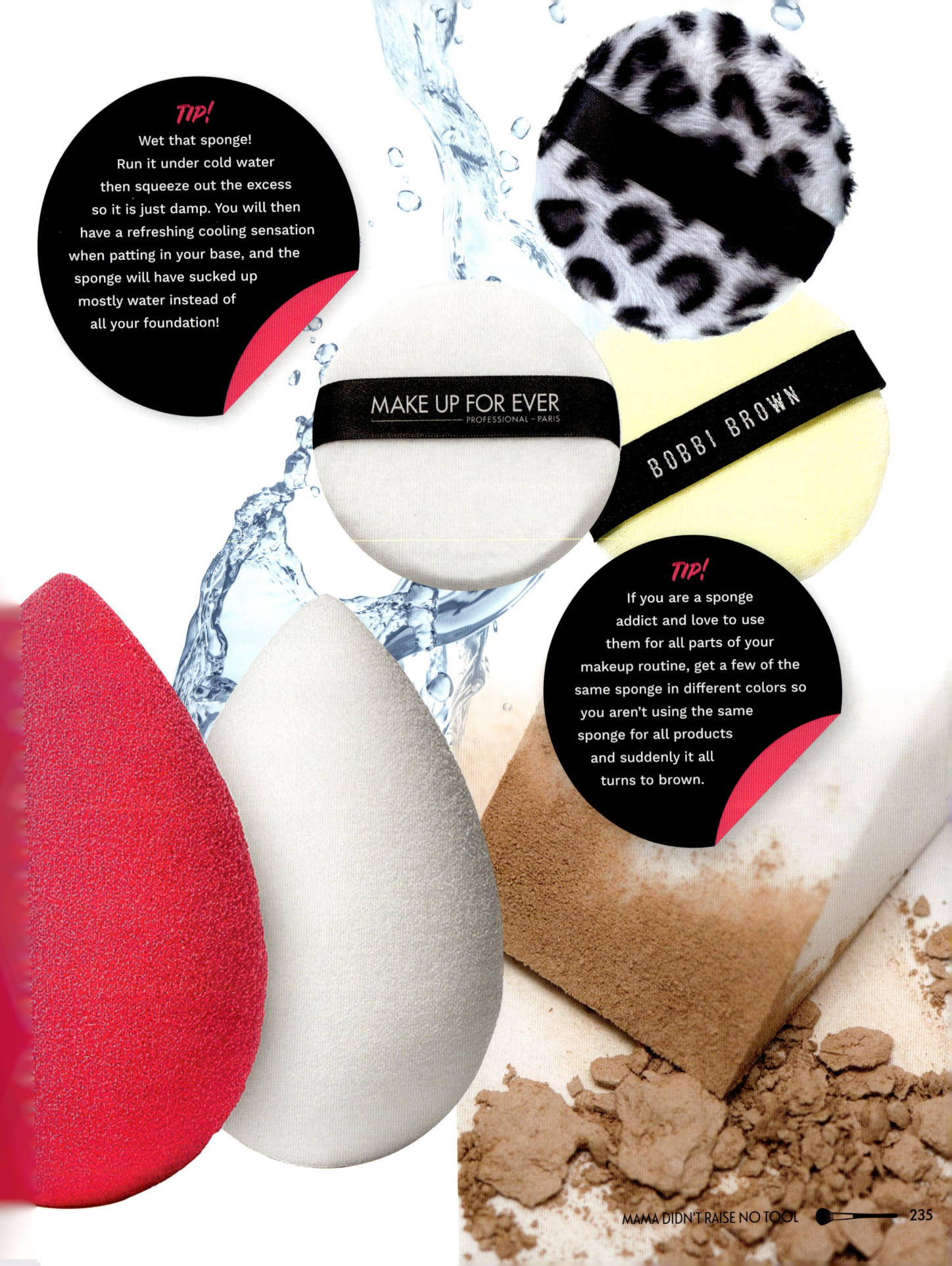

TIP!
Wet that sponge! Run it under cold water then squeeze out the excess so it is just damp. You will then have a refreshing cooling sensation when patting in your base, and the sponge will have sucked up mostly water instead of all your foundation!

TIP!
If you are a sponge addict and love to use them for all parts of your makeup routine, get a few of the same sponge in different colors so you aren't using the same sponge for all products and suddenly it all turns to brown.

MAMA DIDN'T RAISE NO TOOL

Keep 'em Clean!

I cannot be the first person to tell you to clean your brushes! But I hope I'll be the one you listen to. Brushes, like sponges, are breeding grounds for bacteria, dirt and skin cells, all of which will be clogging your pores and probably are to blame for many of your blemishes. I'd love to say, clean your brushes after every use, but that will probably fall on deaf ears. Let's go with once a week because beyond that is, well, gross.

TO CLEAN OUT ALL THE DIRT

I really like using a soap bar to give the brushes a fast, deep clean, because the action of swiping the brushes under the water onto the soap can help keep the bristles aligned. Facial soap works well as it is designed to break down makeup on the face so works on the brushes.

A handy tool I picked up a few years back was a rubber brush cleaning mat! Sounds *ridiculous*, but used in conjunction with cleanser or soap this guy can halve your brush cleansing time!

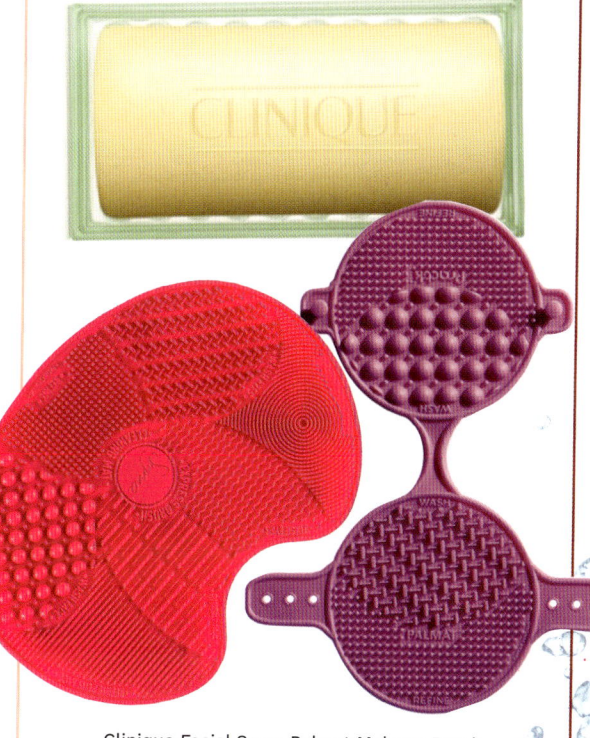

TO QUICKLY CLEAN IN BETWEEN LOOKS

Get yourself a brush sterilizer to purify and disinfect brush fibers without washing. Pour a little into a tissue and stroke back and forth until clean. This will make it super easy to go from applying a smoky eye to blending your concealer color.

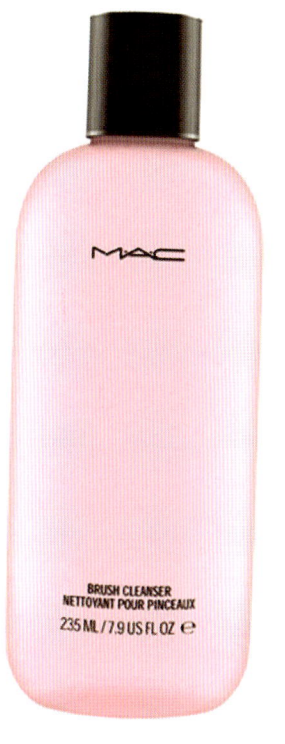

MAC Brush Cleanser

Clinique Facial Soap, Palmat Makeup Brush Cleaning Tool, Sigma Spa Brush Cleaning Mat

FOR TOUGH STAINS

Use a clarifying shampoo. Designed to deeply clean colored hair, these heavy duty shampoos have worked wonders on my white brushes!

For extra, extra tough stains in your brushes, give them a quick cleanse with your facial oil cleanser to break down the heavy-duty waterproof product and then continue with the soap cleaning.

BRING THEM BACK TO SHAPE

The worst thing you can do to your lovely brushes is fuzz them out while cleaning them, it's a little bit hard to give yourself a defined liner with a brush that is no longer pointy! Once washed, remove the excess water by squeezing them flat to retain their shape for years to come.

GIVE THEM AIR

I've saved the most important bit till last! Once you've finished washing the brushes you need to put them out to dry. Stand them up in a jar or glass and the moisture falls down in the brush handle, which will cause damage and rotting if the handles are wooden. Instead lay the brushes down flat with the brush head hanging off the edge of the surface so air can flow freely through. This will mean they will dry faster and be ready to use overnight.

OMG CLEAN YOUR SPONGE!

Right, so we have established that the main function of a sponge is to suck things up, now think about all the makeup and, ahem, dirt your sponge has absorbed in the last few days. Do you really want to pat that all back onto your skin with your next makeup application? Ew. No.

So your cheapie sponges, chuck them away when the color of them becomes gross, and for the sponges you spent a bit of cashola on, like the Beauty Blender, give them a clean. The BB comes with a specific cleaner that dissolves the product without ruining the sponge so you can make use of it for longer. For all your others sponges soap and warm water will suffice!

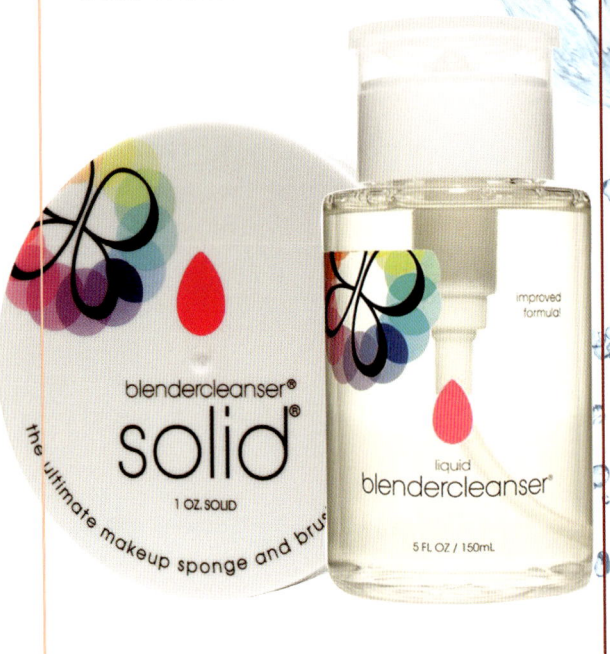

Beautyblender, Blendercleanser in Solid and Liquid

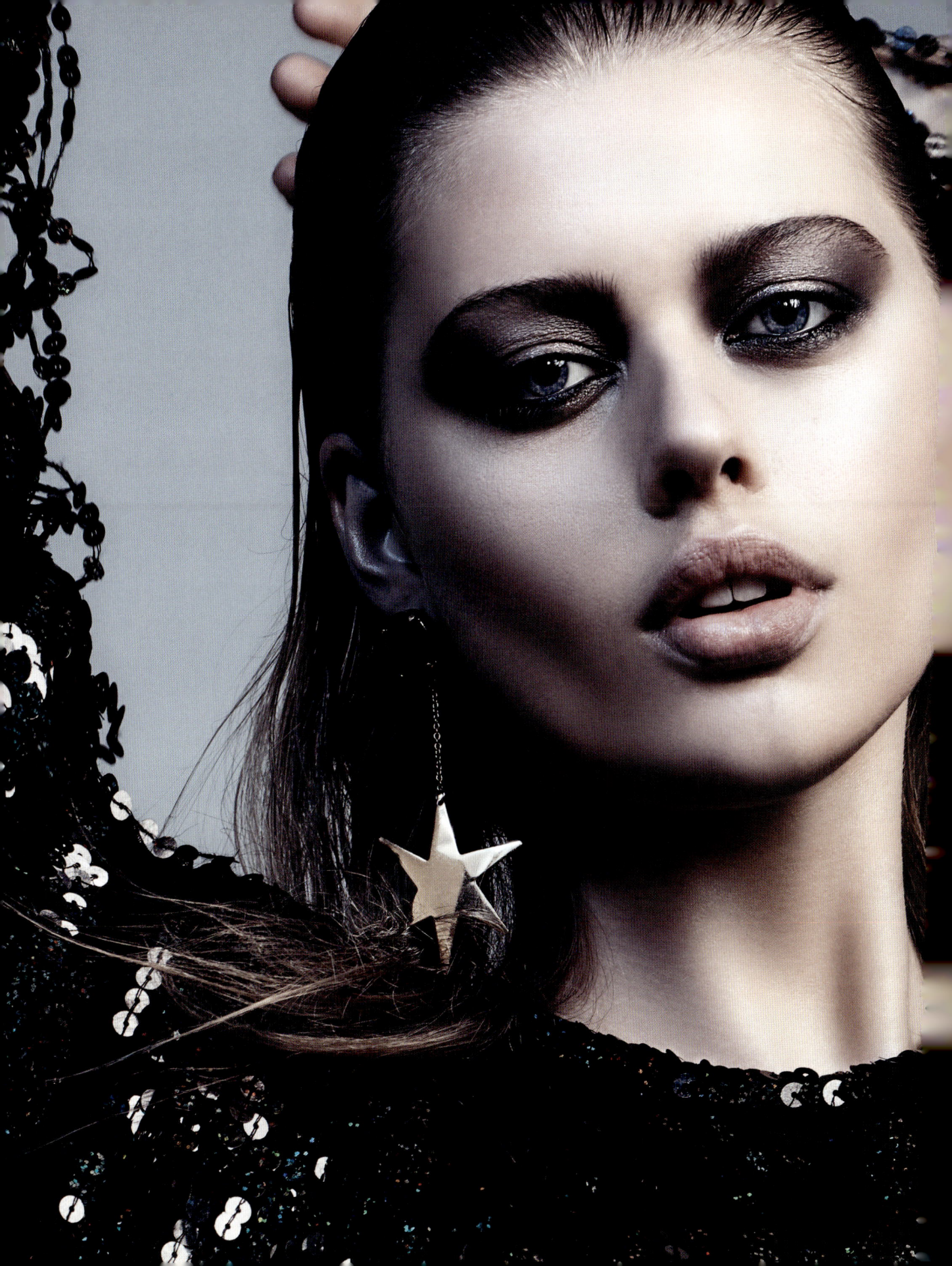

You complete me

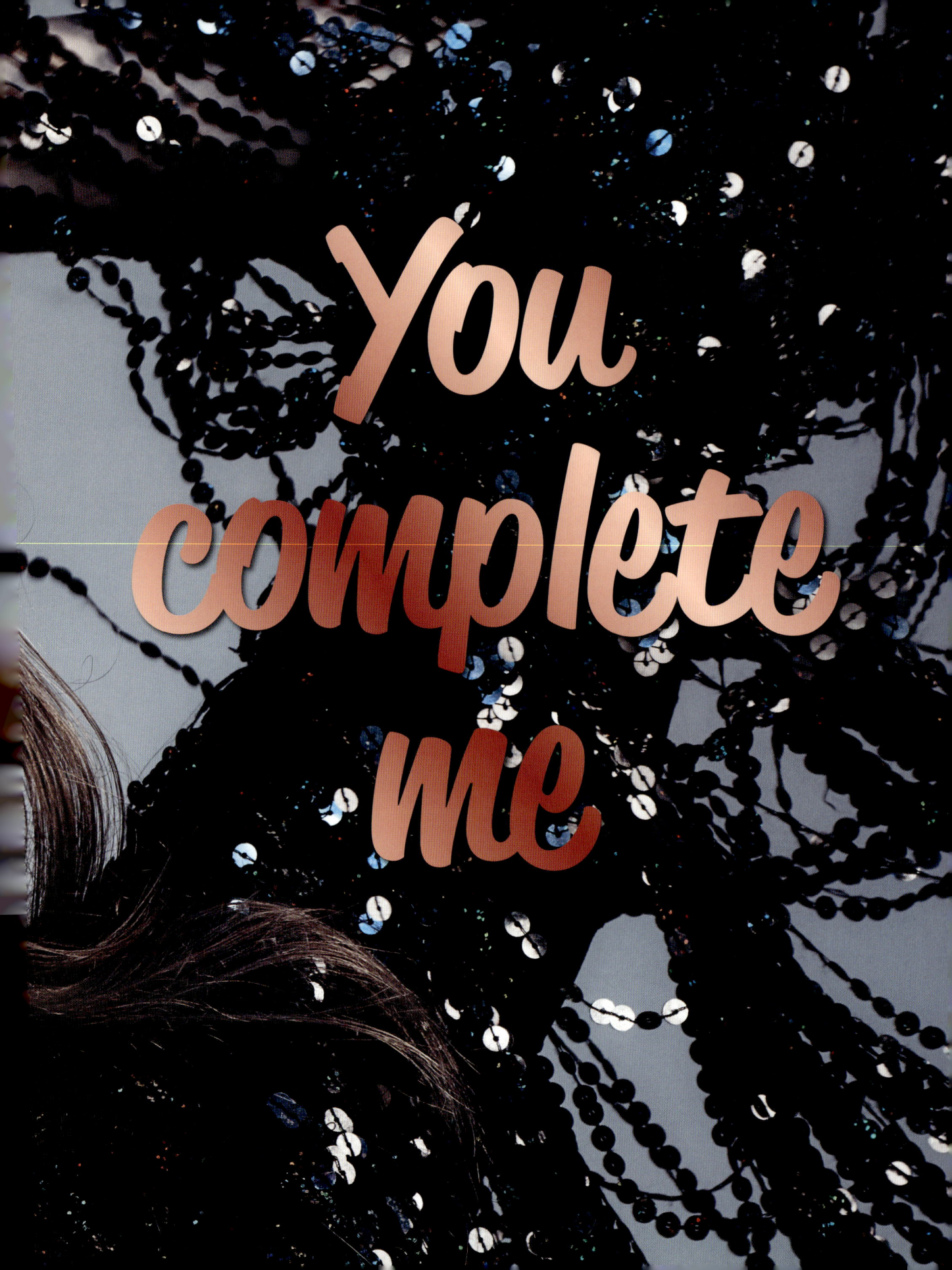

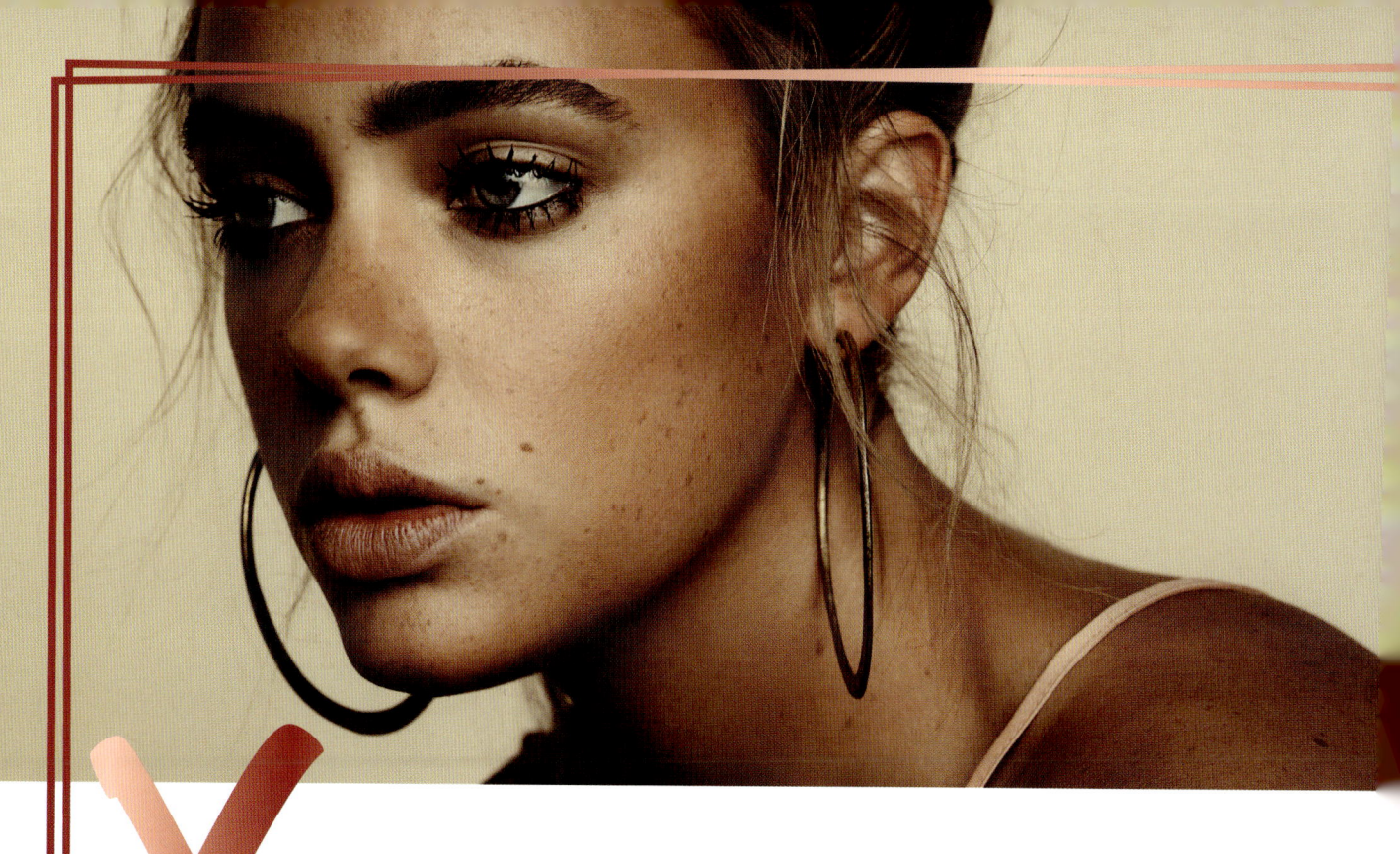

You can have all the designer pieces you want in your wardrobe but that doesn't make putting an outfit together any easier. By this point we have provided you with a collection of makeup techniques so you can put together some complete looks for any and every occasion. The super fun part is mixing and matching and creating your own looks, but to give you a little inspiration I got together with some of my friends to play some dress-ups of our own.

I've been extremely fortunate to have worked with some incredibly talented people over the years, but I consider myself lucky beyond belief when two of them happen to be among my best friends.

Cameron Rains is a hairstylist originally from Australia, now based in New York. When we met it was love at first finger wave! I was so inspired by how he made the most glamorous looks seem so effortless. It wouldn't be long before the worldwide stage would call and now he spends a large amount of his time taking his brush to the likes of Lorde and Kate Hudson.

In my eyes, stylist Peter Simon Phillips (PSP) brings an unmatched creativity, organization and kindness to everything he does. I remember our first job working together and I could not believe the amount of clothing and accessories he laid out ready for the day. It was like all my Christmases had come at once, except I couldn't take the presents home!

Throughout this chapter not only will we break down makeup looks, with references to the techniques we have presented so far, but Cameron and PSP will provide you with some hair and styling tips that help tie the whole look together.

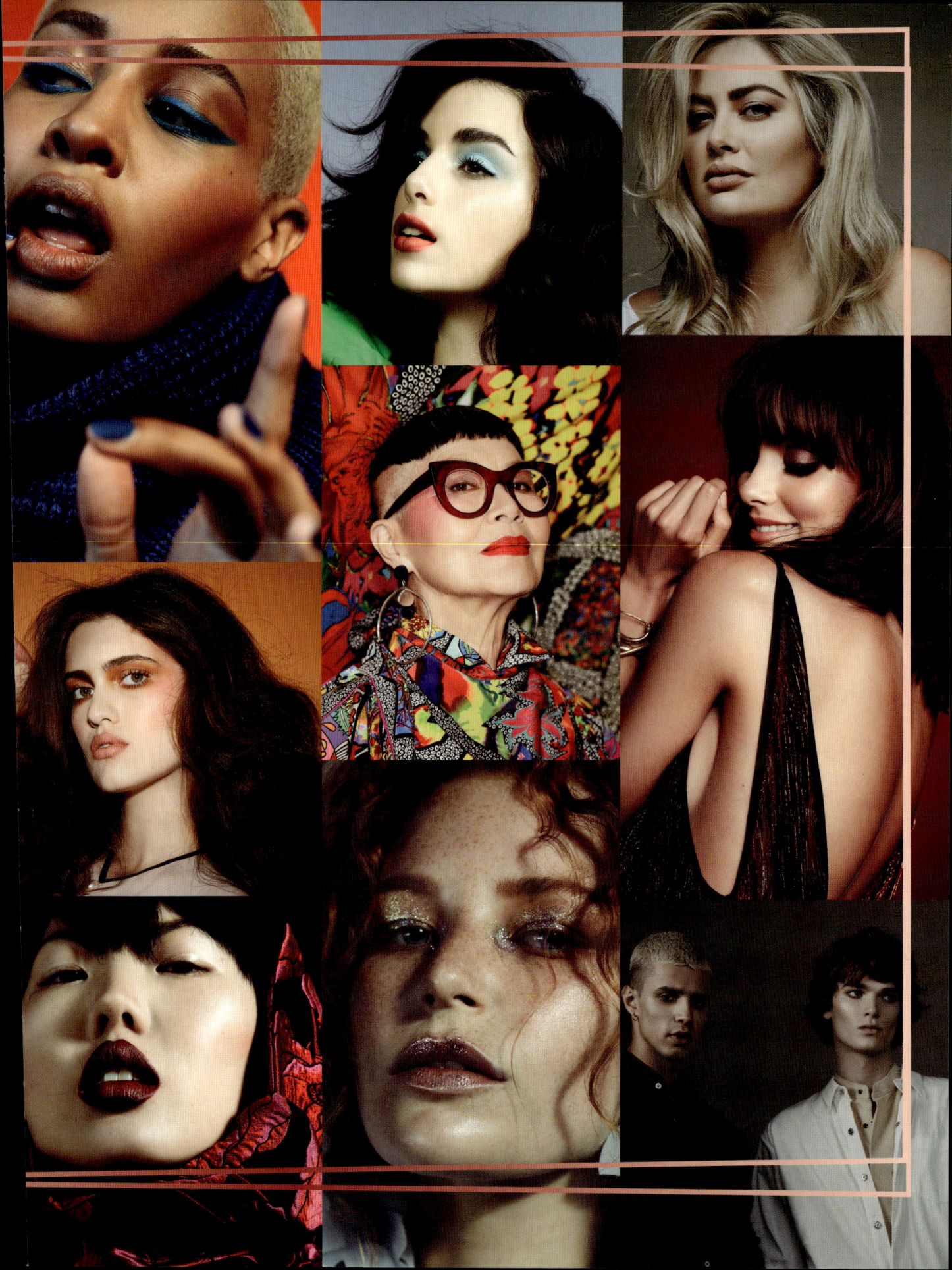

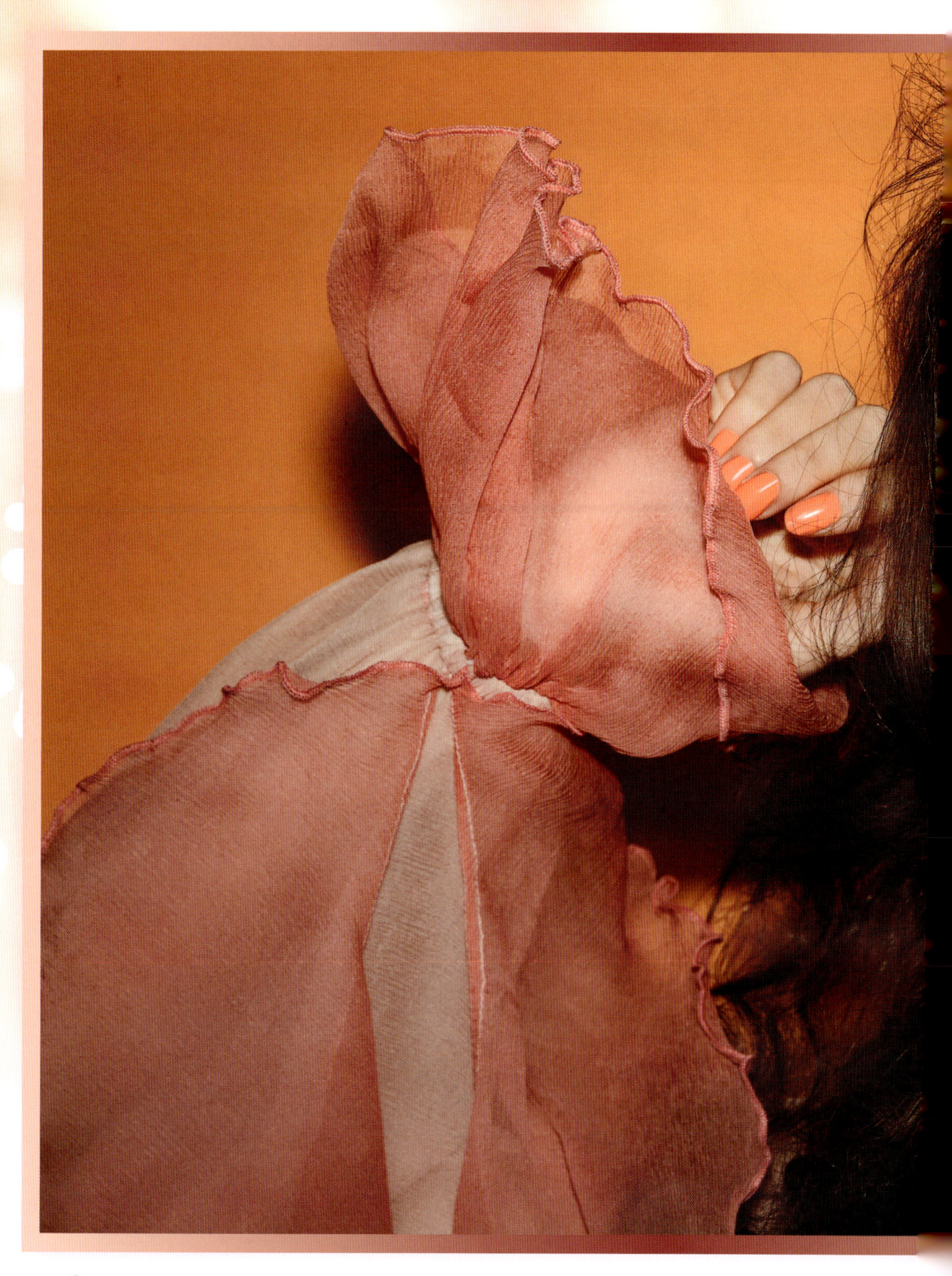

YOU COMPLETE ME   243

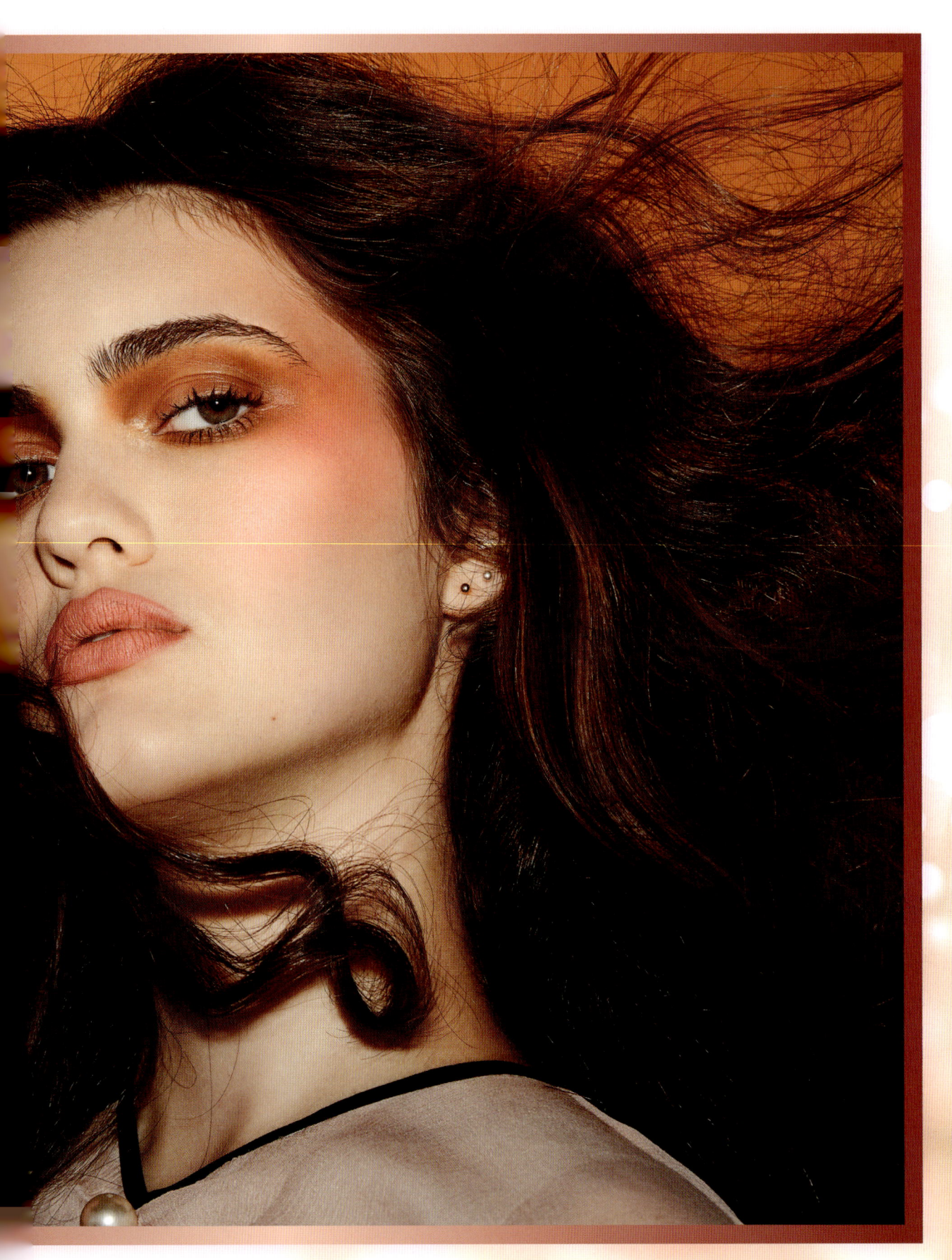

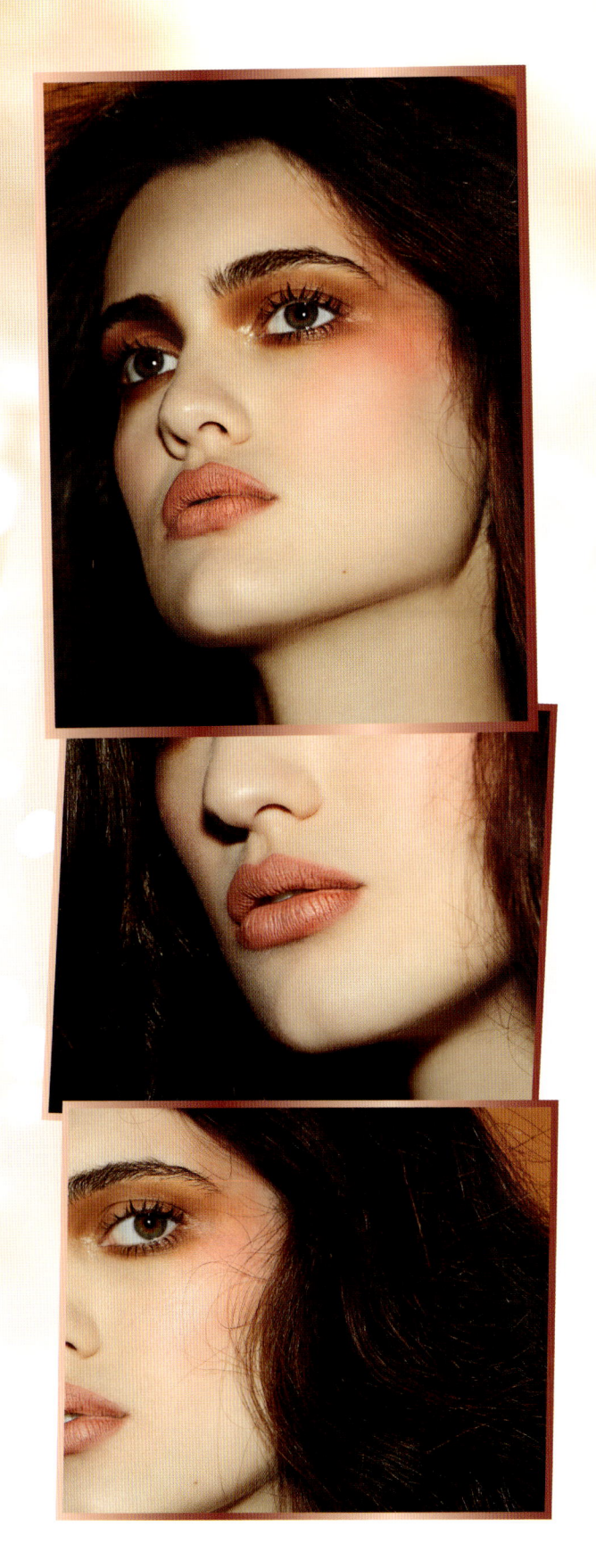

A ROSE HAS THORNS

Creamy coverage (page 58)
Instead of finishing the creamy skin technique with another cream highlighter, I gave the skin the final layer of glow with a shimmering highlighting powder. Highlighting powder sticks instantly to creamy skin and is a great glow option for oily skin.

The not-so-smoky eye (page 118)
Technique stays the same here, just switch up the colors. I used MAC Spice lip pencil as the base, matte shadows in matching shades to contour the eye and a metallic pigment to create dimension through the center. Tap a little light gold pigment on the inner corners with a damp brush for a brightening light on the eyes. Tap a little eye gloss through the center. Elizabeth Arden Eight Hour Cream is a fave for this type of editorial look!

Let your lashes take a back seat
Who said you can't wear makeup on all features at once hey?! It is all about balance. So now that we have balanced eyes, cheeks and lips, a huge black false lash would take this look over the edge. Instead load up your lashes with a brown mascara to keep the look chic.

Nude full lips (page 182)
Swap out the nude lipstick with a dusty pink and complete the steps. This technique can be used with any lip color you would like to create fullness with. Don't be afraid to match your lip color to an element of your outfit for a chic consistent look.

Cream blush (page 218)

I have taken the techniques from cream blush and moved the color placement to the tops of the cheekbones, blending outwards for a romantic, continuous look. Lipsticks can also be used as a cream blush! I have used MAC Please Me matte lipstick here for extra staying power on the skin, and blended it over the cheeks with my fingertips before setting with powder blush for extra color intensity.

Styling tip from PSP: sleeves

Need to hold your sleeves up? Sleeve garters (which is just a fancy name for an elasticated arm band) are a hugely effective tool. If you're lucky your mum might even have some in her jewelry box left over from the eighties. If she doesn't, a good old elastic band will do the trick; I use them on shoots and runway shows all the time to keep sleeves up.

Hair tip from Cameron: seventies disco

Dampen hair with a volume spray, roots to ends, and then hit it with the hair dryer. Once dry, flip back and use the dryer on cool air through the top and around your face. Start to smooth your hair by using your dryer and brush before using a curling iron to curl the ends and create waves. Allow to cool then flip your head and brush for dear life, incorporating a volume powder, and sprinkle the dust throughout. Flip back and add some more powder to create a soft flyway look. A volume powder helps with lift and grip on the hair.

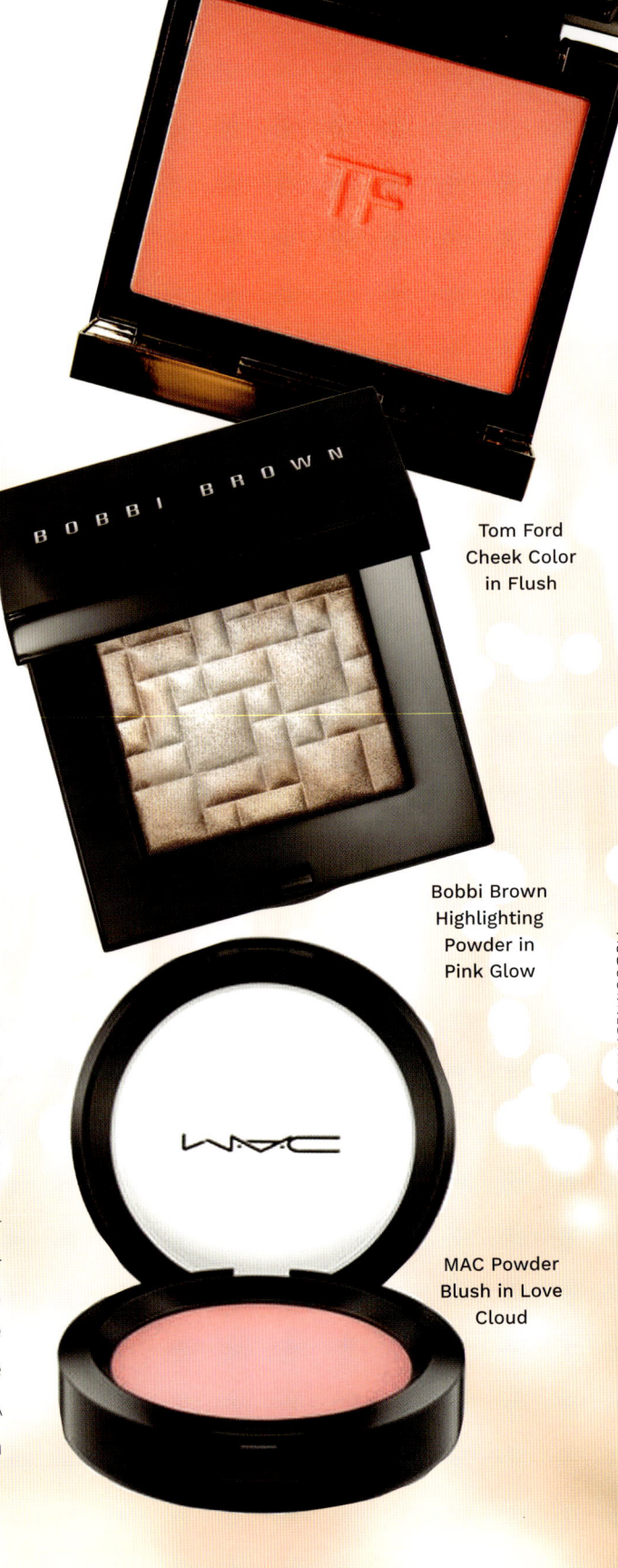

Tom Ford Cheek Color in Flush

Bobbi Brown Highlighting Powder in Pink Glow

MAC Powder Blush in Love Cloud

ALANA MIA FROM CHADWICK MODELS, PINK SHEER BLOUSE, ROMANCE WAS BORN.

BOYS WILL BE BOYS

Tinted skin

For those days when you are in a hurry but still want your skin to look polished and just tinted with color, use a sheer glowing foundation and a large, fluffy round brush to smear on the color with no streaks. Make sure to take the color down the neck and over shoulders before powdering lightly through the T-zone with a super sheer translucent powder. MAC Studio Face and Body Foundation is a makeup artist's fave!

Bronzing (page 78)

Cream bronzer does not always have to give you a dewy finish, it's all in the buff and the brush. You need a lovely soft, medium-sized brush so you have control over the color placement. Hit all the bronzing spots on the face with the color, give your skin a light spray with your hydrating mist and go ahead and blend. Circular motions will avoid patches, then buff, buff, buff for the most naturally bronzed skin!

The perfect smudge (page 154)

For a more grungy look exchange the shimmer eye shadow for matte. Do you feel as though the color is a little messy? Good! This is rock 'n' roll!

Velvet matte skin with highlights (page 66)

Velvet matte skin does not always need to be heavy! I have followed the same steps, but halved the amount of product I have applied to the skin for a more sheer, matte look.

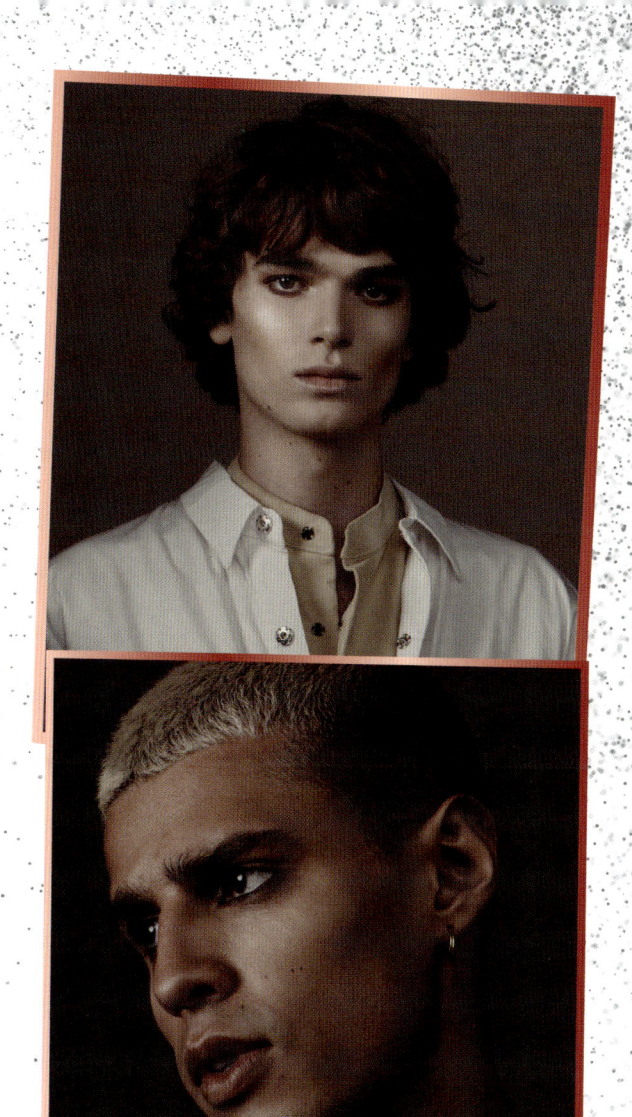

The not-so-smoky eye (page 118)

I have replaced the kohl pencil base with a cream shadow blended right over the lids and under the eyes. I have blended this smoky eye to the crease and slightly elongated at the outer corners to create more of an almond shape – there are no rules to how big or how small a smoky eye can be!

ACE AND CARSON KING FROM KULT MODELS, CLOTHING BY AKIRA

YOU COMPLETE ME

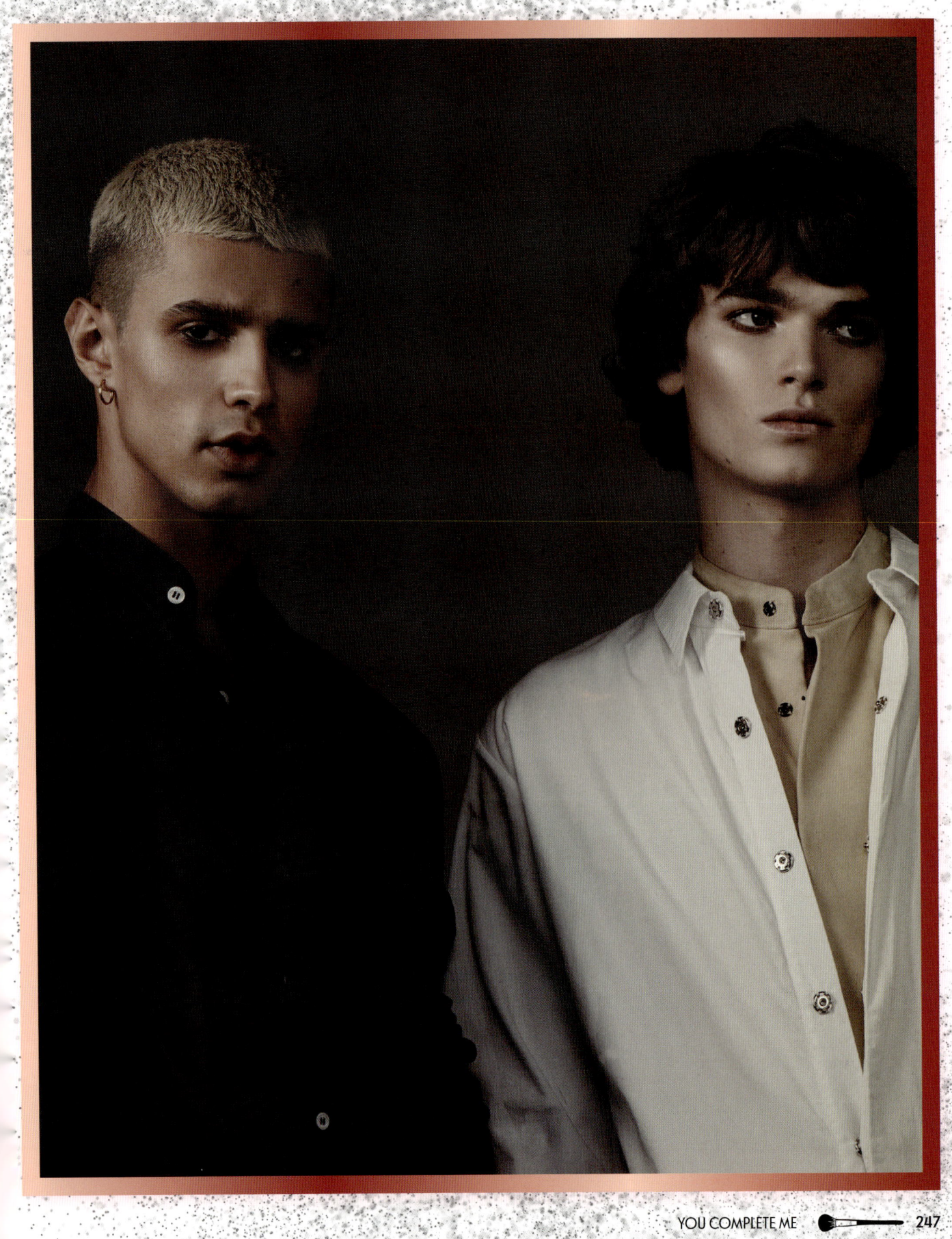

MAKING IT UP

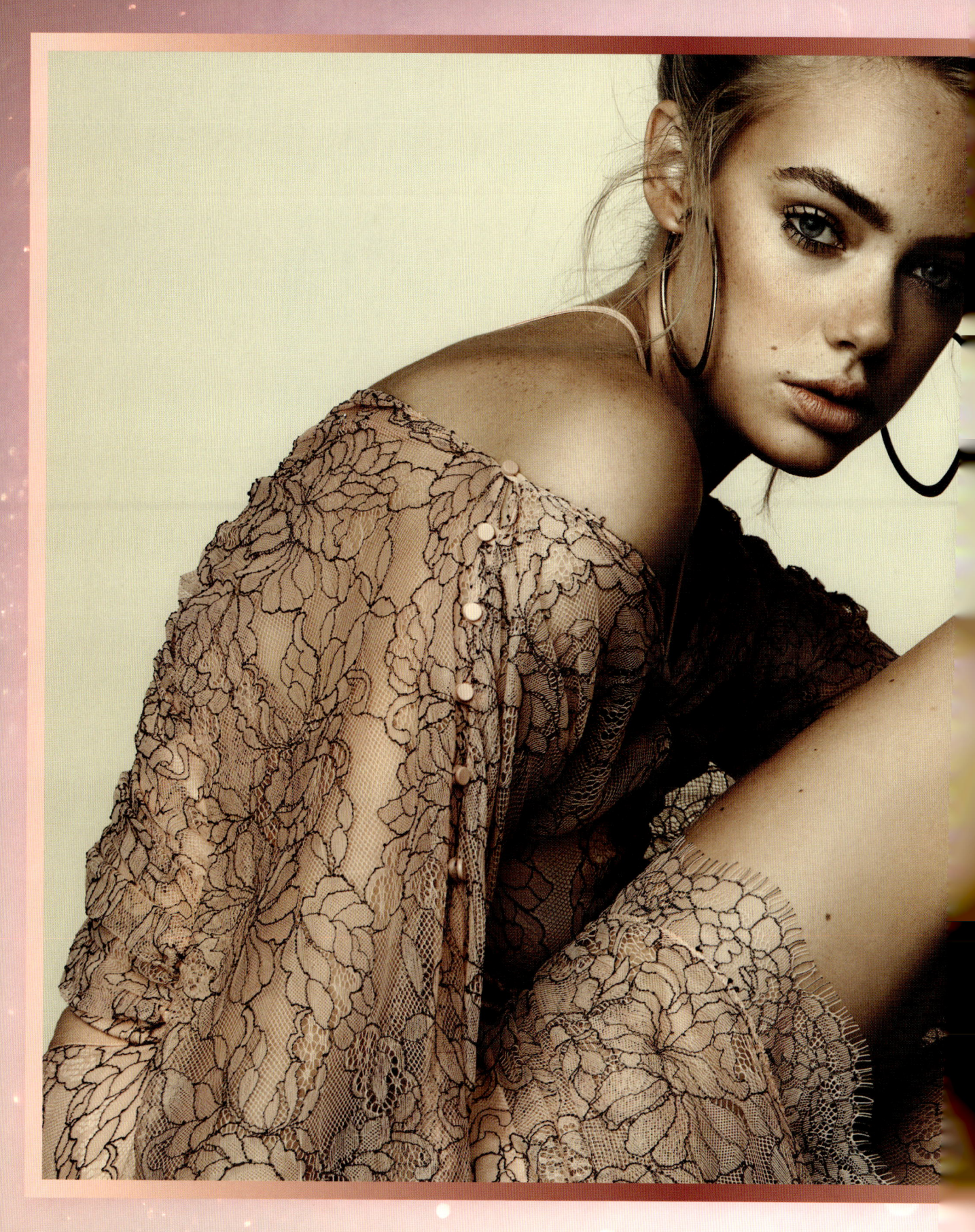

YOU COMPLETE ME 249

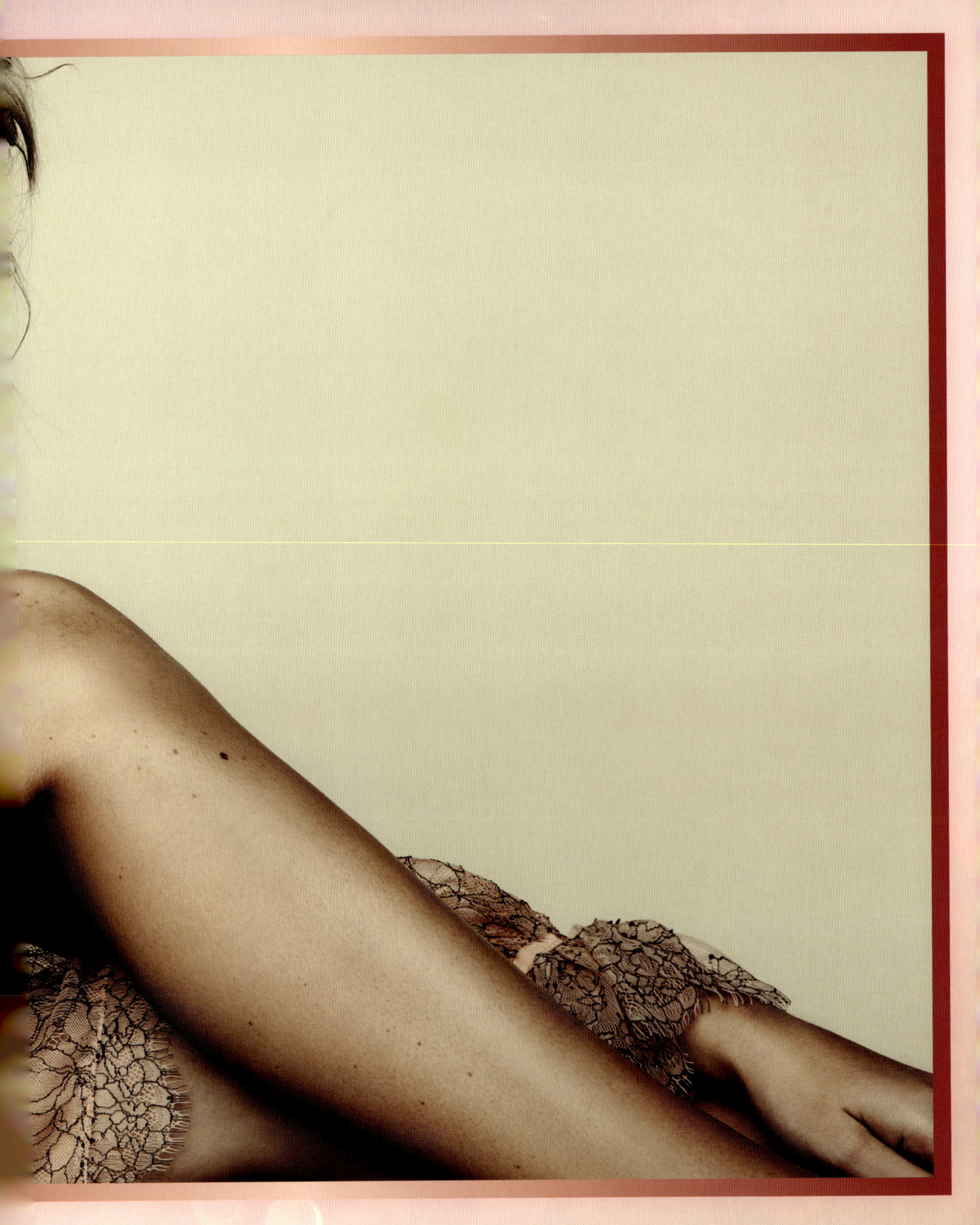

BRONZE IN BOHEMIA

Sheer and glowing skin (page 50)
I have completed all the same steps to get beautifully sheer and effortless skin, and instead of adding more illuminizer over the top to make the surface quite shiny, I stopped at the skin-colored powder step. I have applied the powder with a large brush to give a sheer coverage and then pressed it in with the palms of my hands to seal. Sometimes illuminizer under the foundation is enough glow on its own.

Chunky lashes (page 168)
Change up the color of your mascara to soften or amp up your lash look. Lashes are really fun to make a feature of, as there is no blending at all! Use the primer first to fatten the lashes and give them a slight white tint, making the colored mascara you use on top really pop. I love aubergine mascara to enhance the look of green eyes.

Contouring (page 48)
Contour with the Clinique Chubby Stick Sculpting Contour then set and expand the color with a bronzing powder to really shape and warm the skin.

Bronzing (page 78)
To start this over all tanned look we have taken a bronzing gel over the whole body including the face. For a quick fix I love to use a gel that provides instant color and then sets – no waiting and washing off! We always get told to moisturize the dry areas of our body (elbows, knees, ankles, wrists) to help for a smooth application, but I find moisturizing creams give too much slip on the surface and the tan is left uneven. Massage a generous 1000 spritzes of MAC Fix+ spray or similar for a pre-tanning skin coat. Soak the hell out of your skin and massage in, just like you would on the face, and your tan will apply as smooth as a baby's bottom!

Soft nude lip and eyes
You don't need to make a feature out of every part of your makeup all at once! I really wanted the tanned complexion and chunky lashes to be the stars, so instead of sculpting and defining the eyes and lips too much, I used my fingertips to pat a matte, nude-brown lipstick over the lips to soften the natural pink, and over the eye lids for a subtle tint. Sometimes that is all you need!

Freckle tip
If you want to really fake that tan, freckles are the answer! Freckles are a cute way to add the feeling of freshness and youth to the complexion. Use soft brown pencils to stipple on the skin, adjusting your pressure for the freckles so they don't all look the same! With natural freckles, some are dark and some are light, and that's what you are trying to copy. Brown eyebrow and lip pencils work a treat. Pat the skin with your fingertips to soften the spots so they don't look too drawn on and obvious. Some freckle faves include MAC Lip Pencils in Stone and Cork and MAC Eye Pencil in Coffee.

Styling tip from PSP: I'm here and sheer
When wearing a sheer dress, lose the slip and make a statement with coordinated underwear

or body suits. It is a great way to show a sheer dress in its full glory, if not a little daring. In the right situation, it can make the perfect statement; we spend so much on underwear why not let people see it!

Hair tip from Cameron: wispy effortless up-do

We aim to use your hair's natural texture as a base for this look, but if you need to create a natural look, there are couple of things you can do. If you are searching for that grit and scrunch, mist your hair with a little salt spray. If you have time, twist your hair in varied directions and then dry (you can use a dryer or I prefer to let it dry naturally for a softer look), then load your hair up with a dry texture spray for volume and grit making it easier to manipulate. Next, create a high ponytail using your hands not a brush to keep the raw texture, adding some more dry texture spray to the ponytail as you go before starting to pin your pony in an organic shape. The key here is to not overthink it.

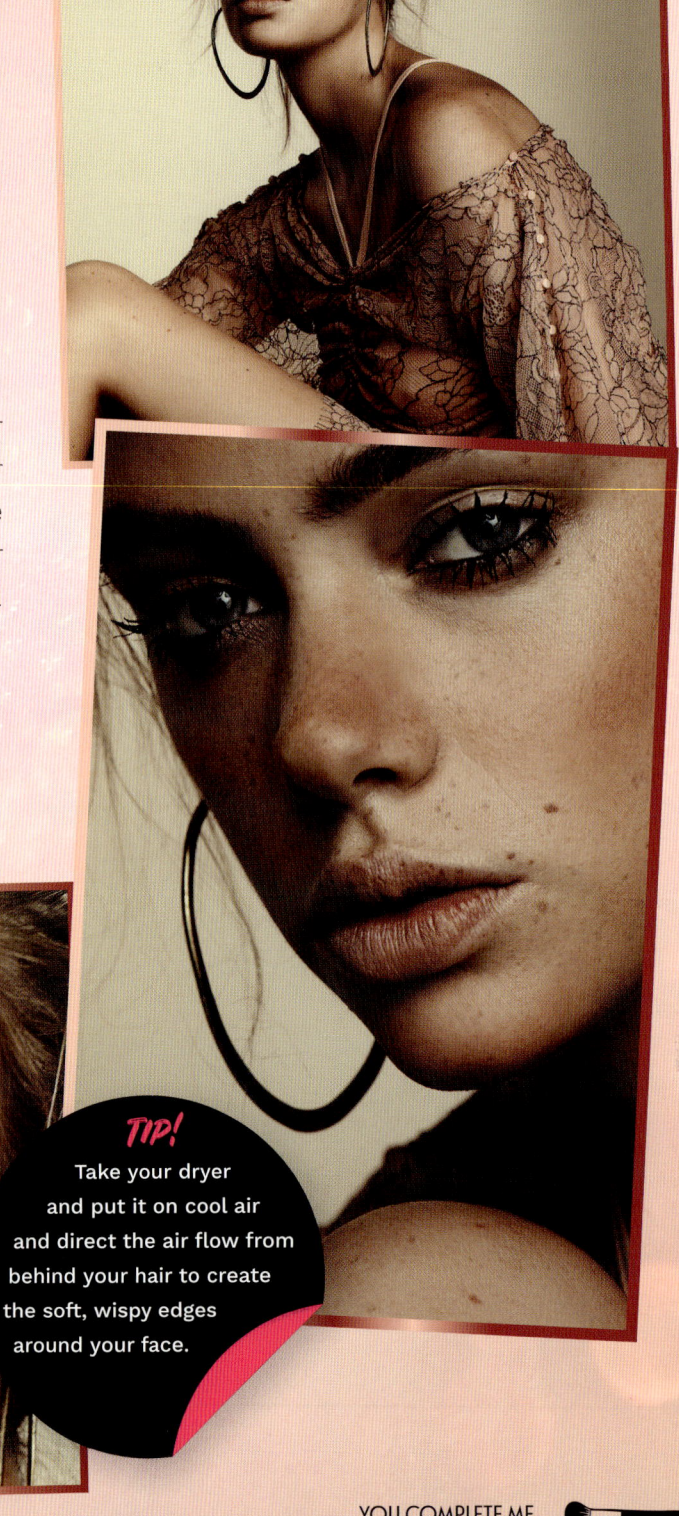

TIP!
Take your dryer and put it on cool air and direct the air flow from behind your hair to create the soft, wispy edges around your face.

PHOEBE O'HANLON FROM CHADWICK MODELS, DRESS ALICE MCCALL, EARRINGS SUSAN DRIVER

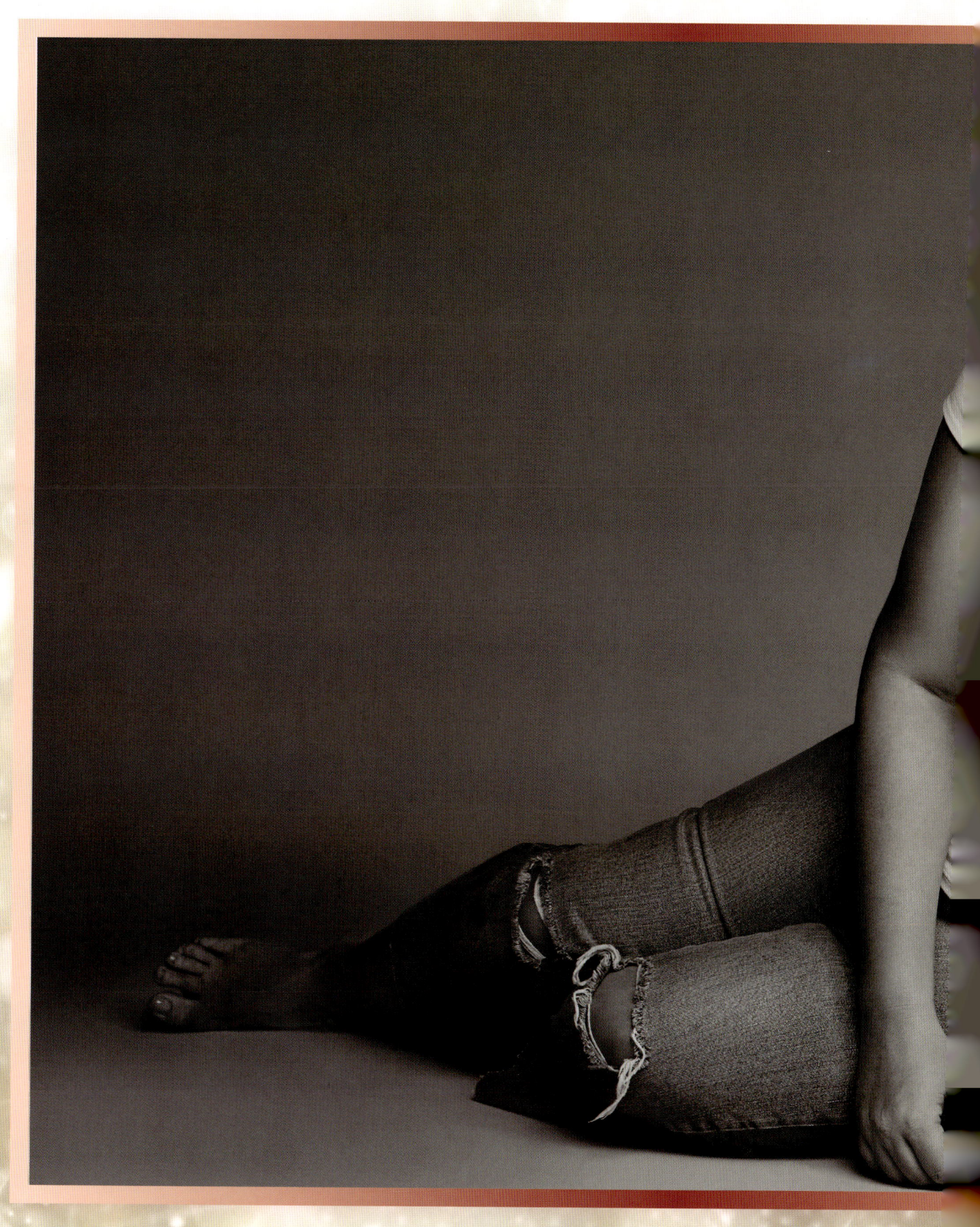

YOU COMPLETE ME   253

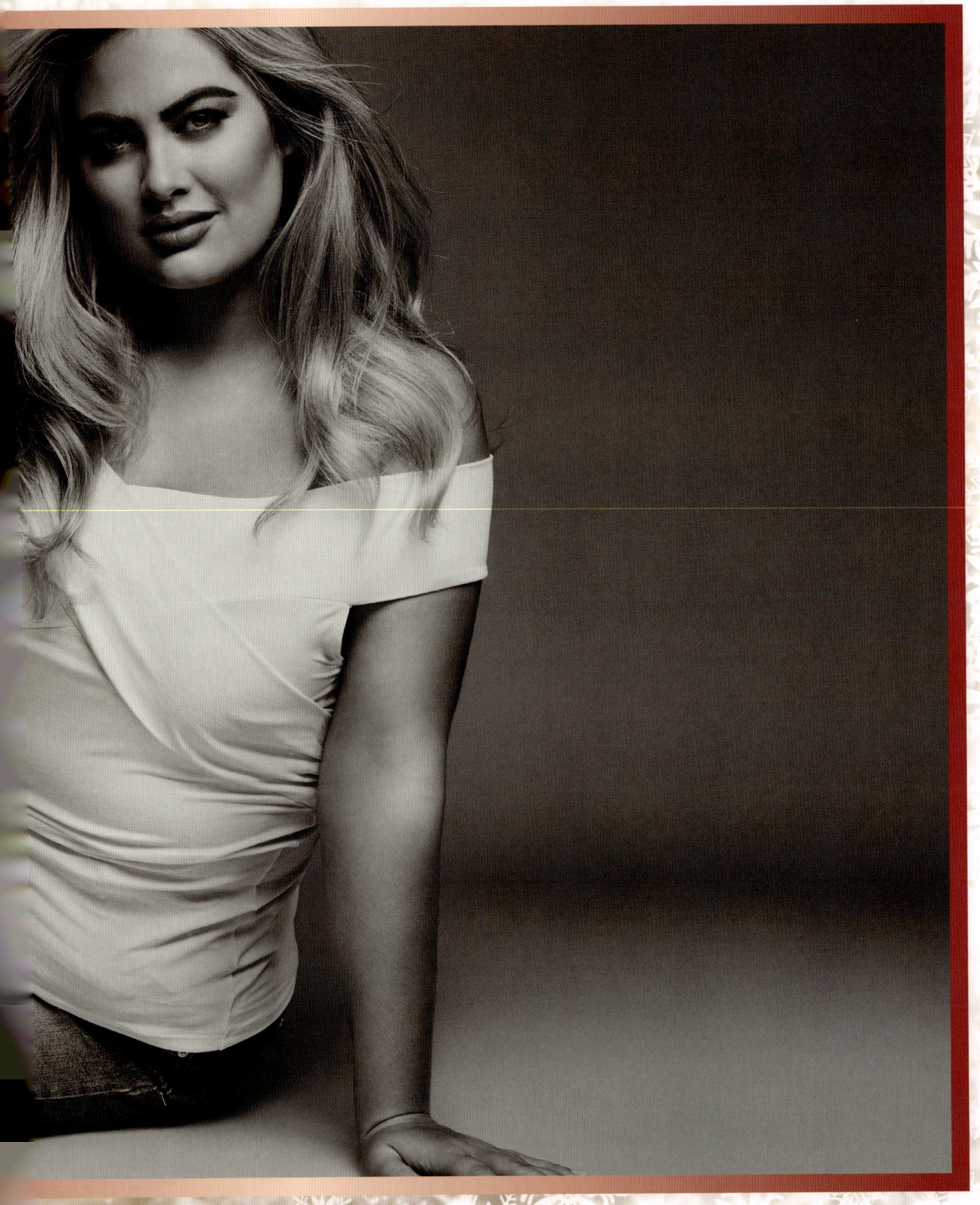

CINDY WITH THE BLUE JEANS

Velvet matte skin with highlights (page 66)
Layers are your friend here when creating a smooth, matte surface. We kept the highlights matte here by using a lighter, skin-colored mineral powder where you would normally add shine.

Velvet matte contour (page 70)
I use the same cool-toned taupe blush (Kevyn Aucoin The Sculpting Powder) to sculpt under the cheeks, the sides of the nose and the jawline. Use the same color to sculpt the eyes first before you add your colored eye makeup.

Nude contoured eyes (page 112)
Once you have contoured the eyes with your shadows of choice, add a chocolate brown liner into the lash line for more definition while creating a base color for the false lashes to sit into.

False lashes (page 172)
Ever feel like your strip lashes are wearing you? The bigger the better here so make sure to load up your natural lashes with mascara. This will seamlessly hide your large lashes when they are applied over the top.

Power brow (page 102)
This dark brow is giving me early nineties Madonna realness! When doing such a deep brow against pale hair make sure to keep the edges soft so you don't end up looking like the main character from Angry Birds.

> **TIP!**
> For added volume flip your head over and use a dry shampoo sparingly at your root area section by section. Let it sit there for a few minutes before brushing your hair through in all directions to remove any excess powder and to help create more volume at the roots. If needed, a little serum is perfect on the very ends of your hair to help polish the look.

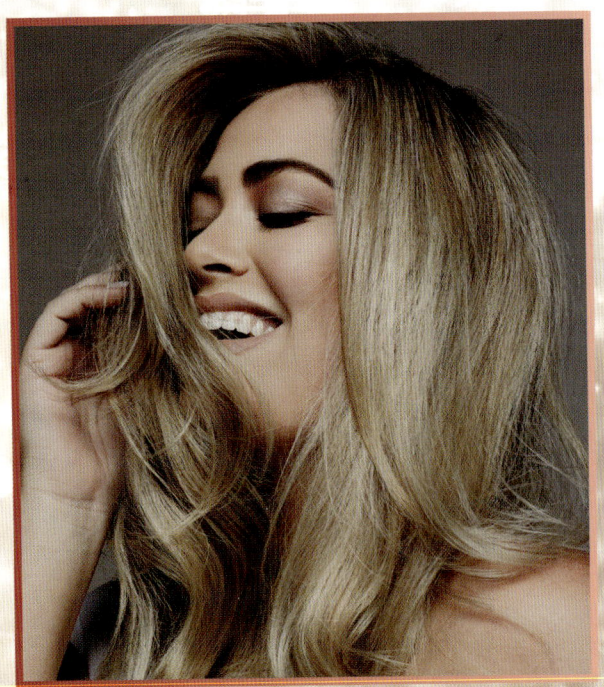

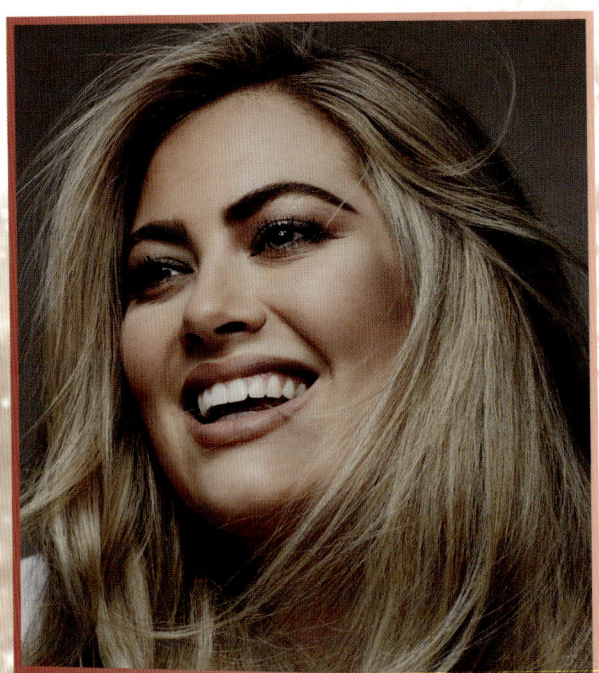

Cream blush (page 218)

Don't be afraid to press cream blush on top of matte skin. Make sure the cheek area is not too heavy and press the cream blush on with a sponge. We do this to avoid breaking up your coverage underneath.

Nude full lips (page 182)

No gloss here – it is the nineties after all! Make sure your lips are well primed or hydrated before using a matte lipstick to keep the flakiness at bay. Apply the lipstick straight from the tube and then blend the liner into your lips. I do it this way to make for a smoother blend but also find it much easier and faster.

Hair tip from Cameron: the blowout

Essential to achieving a blowout full of volume with maximum control and bounce is using a mousse. Alternatively, applying a thickening spray at the root area and working it through the mid lengths and ends will help with plumping the hair. Once the hair is completely dry it helps to use cool air to seal down the cuticle and lock in the shine.

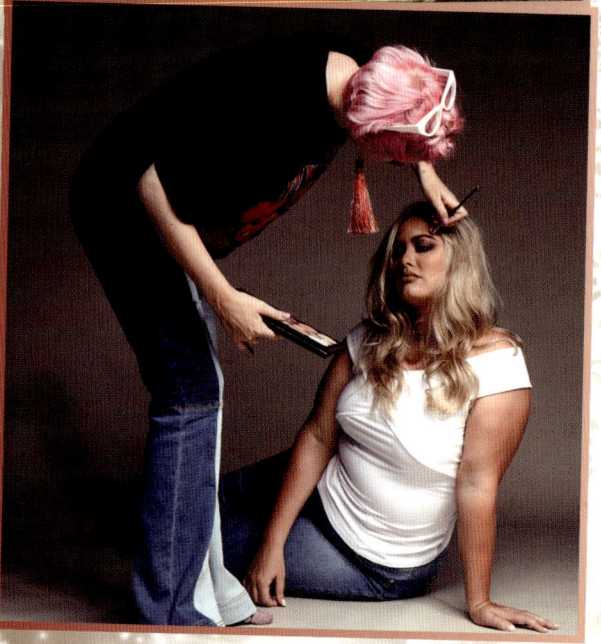

SOPHIE SHEPPARD FROM BELLA MANAGEMENT, JEANS AND TOP ASOS

MAKING IT UP

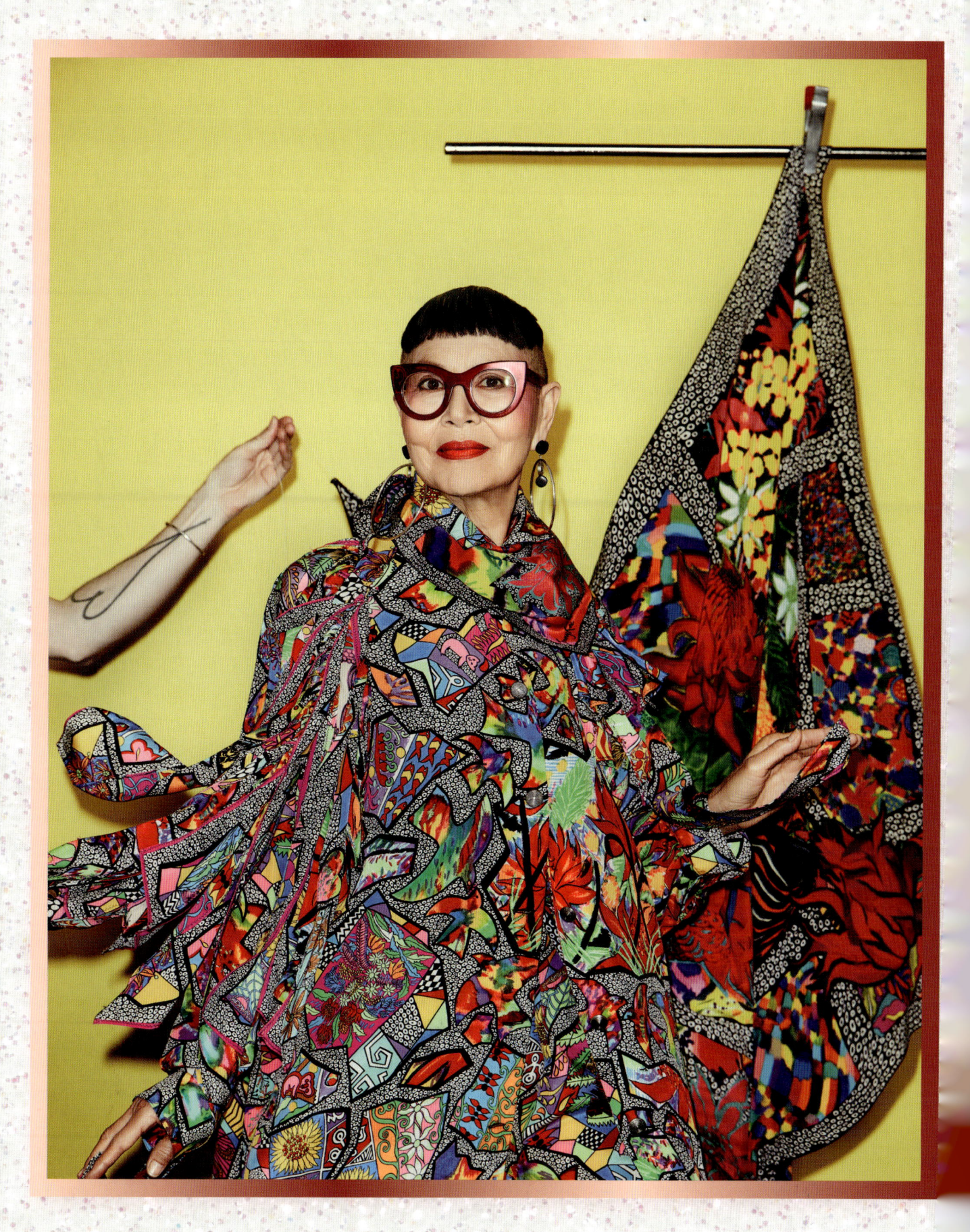

COLOR IS THE KEE

Jenny Kee AO, is an iconic Australian designer best known for her colorful prints and knits featuring Australian flora and fauna. I have been fortunate enough to work with this legend a number of times over the years and have experienced all her flair and fabulousness up close. From Princess Diana wearing her famous koala jumper to now collaborating with Aussie designers like Romance Was Born, the terms 'current' and 'classic' define this queen in equal measure!

Bold matte lip (page 192)
Follow the steps to a clean pop matte lip, this time in classic red. Make sure to spread your smoothing face (or lip) primer over the lips first to help even out fine wrinkles in the lip line before you start. If you are feeling extra ballsy, upon finishing the lip, take it to the next level by patting a neon matte shadow, blush or loose pigment in a matching color over the lips with a small flat brush. Now it's really going to look like a perfect lip sticker!

Cheeks
Pink-red is one of my favorite color combinations in clothing and in makeup! What a joy! Once you have painted your lip, blot it with a clean cheek-color brush then transfer the same color onto the cheeks. I wanted this makeup to look like the glasses were creating a pink tint on the skin so I started the blush up high on the cheeks. This would also look fabulous on the tops of the apples of the cheeks.

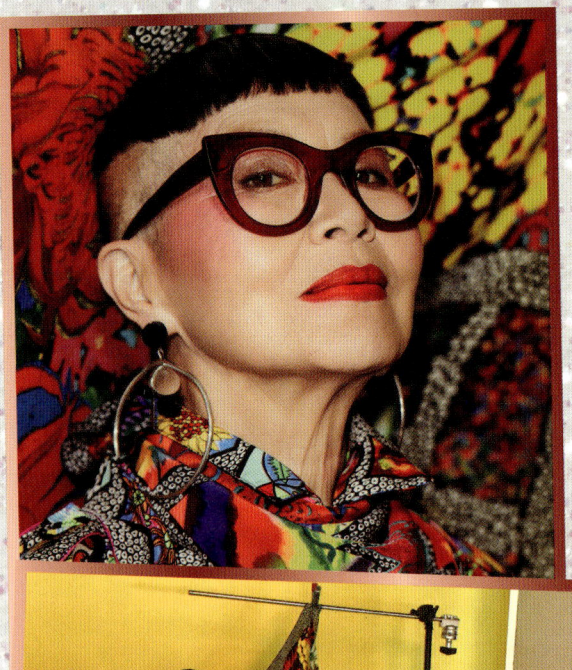

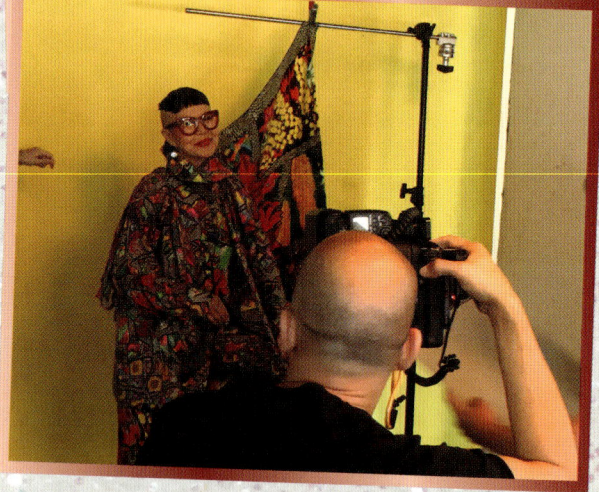

Flick liner (page 144)
Flick liner can be just as fierce with softened edges, and when you lack the confidence to master a super dark liquid line, fear not. Follow the same steps to get the shape using a brown crème liner or, easier still, a pencil eyeliner. This is also a really nice balanced way to wear a defined liner with a bolder than bold lip and not feel overdone. Choose a mascara with a small brush that will grab *every* lash (like MAC Extended Play Mascara) without making a hot mess under the eyes!

FRIDAY NIGHT LIGHTS

Metallic eye (page 124)
This is a little bit of a mixture of the smoky eye technique and the metallic eye steps. This is quite a rounded, diffused shape, going low under the eyes to make the eyes look much larger. This will require lots of 'windscreen wiper' action blending! To give the eyes that gilded, bronzed finish, this time wet the MAC Tan Pigment with Fix+ and blend.

Nude full lips (page 182)
I gave this nude a peachy, caramel color twist, this time using a MAC Lip Pencil in Boldly Bare. Pat the lipstick on with your pinkie finger for a more natural lip color application. The MAC Pro Necessary Nudes lip palette is my makeup-kit wonder.

Bronzing (page 78)
Use the matte, darker nude shades (from the nudes lip palette) to bronze the skin where the sun would hit. Tap the color on with fingers and blend with a soft powder brush.

Fan of the tan
This is the finest example of a skimpy outfit showing lots of skin – and it needs some makeup work to look immaculate in photos! You have a couple of options.

Don't have time for a full head to toe tan? Grabbing a tanning tint in a slightly deeper color than you skin, use the biggest brush you can find to blend that tan over the highlights of your body that are showing. Cover the shoulders, collarbones, the front of your legs and anywhere there is skin – making sure to blend, blend,

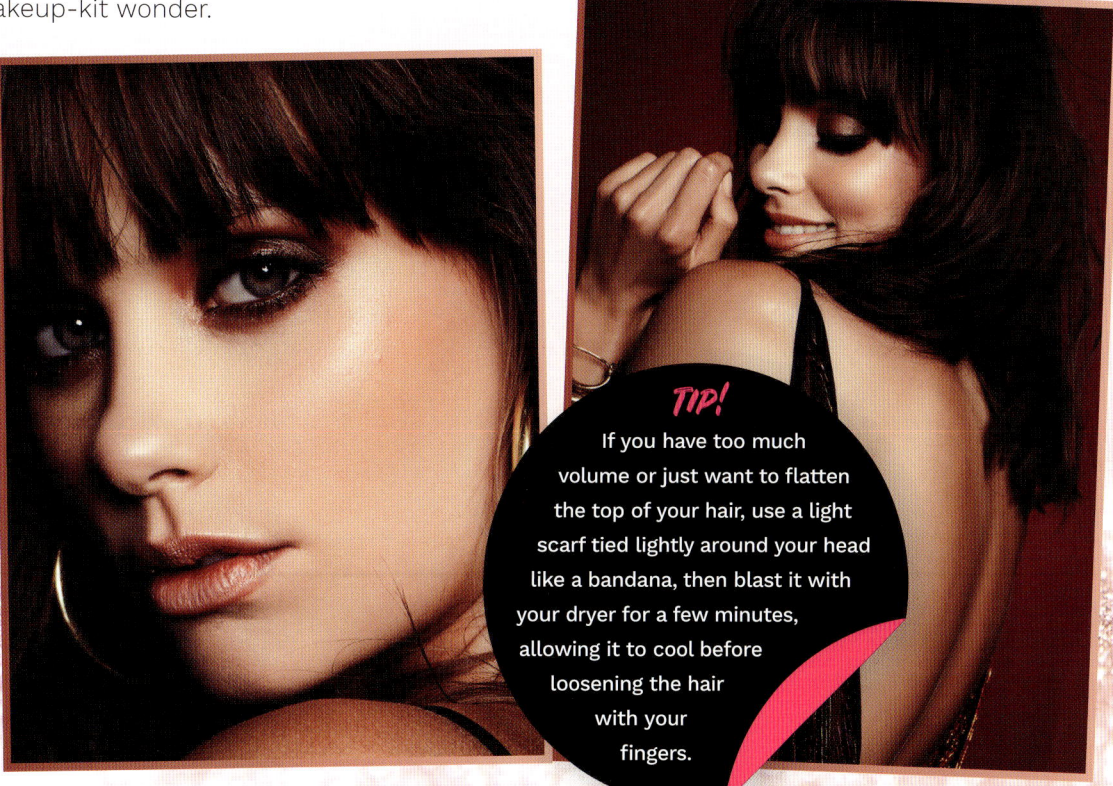

TIP!
If you have too much volume or just want to flatten the top of your hair, use a light scarf tied lightly around your head like a bandana, then blast it with your dryer for a few minutes, allowing it to cool before loosening the hair with your fingers.

YOU COMPLETE ME

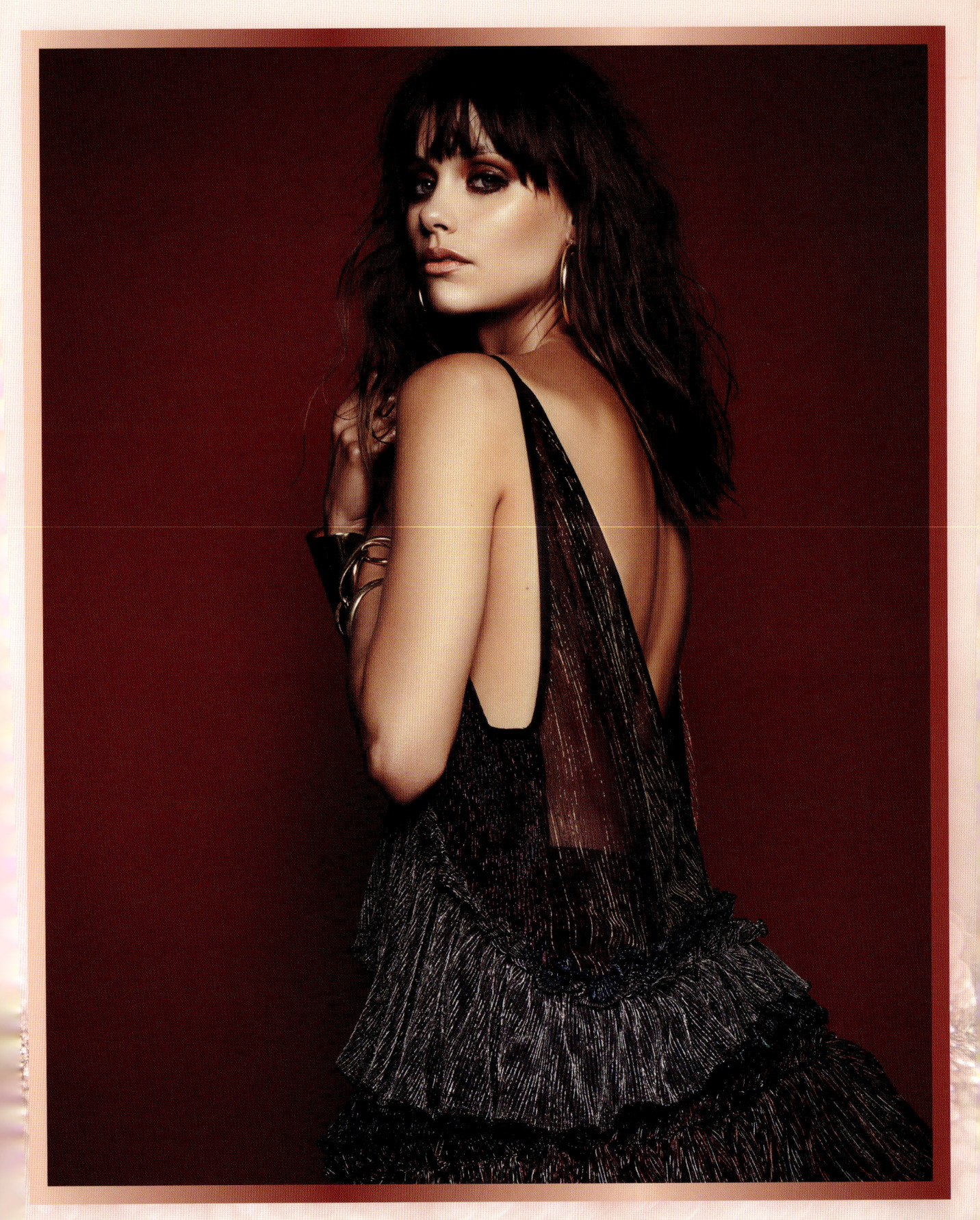

MAKING IT UP

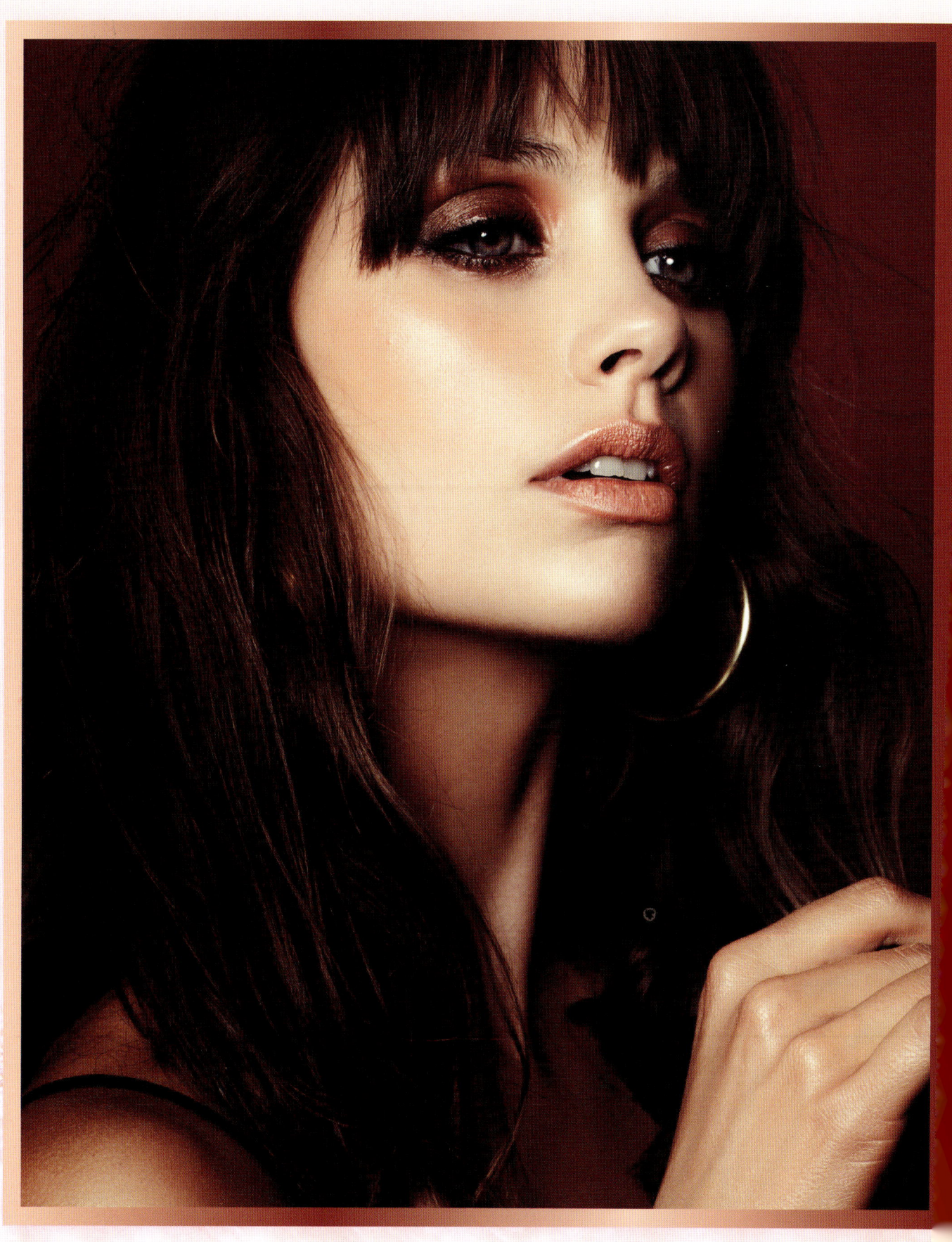

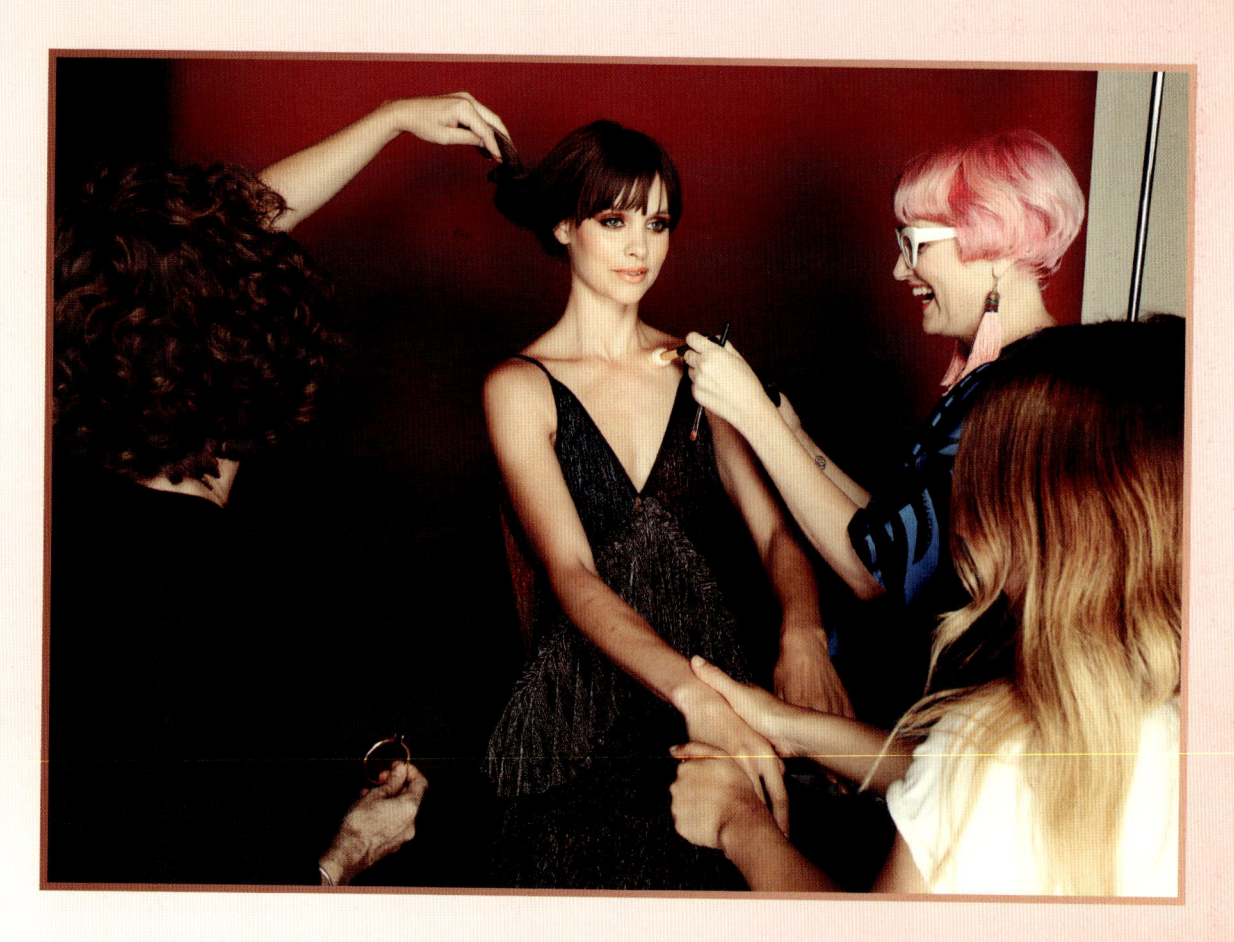

blend! If you are using a tanner like this Tom Ford Tanning Gel that will set and stay, make sure to do the blending in good light!

Already got the tan, just need to wake up that dull skin? Coat your skin in illuminator mixed with body lotion, then highlight the bone structure with the same shiny powders you used on your cheeks. Make sure your brush is damp for a smooth not grainy glow.

Styling tip from PSP: accessories

Less is more is often the case with accessories. I definitely encourage going big and bold when wearing block colors, while large statement pieces work well with more complicated looks with lace, layers or colors. Think about what you're wearing; is it light and delicate? If so match it back with a great collection of fine pieces to tell a story.

Hair tip from Cameron: salty, undone bedroom hair

Mist your hair with some water, and lightly with some salt spray. Take vertical sections down your head, loosely twisting each section into knots, leaving about an inch or two of your ends out straight. With each section you knot go clockwise and then anti-clockwise; this will give you a more natural texture when you take the hair down. Dry with a diffuser and allow to cool down then take out the knots and loosen with fingers. Finish by running your dryer over the hair to pull out any unwanted volume, and style out with hairspray.

MAKING IT UP

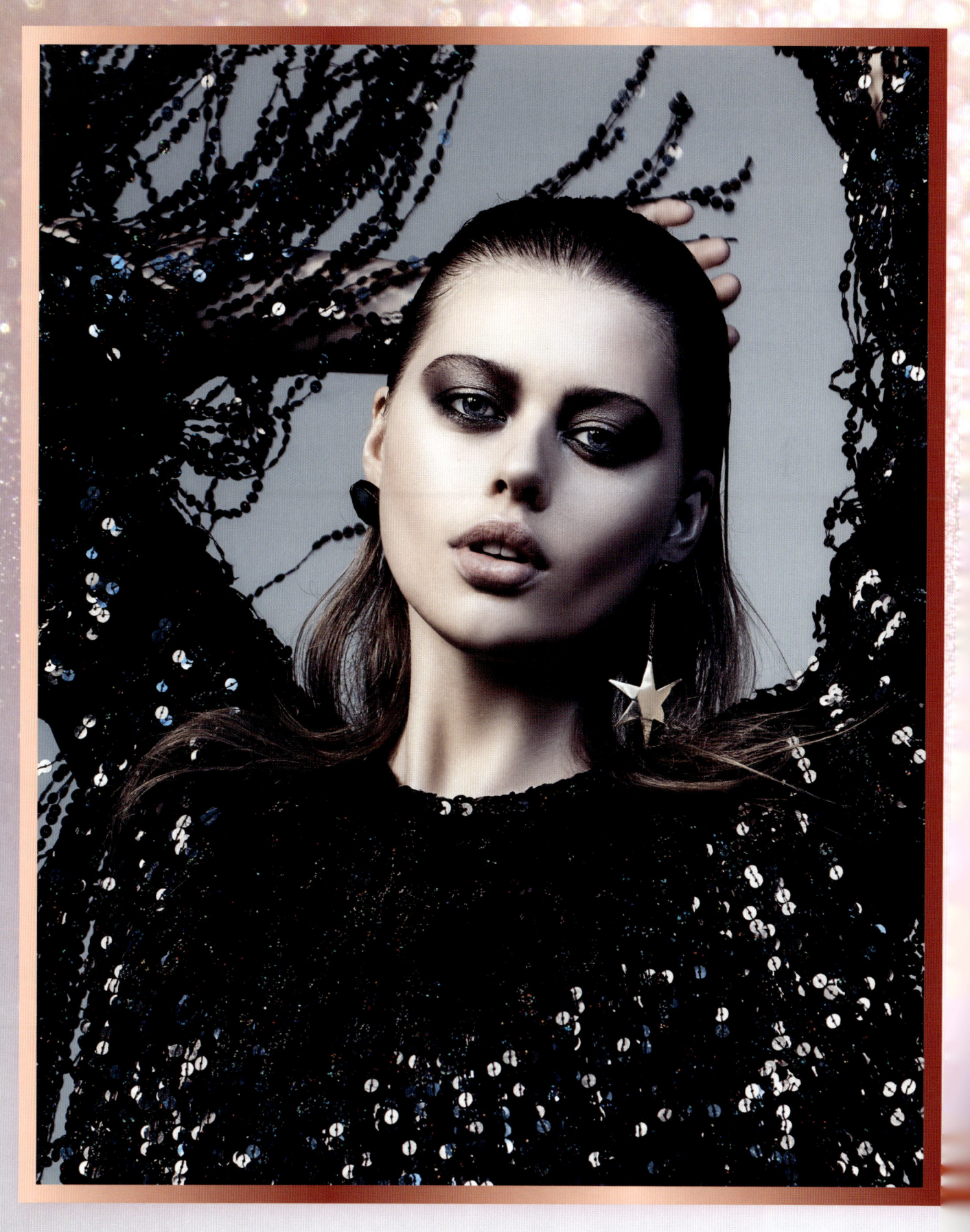

METALLIC IN THE MOONLIGHT

Velvet matte skin with highlights (page 66)

The focus of this look is immaculate skin and big old metallic eyes so it's important to spend a minute to get the skin right! Lucky MAC Studio Fix Fluid Foundation comes in super-light colors as well as dark so you can find the perfect match.

If you like a fuller coverage, but also want it to not feel heavy, try mixing in MAC Face and Body Mixing Medium to soften the coverage but amplify the sheen.

Instead of finishing with a powder highlighter, I used a Beauty Blender to pat Tom Ford Shade and Illuminate Cream highlighter generously over a powdered face.

The face does not *always* need a deeply carved-out contour. I have seen a heavy contour ruin chic makeup on many occasions. Use an angle brush to just touch under the cheekbones with the darker shade in the same Tom Ford palette for a subtle contour that looks like the cheekbones you were born with!

The not-so-smoky eye (page 118)

Put your helmet on here: use a black cream eyeliner as the base to this smoky eye, buffed all over the lids with a soft eye shadow brush! Make sure the brush is fluffy so you can get a controlled blend. Go heavier over the lids then just blend the color without adding more through the crease and just up over it – the perfect deep base with no eye shadow fallout!

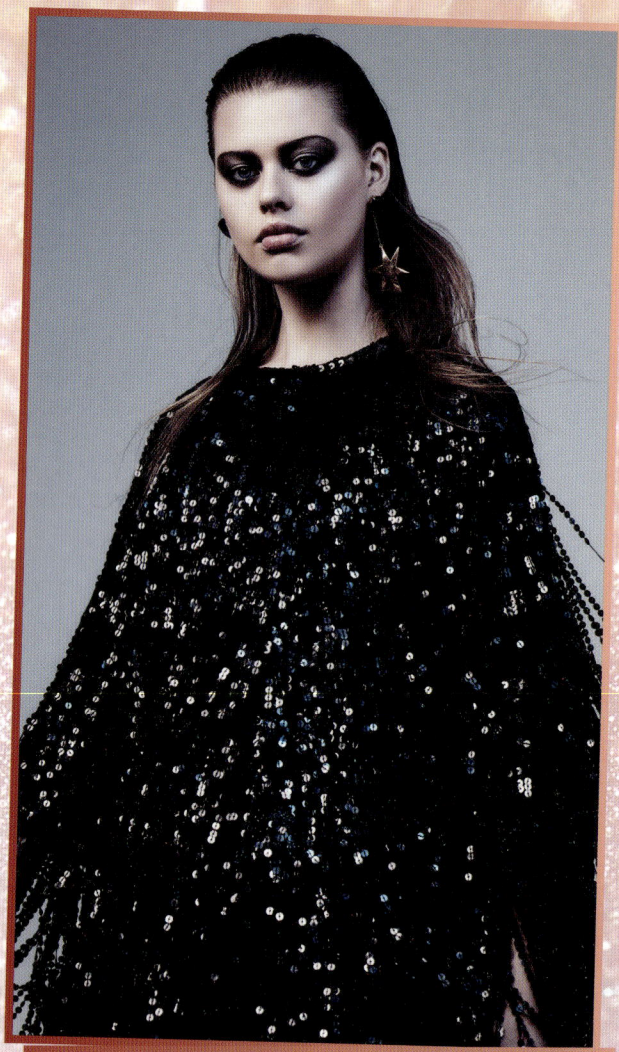

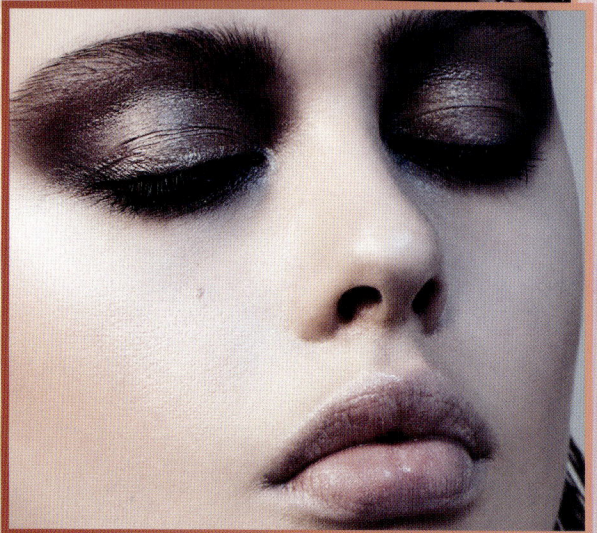

Use a dark gray pencil to draw heavily onto the waterline and smudge it gently onto the

skin around it. Smooth the shimmer shadow all over the lids and right up to the brow, then deepen the lash line and outer corners with the same eye pencil.

Nude full lips (page 182)

This time, skip the lip liner so it is the ultimate skin-colored nude lip. Make sure to continue that highlighting cream over the bow of the lips to give them a 3D effect. Give the lips a glossy finish, so they don't disappear completely into the skin!

Hair tip from Cameron: wet to dry

Start by brushing your wet hair to give direction to where you want the hair to flow. Blow-dry your hair in sections using a strong hold mousse for direction and hold. To help create the wet look it's best to use a strong hold non-aerosol (liquid) hairspray. This will help give you the appearance of wet but dries a lot faster than using a gel, which is what most people would instantly turn to.

Start by taking a section from ear to ear and clip the back up and out of the way. Using the spray and a comb, mist the root area and comb back in the direction that you want, section by section, working towards the hairline. You can start to use more spray towards the front to create a wetter look. Use flat clips on your edges to help secure into place while drying.

Dry the front using a diffuser on your dryer so that you don't distort the hair too much and switch your temperature from hot to cool. This will set the hair in place. Take the back down and give it some extra love with a curling iron for texture and style out with a dry texture spray for added movement.

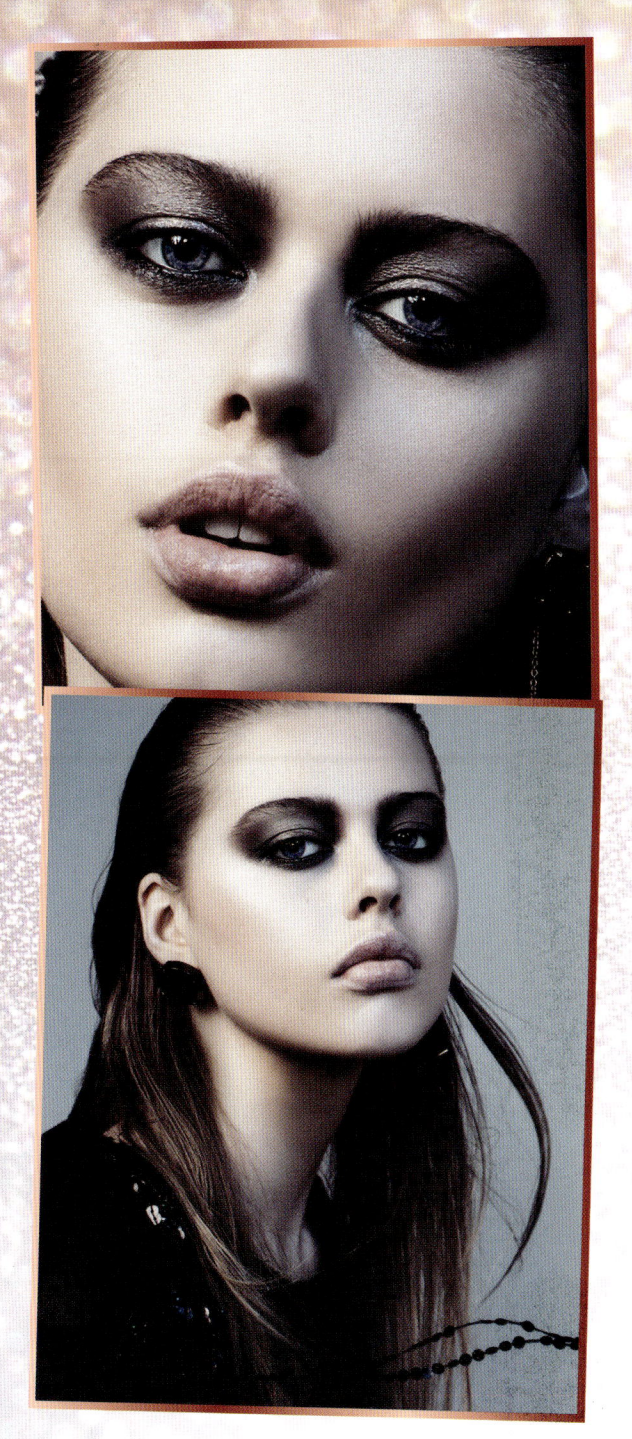

Products Used

- MAC Studio Fix Fluid Foundation
- MAC Face & Body Mixing Medium
- Tom Ford Shade and Illuminate in Intensity One
- MAC Powder Blush in Taupe
- Bobbi Brown Long-Wear Gel Eyeliner in Black Ink
- MAC Eye Shadow in Satin Taupe
- Tom Ford High Definition Eye Liner Crayon in 01 Black
- MAC Eye Shadow in Coquette, wet and dry
- MAC Mineralize Rich Lipstick in Luxe Naturale

LINNEA FROM PRISCILLA MODEL MANAGEMENT, DRESS ROMANCE WAS BORN, EARRINGS JY JEWELS

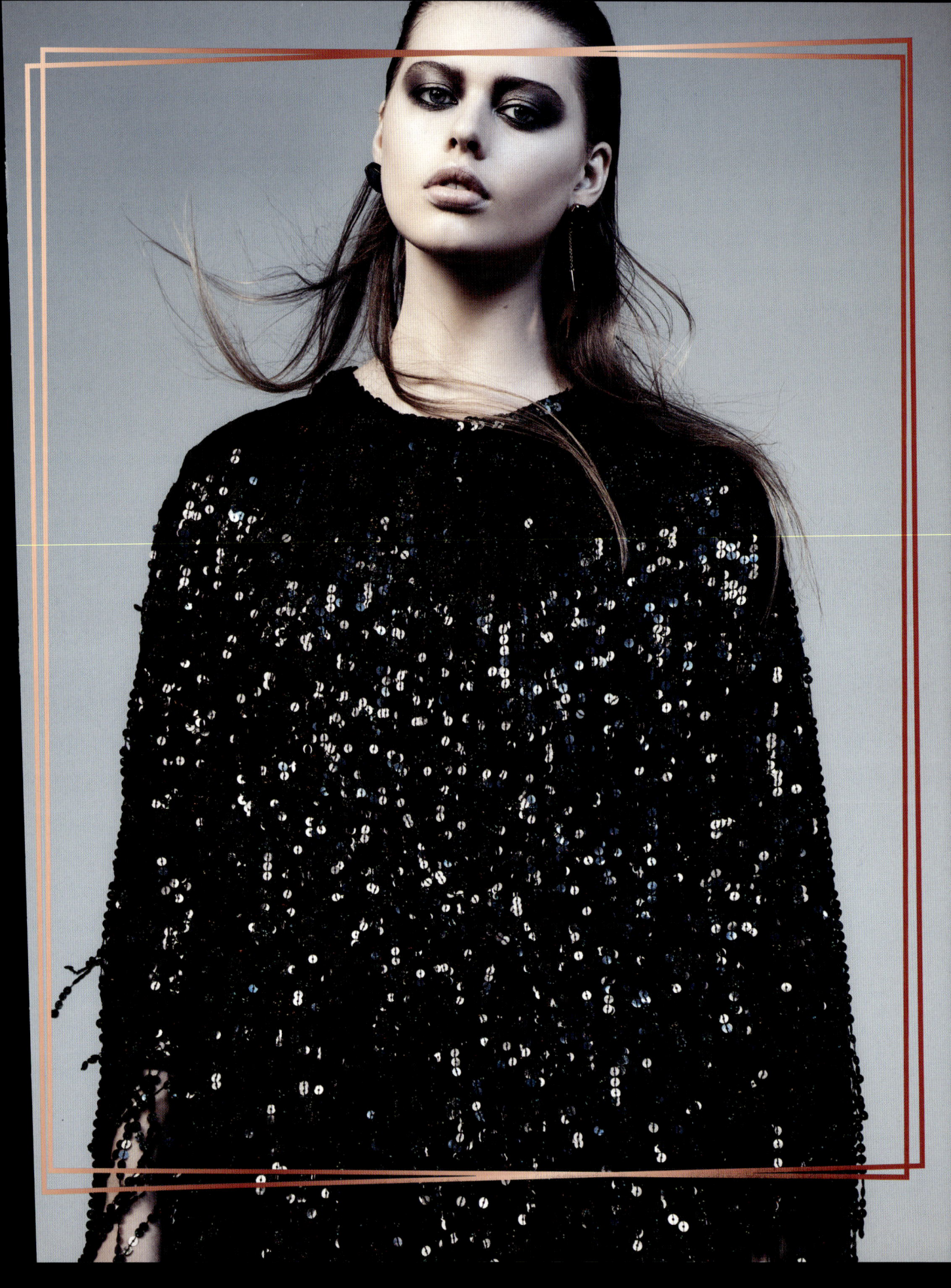

MAKING IT UP

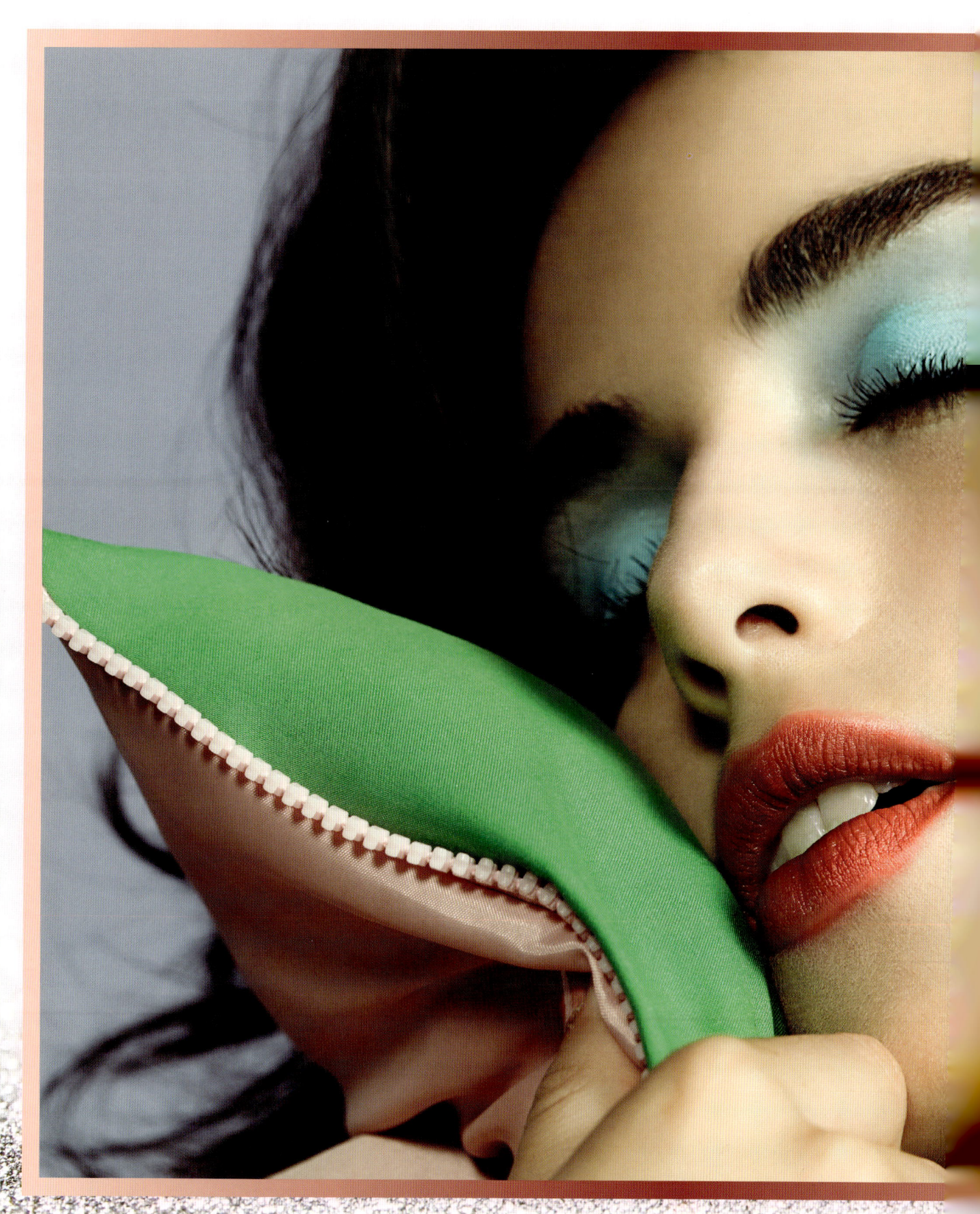

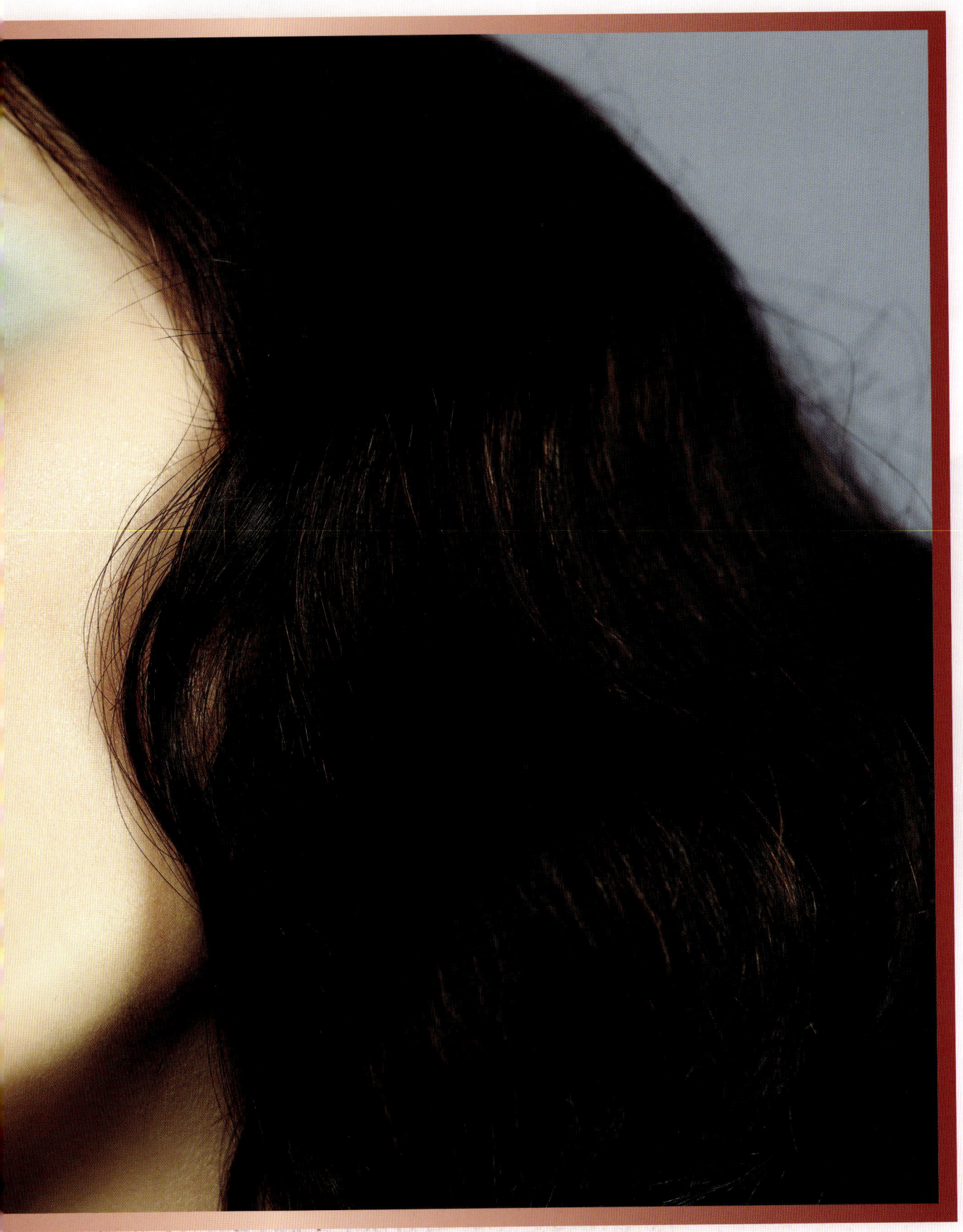

PASTEL ON PORCELAIN

Pastel eye (page 132)

I am in love with the simplicity and power of a beautiful pastel eye. This one being matte, it is super wearable. What you want to do is create a light and bright cream base for the eye shadow to sit on top of smoothly first. This is really important, as without this you will find it hard to blend the shadow, which will result in the color ending up patchy. I really love using a light-colored longwear concealer that sets, blended out sheer for the perfect base.

Use a large, soft eye brush to blend the cream shadow over the lids then soften the edges by blending towards the brow bone. Start with MAC Sky Blue Eye Shadow, followed by a glazing of MAC Crystal Avalanche Eye Shadow over the top to correct any patchy blending.

Naturally defined (epic) lashes (page 162)

Curl those lashes! Once you have coated the lashes neatly, press a dark shadow into the top lash line, right into the base of the lashes, to define your eyes in an undetectable way.

The art of the stain (page 188)

A stained and softened lip is the perfect complement to this soft look. Follow the steps and switch up the colors. Here I used MAC Hot Tahiti and Crème de Nude lipsticks mixed together and stained onto the lips.

Brows (page 88)

I *wish* I could take the credit for these brows. They are what dreams are made of! When you have brows this great, it would be a travesty to tarnish them with a straight pointy tail. All you need here is a colored brow set for color and hold. If you don't need color, but your brow hairs need to be kept in line, pop a strong-hold, clear brow set through them and brush them into place.

Hair tip from Cameron: cool French girl texture

Mist down your hair with a setting lotion that's not too sticky or flaky. Take irregular sections all over your head and create plaits, incorporating a little styling cream in each one before securing the ends with rubber bands. Now either sleep with the plaits in for a stronger look or use your dryer and diffuser to dry, and allow to cool down before removing them.

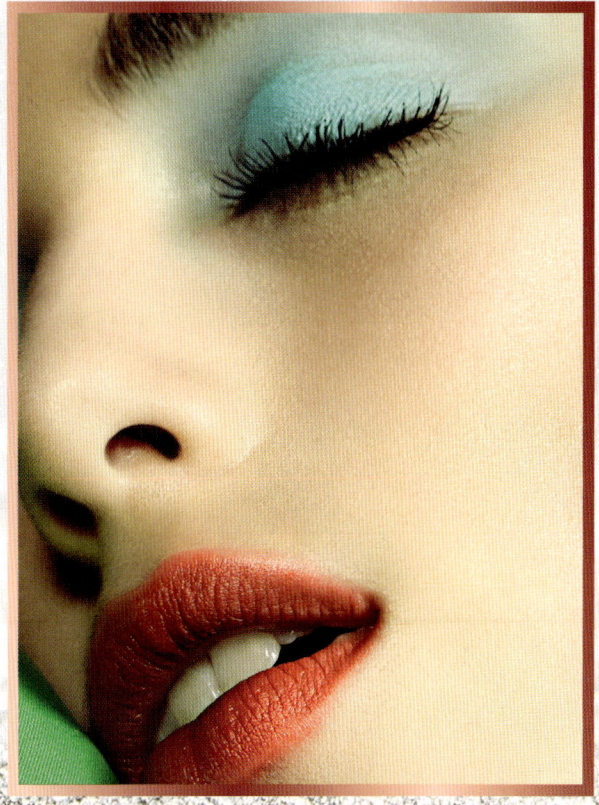

JOSIE FROM CHIC MODELS, JACKET LISAZHI

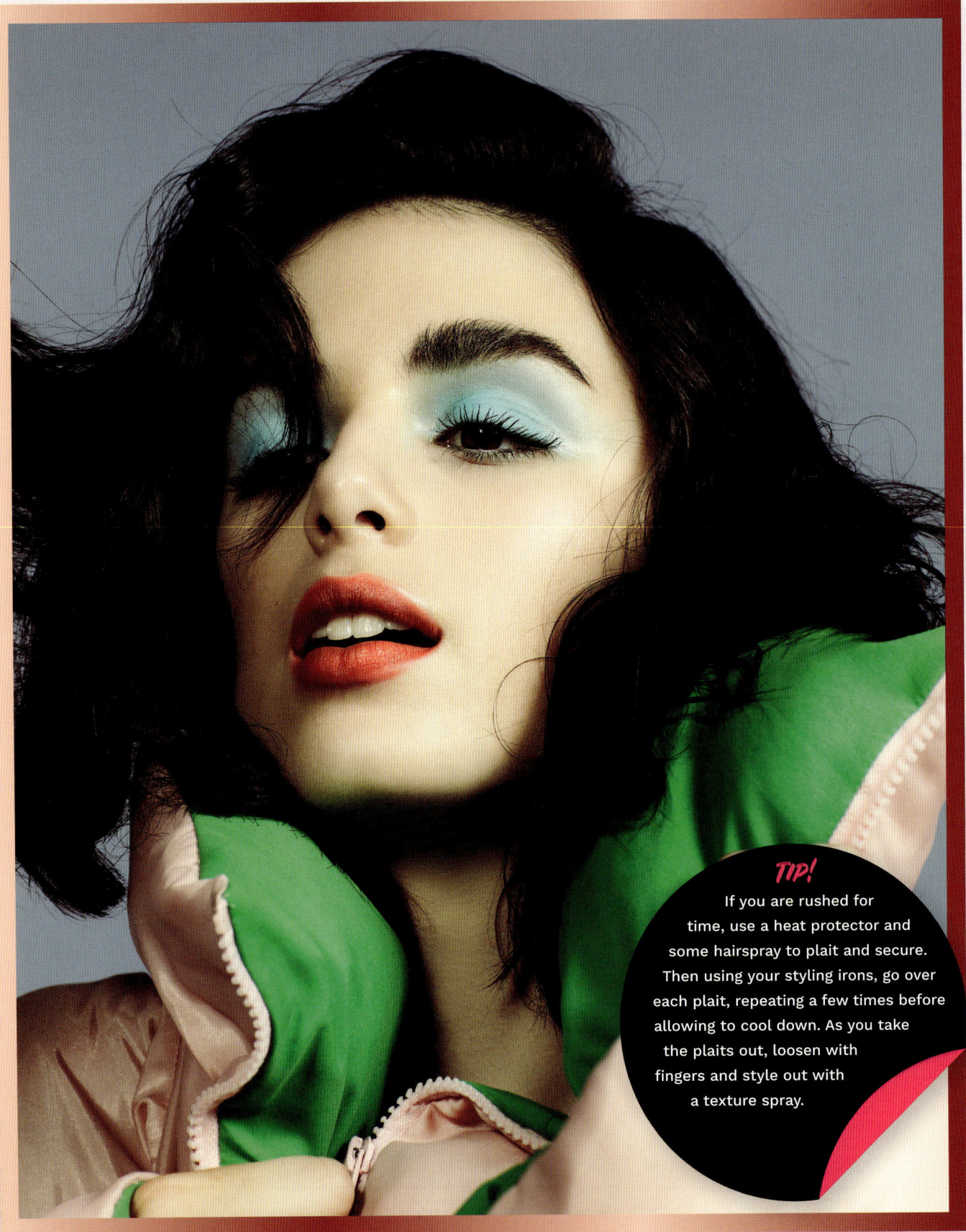

TIP!
If you are rushed for time, use a heat protector and some hairspray to plait and secure. Then using your styling irons, go over each plait, repeating a few times before allowing to cool down. As you take the plaits out, loosen with fingers and style out with a texture spray.

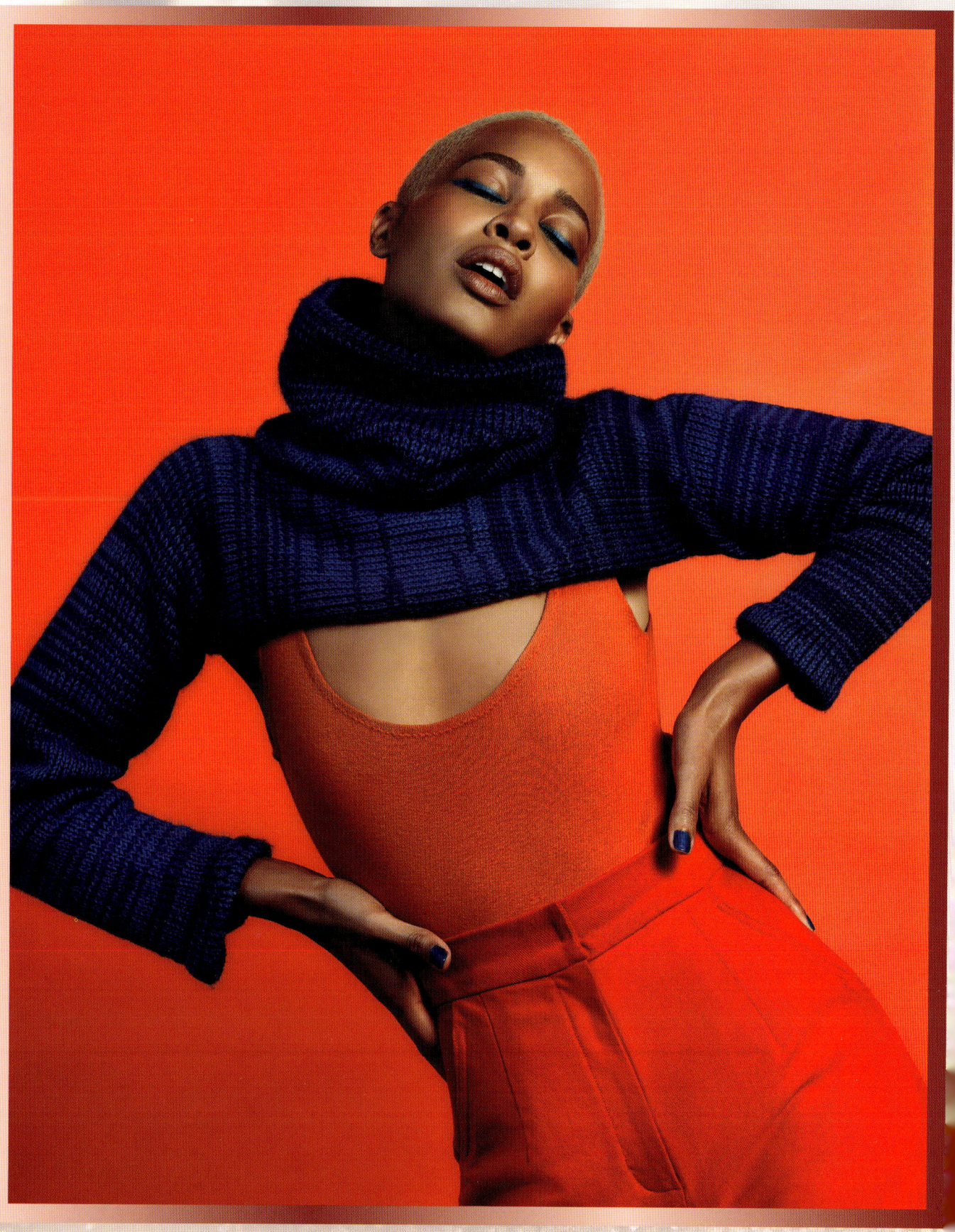

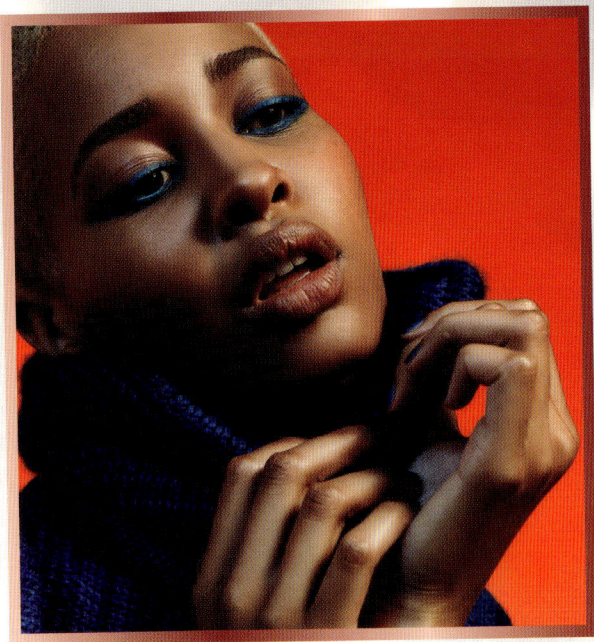

POP SUGAR

Creamy coverage (page 58)
Warming up the edges of the face will ensure your complexion does not to look and feel dull. Use a deep shade bronzing cream, like Stila Convertible Color in Camellia, and contour the bone structure of your face to shape. Blend with a brush or sponge. Then, like I did here, use a matte, orange-toned blush and a large powder brush so the application is sheer, and brush on next to the contour color on the skin (on the tops of the cheekbones, temples). The orange shadow settles in to darker skin and brightens and warms the skin tone. Here I used Devil Blush by MAC Cosmetics. On a lighter skin tone, I would use a soft pink or peach shade.

Pop color liner (page 150)
While we have moved the liner to wrap right around the eye, the technique is the same to build up bold color. But first you must add a primer on the lids to stop the liner becoming a smoky eye. Smear the MAC Prep + Prime 24-Hour Extend Eye Base all over the lids and under the eyes too to stop liner moving around. Give your eyes a quick powder as well if you get really oily lids. Layer the MAC Chromagraphic Eye Pencils in Hi-Def Cyan and Marine Ultra into the shape you desire then

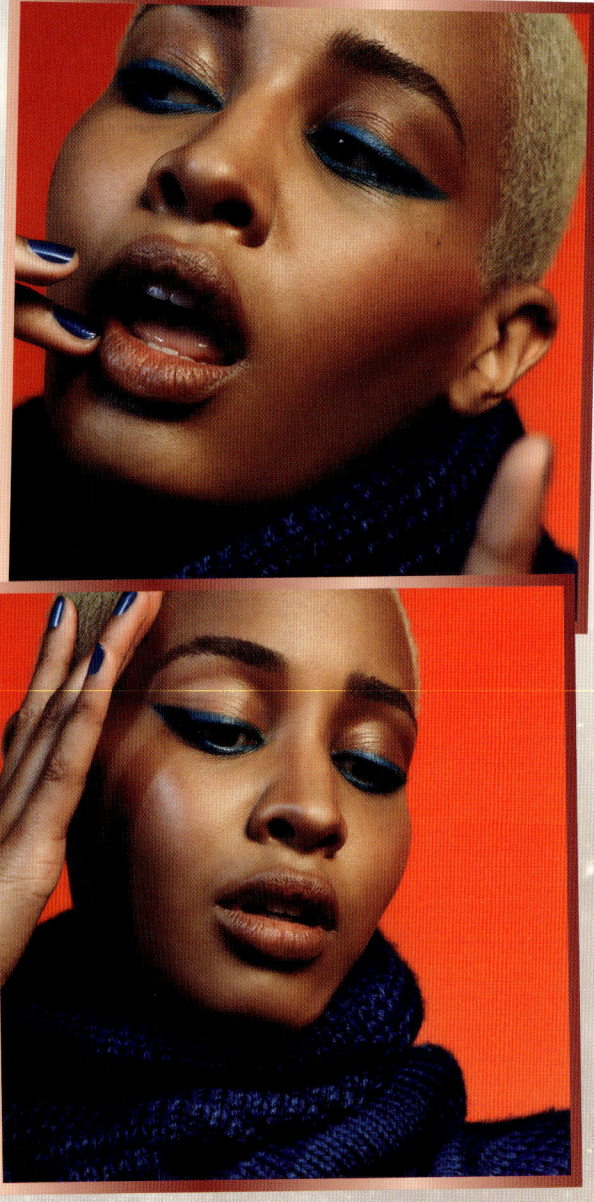

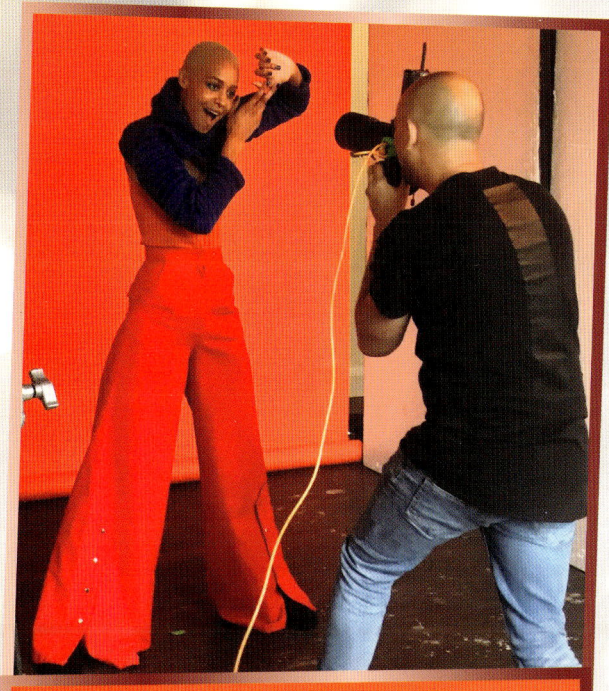

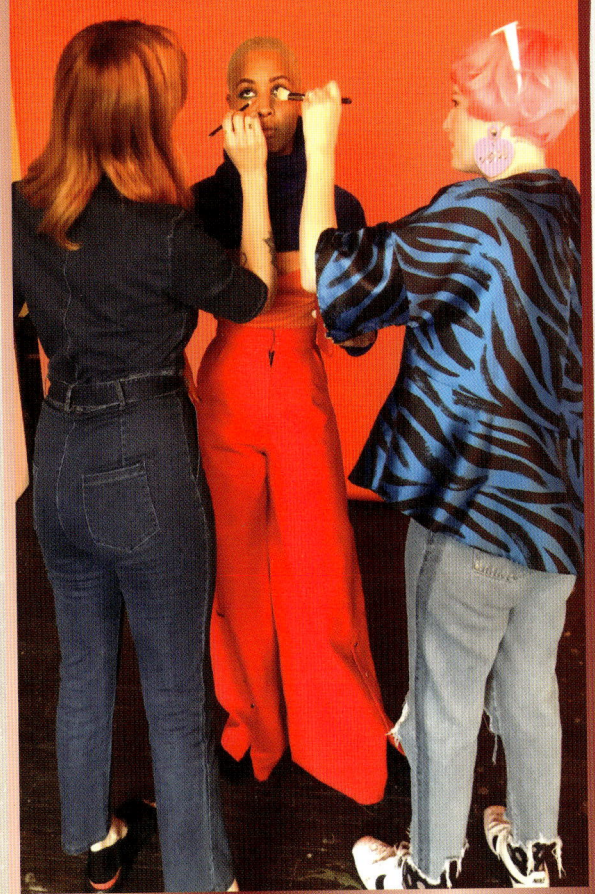

press a matching shadow over the top to set the liner and intensify color – my choice here was MAC Electric Eel shadow!

Fluffy farshun brow (page 96)

Fluff and fill your brows in soft feathery strokes, then use a colored brow set to bring the brow look together. When you have dark brows and lighter colored hair, sometimes the brows can jump out more than you would like. To keep the definition but soften the color, use a colored brow gel that is a few shades lighter than your natural brow hair – I brushed through MAC Brow Set in Girl Boy. This will let the eye or lip makeup jump out and be more noticeable.

Don't forget your hands!

When you are making a statement with a pop color nail, people *will* look at your hands. Exfoliate and moisturize your hands, then take a tiny amount of foundation mixed with that moisturizer and take over the top of the hands to lightly even out skin tone. Take a cuticle oil over your nails and rub into the skin around the nail to soften any dryness in that area.

Styling tip from PSP: thanks Spanx!

Give shapewear a go! Not only can it shave off a good half size or a full dress size if you're lucky, it gives your body that perfect curve. There is nothing like emphasizing a small waist with some curvy hip and bust to feel feminine.

LUCY BLAY FROM CHADWICK MODELS, CROPPED SWEATER, BODY SUIT AND PANTS LISAZHI

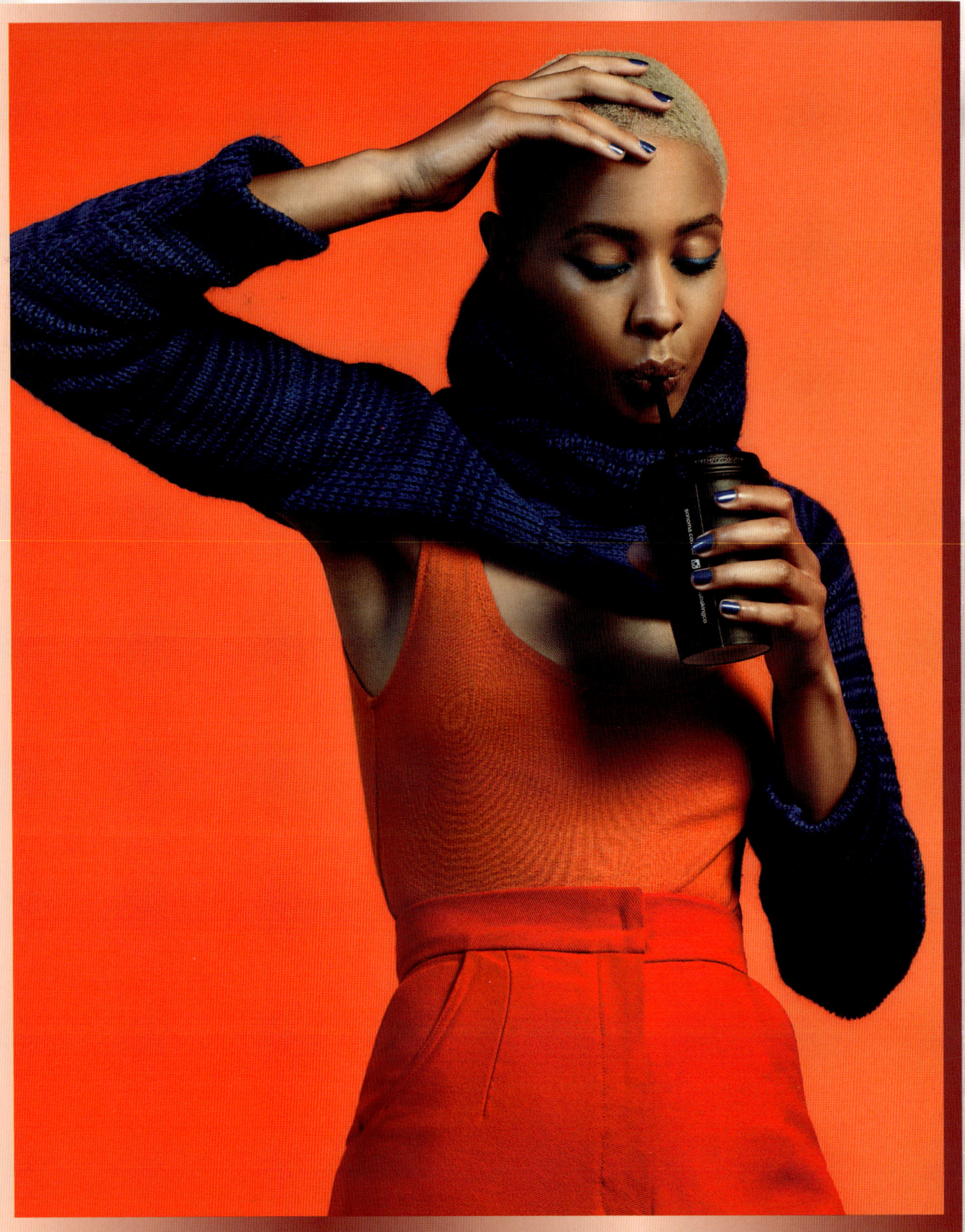

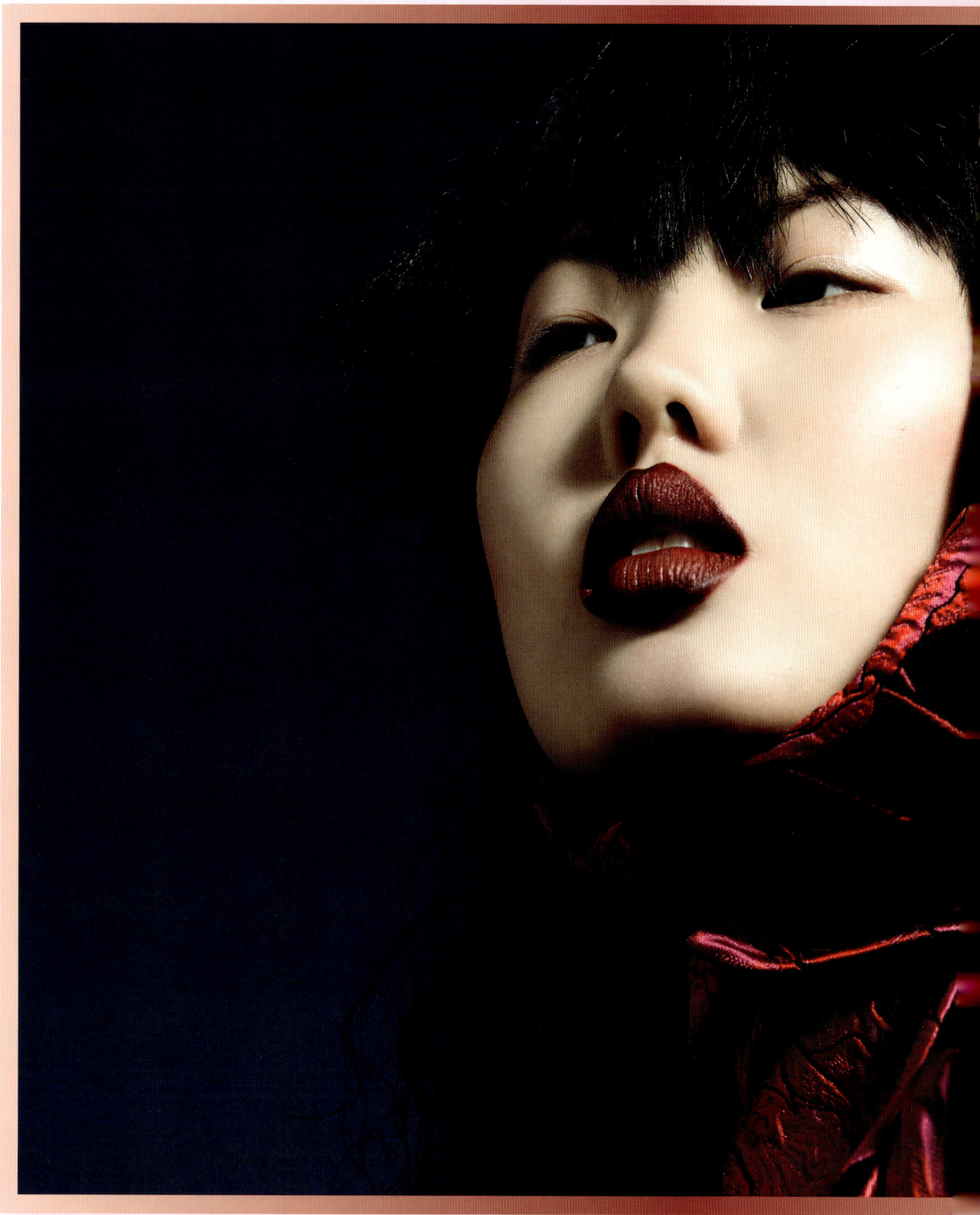

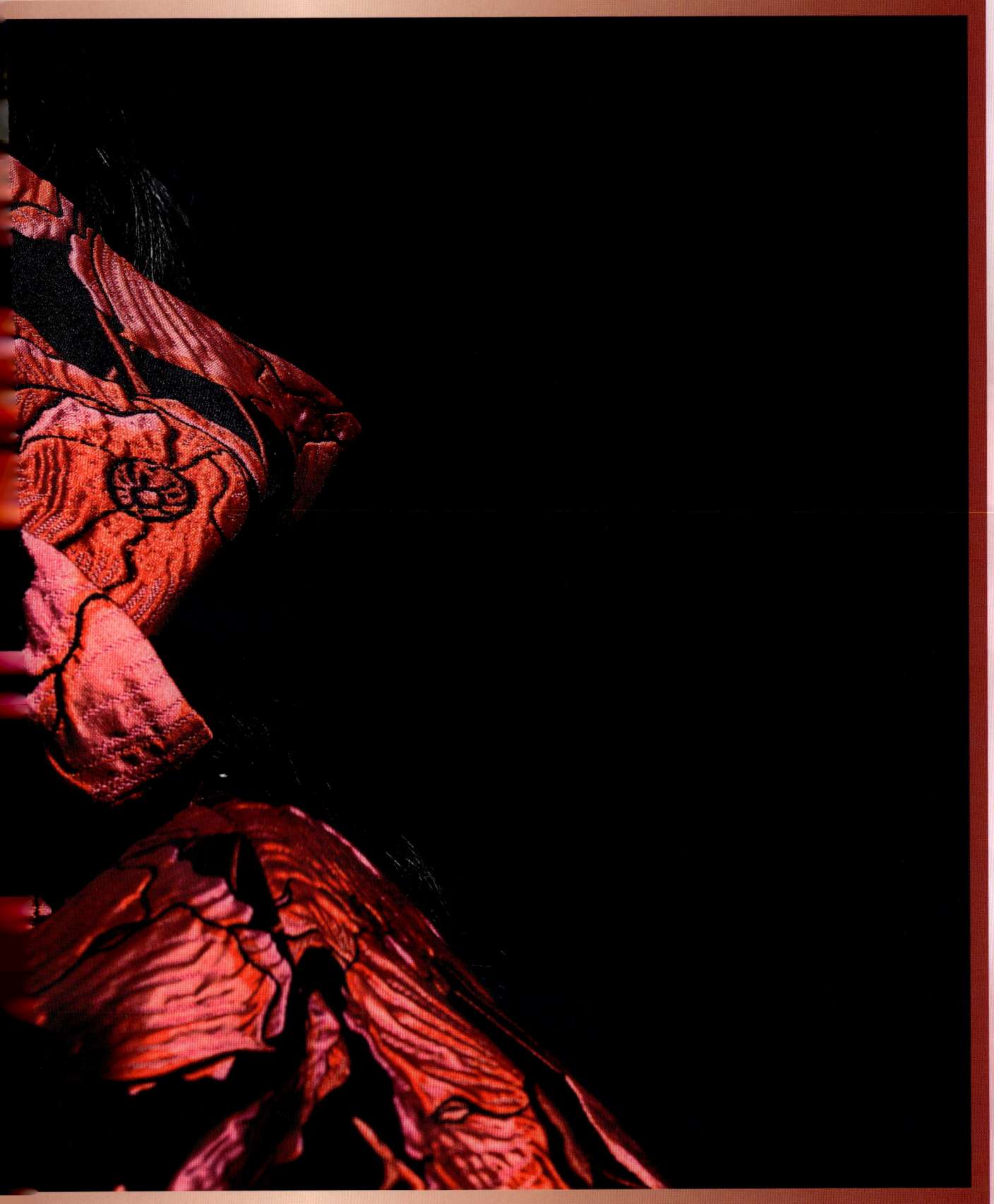

YOU COMPLETE ME

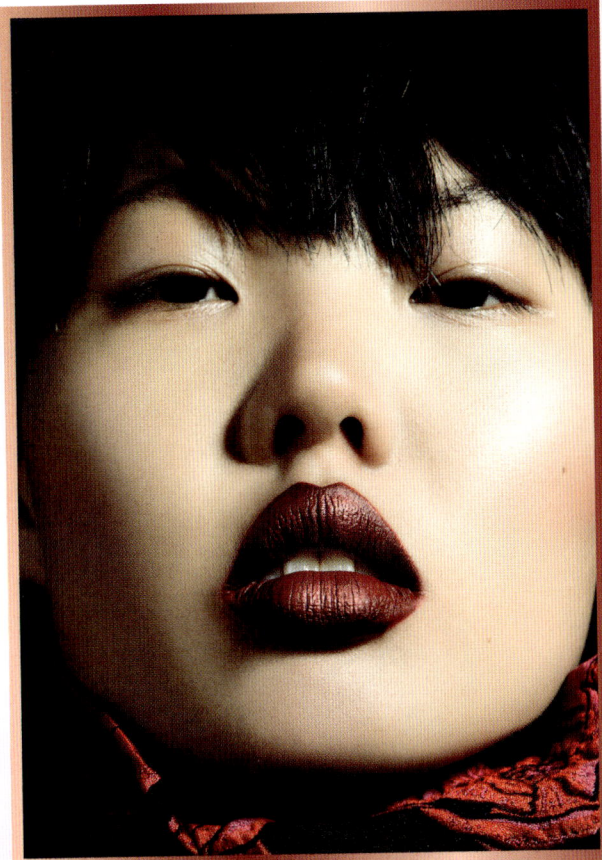
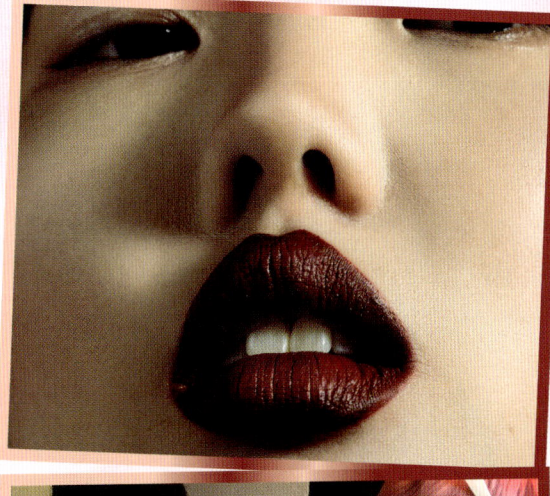
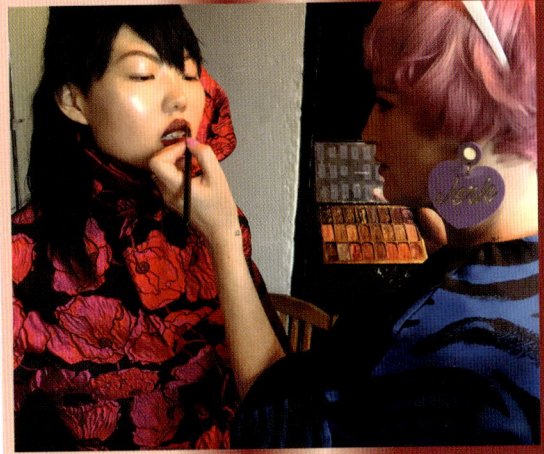

READ MY LIPS

Metallic lips (page 202) & dark lip (page 196)
We have combined the two techniques together here to create this perfect pout. When the lip color is this good all you need to wear with it is impeccable skin and softly defined features. Let this killer lip be the star! I've used Tom Ford Lipstick in 28 Nicholas and MAC Heritage Rouge Pigment over the top.

Velvet matte skin with highlights (page 66)
If you are really pale, you may find it hard to find a pale enough foundation shade for your skin. I love to mix MAC Face & Body Foundation in White, which is sheer and luminous, into any type of liquid foundation to pale it out and perfectly match my skin. Just a few drops will be enough to adjust the color.

Highlighting was so important to achieve this perfect skin. Use a sponge to really work the NARS Illuminator Cream in Copacabana over the high points of the face before brushing on Bobbi Brown Highlighting Powder in Pink Glow to set. Again, dampen your brush to apply for the smooth effect.

Powder blush (page 222)
Blush really can move around the face to where the heart desires! For this look, I wanted to have

her amazing cheekbones stand out so didn't want to cover them with blush. I sat the blush just on the underside of the cheekbone, to softly sculpt. Just a soft sweep of blush in a similar tone to the lips can really enhance the overall look!

Soft eyeliner

Softly press a brown matte shadow into the lash line to define eyes before slicking mascara on.

Styling tip from PSP: clean up that makeup!

The best thing I have ever found to remove makeup from clothes is a 'brush cleaner'. Be delicate and only spot clean as it can be harsh on fine fabrics, but it is the perfect quick fix if you notice something as you are rushing out the door.

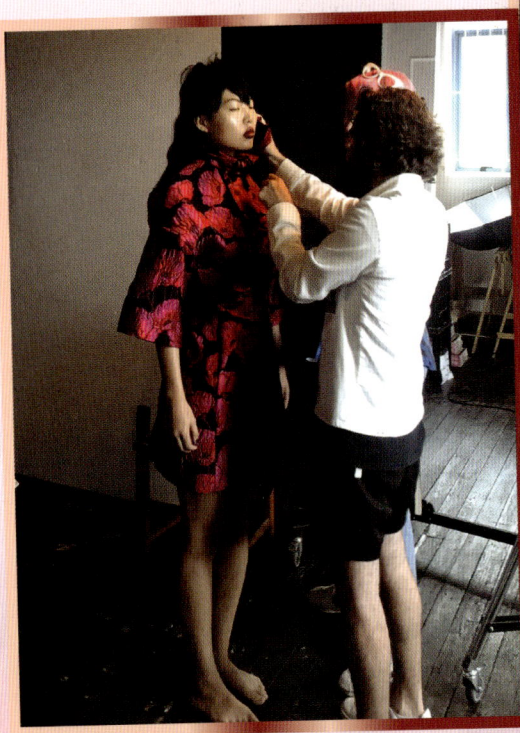

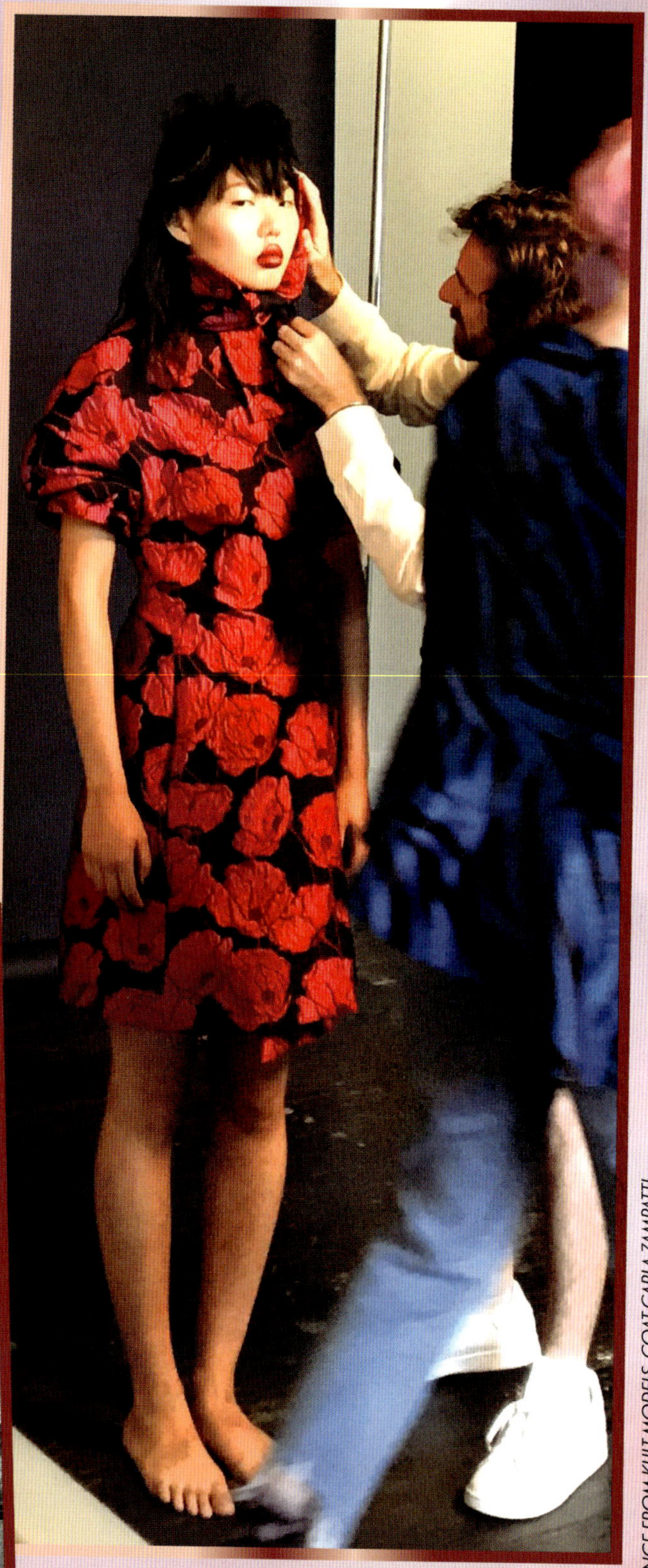

ANGE FROM KULT MODELS, COAT CARLA ZAMPATTI

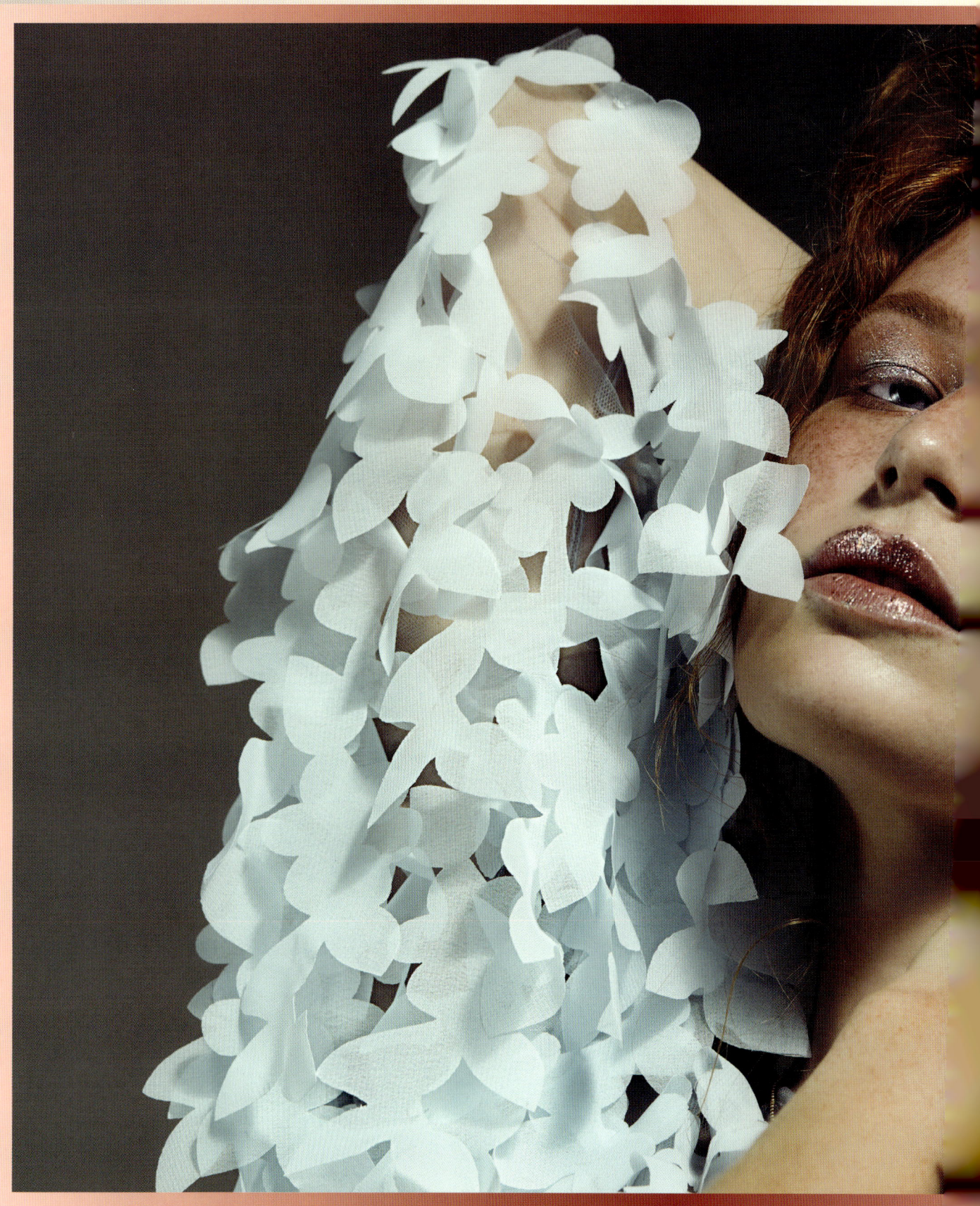

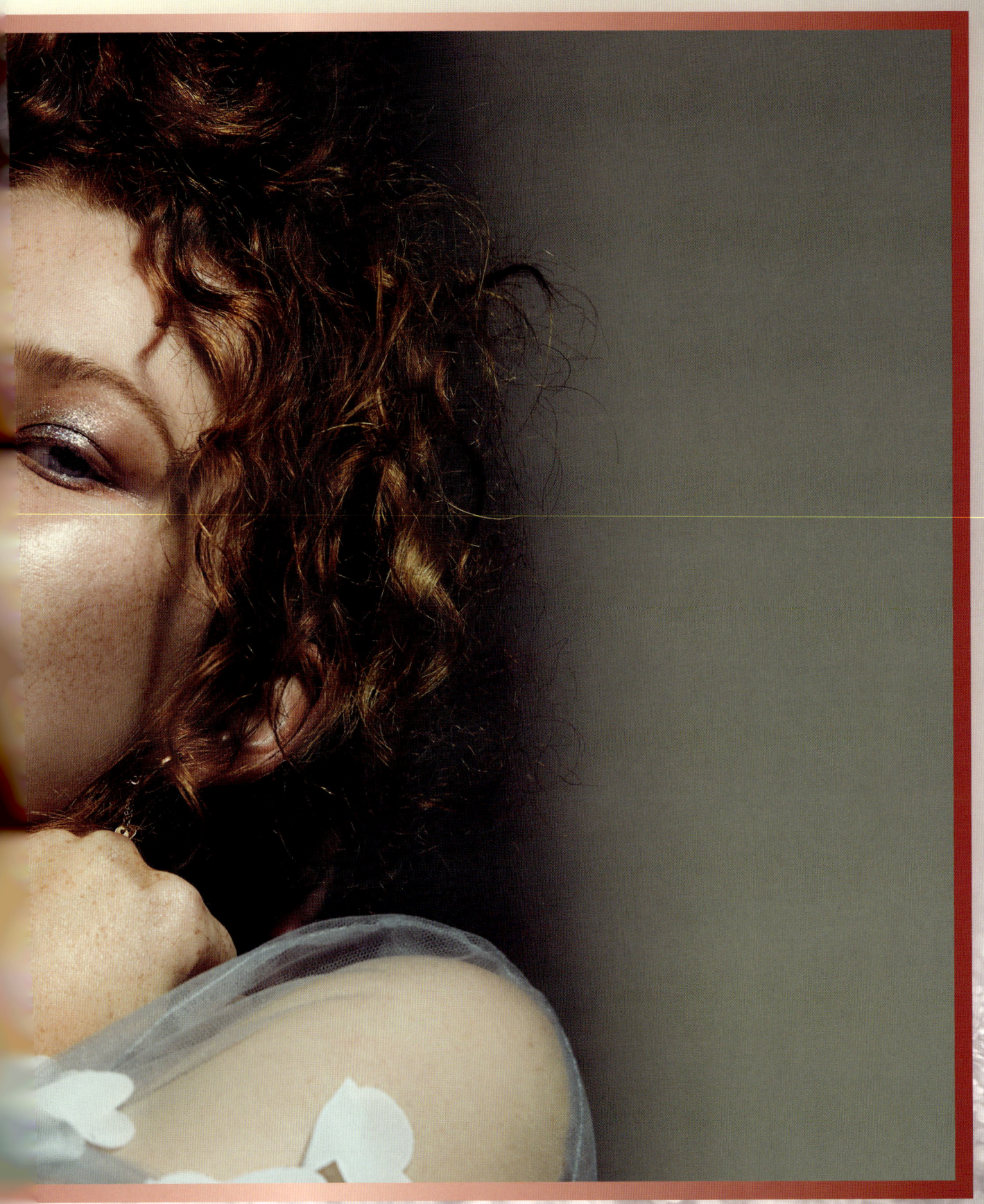

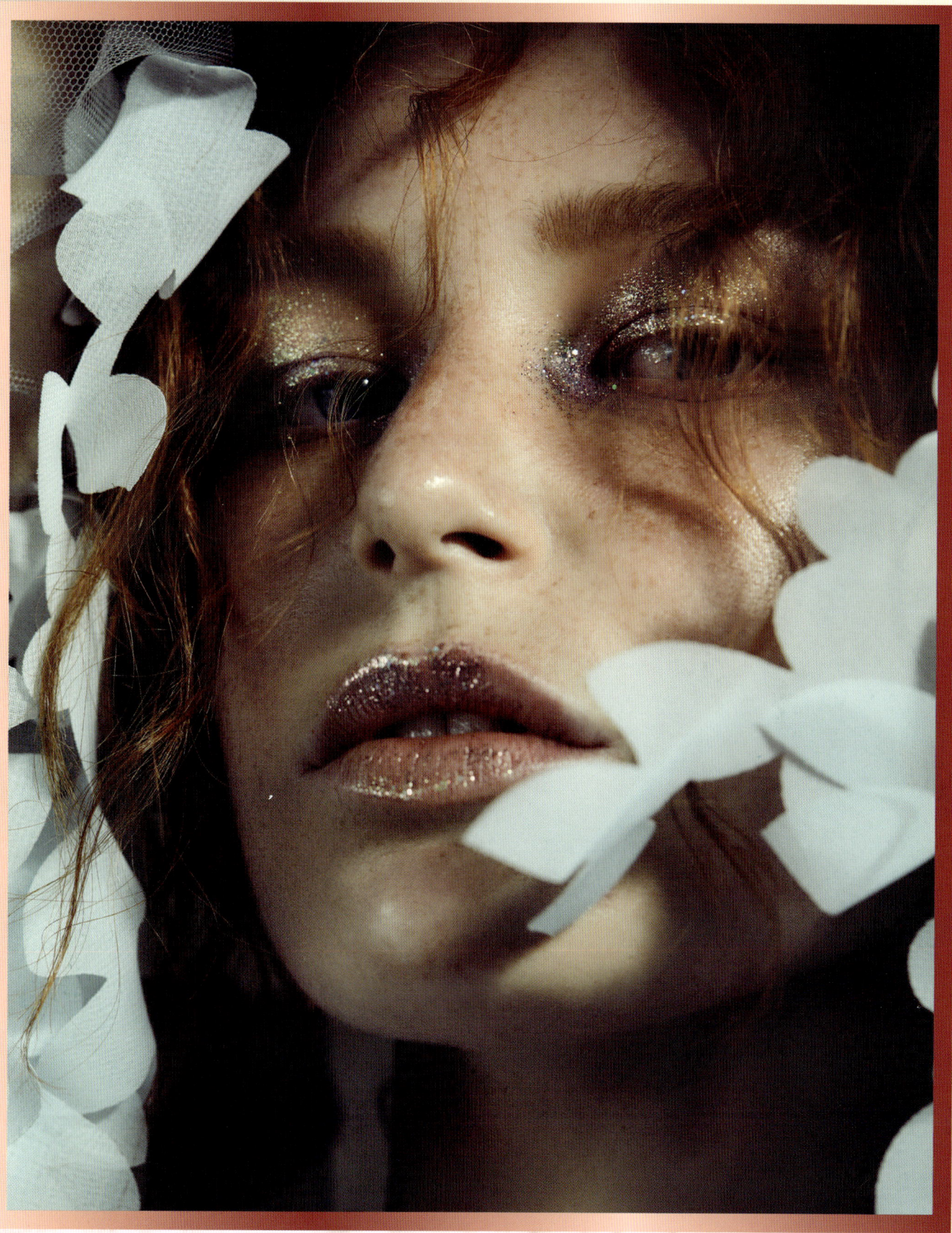

SHINY DISCO BALLS

Glitter eyes (page 136)

Blushes can double as great eye shadows! Often, they are a little more sheer in color so can create less stress with blending. Here I used MAC Mineralize Blush in Warm Soul across the lids and cheeks. Wherever the glitter is being applied I like to add a metallic shadow in the same color to help disguise any patchy glitter. Tap on your mixing medium or glitter glue and then tap on your glitter across the lids, making sure the edges are blended. This will avoid the glitter ending up with a hard edge. Pop the lightest glitter on the inner corners of the eyelid to brighten. A small amount of glitter goes a *long* way!

Glitter lips

Glitter will stick to anything. Seriously. With a soft, glossy lipstick coating your lips, tap the same glitter mix from the eyes through the centre of the lips for a little extra bling. Have you ever tried mixing glitter in with your clear gloss? It will put the POW in POUT!

Custom mix your shine

It is so fun having a color that no-one else has. Loose glitter and loose powder pigments are the easiest things to mix and make brand new colors that are you own. It's especially fun to mix up completely opposite colors in glitter, like blue and pink, and make your own 3D holographic shade. Drop a little of each glitter into the centre of a tissue, fold up the sides and shake to make magic!

Glitter clean up (page 139)

Check out these tips for easy clean-up of the dreaded glitter spill.

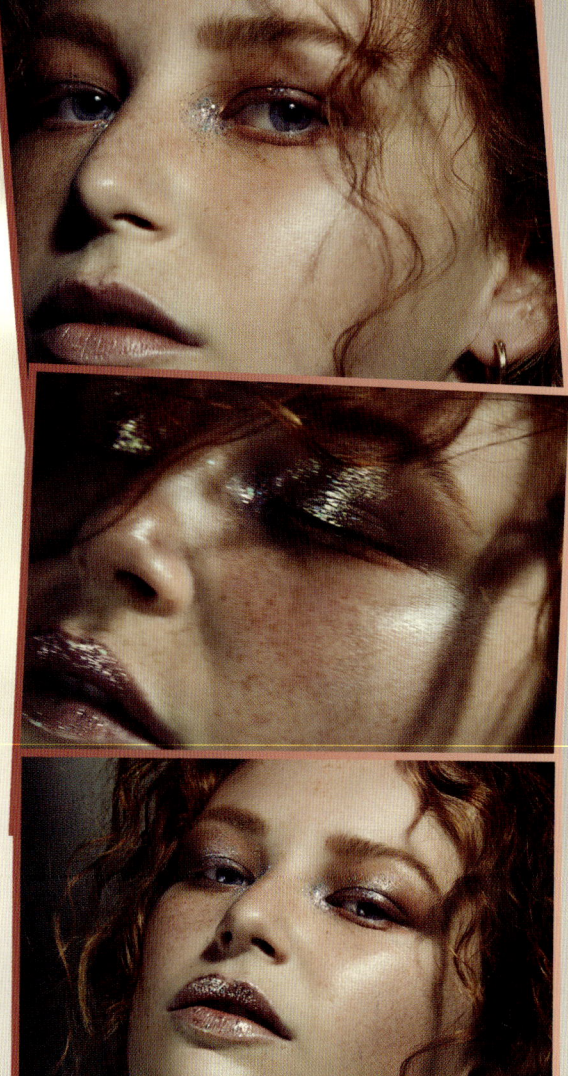

GEE GEE FROM KULT MODELS, CLOTHING GINGER AND SMART, JEWELERY MODELS OWN

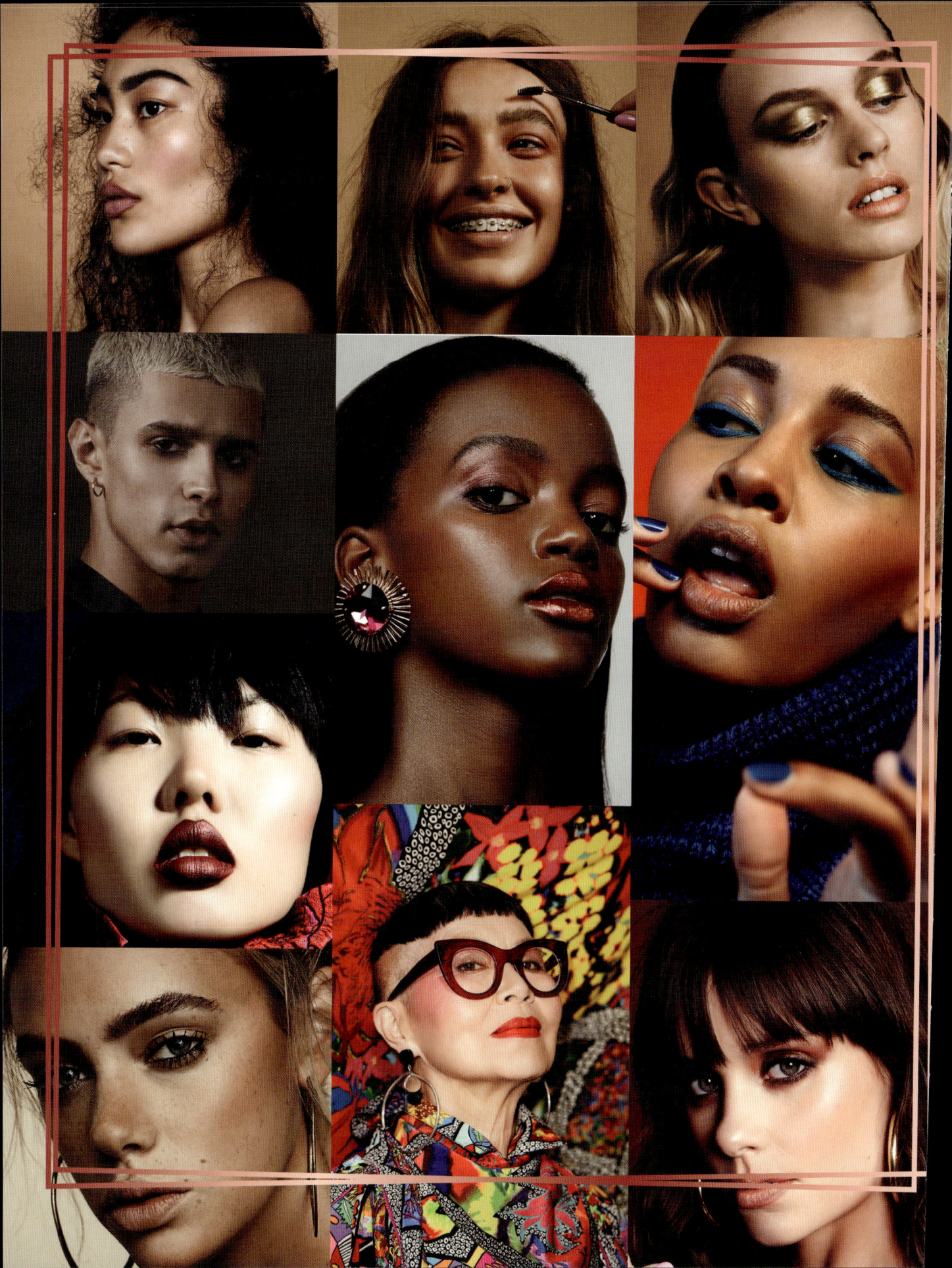

Acknowledgments

Steven: thank you, thank you, thank you!! We did it! When I asked if you wanted to join me on this crazy journey of a book, you said YES without hesitation and I appreciate you so very much. I'm sure you may have regretted your decision along the emotional journey, but your enthusiasm never wavered. You encapsulate talent, professionalism, speed, and quality all wrapped up in a big smiley bow and it was a pleasure to work so closely with you. I knew my vision was safe in your hands.

Cameron, what a perfect storm. Cannot believe how the universe works! Having you magically land in the country at just the right time to work on this with me; you and I have always been kindred spirits in work and play and I couldn't have done this without your love, cuddles, dancing, hair flicks, your beyond incredible talent and of course you snapping me back to reality with a sarcastic quip or joke at just the right time. Love you.

PSP, when I first met you and you unloaded masses of jewelry and clothing, like the Mary Poppins of styling, all with a smile, I knew we were going to be friends, whether you liked it or not. I admired you and your work before that moment, and boy has that admiration grown ever since. I feel lucky to have been able to work with you on so many special projects since then, this one is another box ticked. Just a couple of kids from the burbs making some magic.

My girls! Sanaz, you were literally my right-hand woman for the entire shoot and I can't thank you enough for the sunshine and skills that you bring! Rochelle and Rosie, how lucky am I to have such amazing makeup artists give up their time and travel from afar to help me?! You gals are incred. Cat, my original ride-or-die – could not have done this without you.

Jordie and Anna, thank you for jumping into this madhouse of a shoot! Thanks for being Cam's skilled wingman and wing-woman Byron, big hearted and full of surprises. Your creativity knows no bounds; you think so far out of the box it's actually a circle. Thanks for creating some wizardry. Jarred, always a GIANT smile behind the camera, I catch your enthusiasm when I am around you. Thank you for capturing the most special moments of the shoot. Dale, thank you for your encouragement and support from across the globe.

To the icon Jenny Kee, your courage to use color is such an inspiration. It was an honor to have you as my blank canvas for the day,

thank you for embracing it. The only thing that lights up the set more than your signature prints is your spirit, and it spilled far beyond your photos in this book.

All the Models from Chic, Chadwicks, Priscillas, Kult and Bella and their management teams – thank you for your support of this project!

The shoot crew from heaven – #strictlynodickheadsallowedonset.

Val, I consider myself beyond lucky to have shared many amazing moments with my absolute makeup idol over the years we have known each other. Having your words open this book perfectly sets the tone to celebrate creativity and your individual journey. THANK YOU.

Mum and Dad, you raised me to work hard and grab what I want. Having your loving, non-judgmental (even through all of my looks) safety net in life has made it that much easier to leap into the unknown without fear. Tania, your ingenuity made me realize that regardless of the challenges there is nothing that can't be achieved through love and resilience. That is very inspiring. Thank you parental gang for helping us hold down the fort during this crazy busy time.

Jodie, years of your belief and unwavering support have pushed me forward – lest we forget that without you, there would be no PINKY!

Raelene, Ciara, Kia and the UNION Management gang, I adore working with such a supportive, empowering group of women. Nothing is ever too much, and this quite simply wouldn't have happened with your support. Can't wait to see what the future will bring. You can't get rid of me now!

Terry, Kate, Carolyn and the many incredible Estée Lauder brands, thank you for always being in my corner.

All my MAC peeps past and present. I am constantly inspired by the colorful, creative chaos that is MAC. Thank you for accepting me as I am and affording me some of the most memorable life and work experiences EVER over the past 15 years.

Thank you to Monique, Victor and Fiona at New Holland Publishers for pushing for this project from day one. Liz Hardy you legend. Thank you for joining forces with Sara Lindberg to help turn my words into magic.

Adam, living life with you is living a life of encouragement. Get ready for some cheesy stuff here. You are not my rock, you are my wings (there may be some wind beneath them!). Nothing is ever out of reach, whatever I'm doing, as ridiculous as it may be. You aren't standing behind me pushing me forward, you are holding my hand every step of the way. Fifteen years ago you made the best passing comment ever: why don't you think about doing makeup for a job? Where would I be without you? Cheers, we did it! I couldn't love you more.

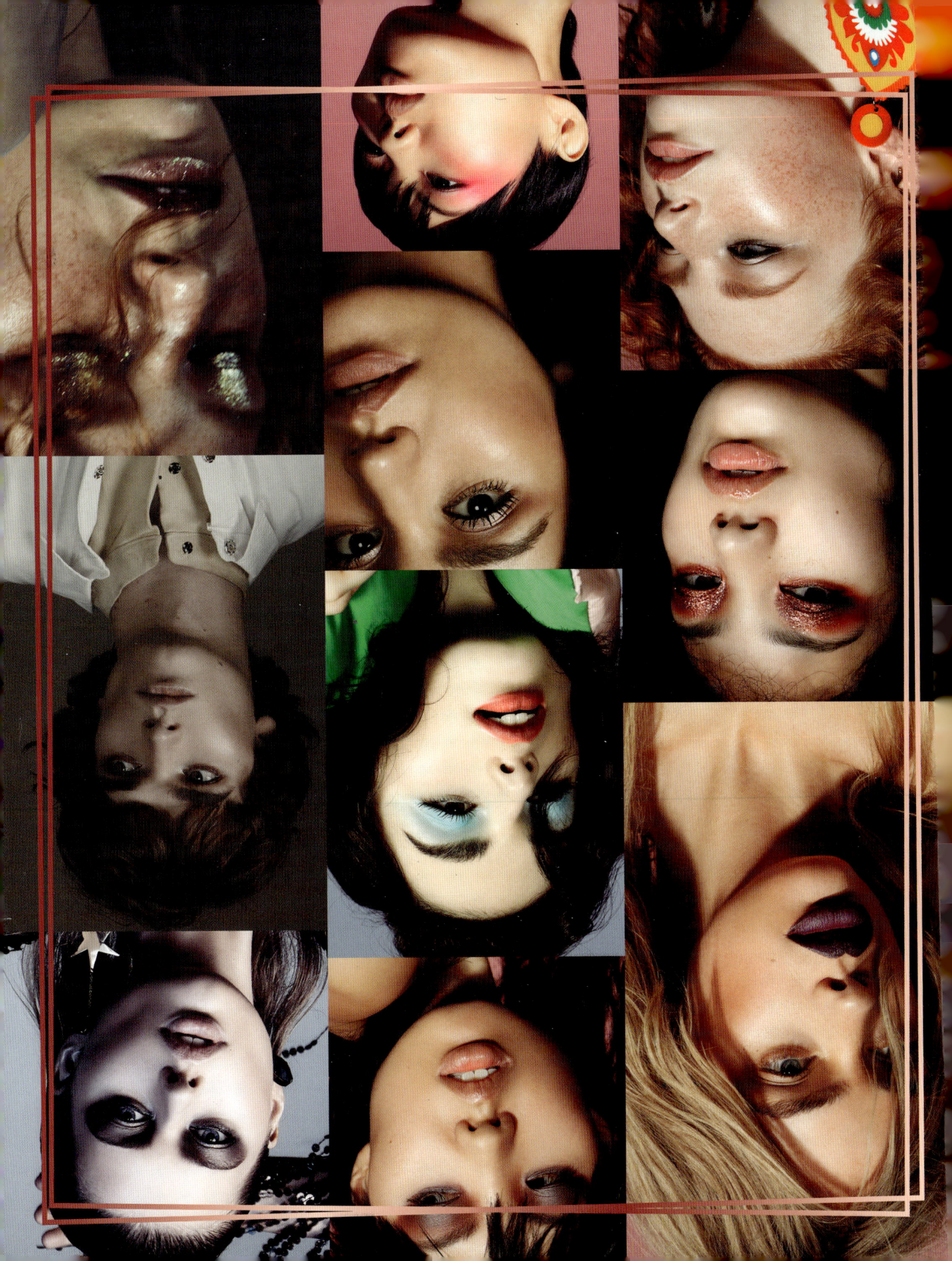

Credits

Photographer: Steven Popovich (Network) @stevenpopovich
Makeup: Nicole (Pinky) Thompson (Union Management) @pinkiiieee
Hair: Cameron Rains (The Wall Group) @cameron.rains
Styling: Peter Simon Phillips (Company 1) @petersimonphillips
Makeup Assist: Sanaz Fakhra @sanazfakhramakeup, Cat Smith @catsmithmakeup, Rosie Humphreys @rosiehumphreys_mua, Rochelle Spotswood @heyimrochelle_
Hair Assist: Anna Rose @annarosemaney, Jordan Robertson @jordanrobbohair
Photography Assist: Alisha Gore @alishagore
Production: Union Management @union_management

Models: Jenny Kee – Jennykee.com @jennykeeoz
Bella Management @bellatalentmanagement – Sophie Sheppard, Tiare, Ashlee
Chadwick Models @chadwickmodels – Phoebe O, Alana Mia, Lucy Blay, Madeline Hotznagel, Marlo, Emilie R, Azlin
Priscillas Management @priscillasmodels – Linnea, Ella
Kult Models @kultaustralia – Ace, Carson King, Ange, Gee Gee
Chic Management @chic_management – Hannah Wick, Rosie, Sameerah

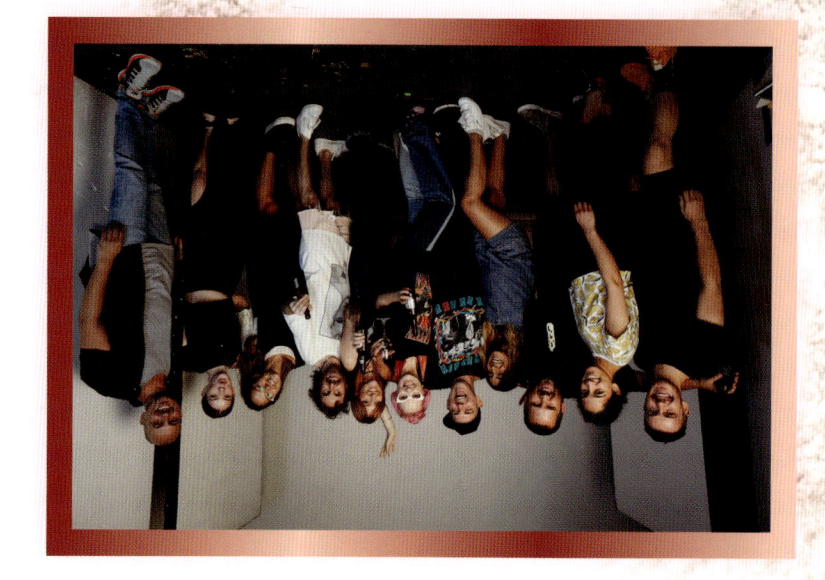

About Pinky

Nicole Thompson was born in 1982 in Sydney, Australia. Following an adolescence dominated by liquid liner and mauve lipstick, she completed high school in 1999. After graduation, she studied visual merchandising and worked within the retail sector for three years. Away from work Nicole was a passionate artist who had painted and sketched from a young age. Looking for a way to combine both her love of art and makeup, Nicole enrolled at the Australian College of Make Up and Special Effects in 2003.

With her studies completed, Nicole began assisting acclaimed makeup artists such as Linda Jefferyes and Liz Kelsh. An exposure to high-profile projects fed Nicole's desire to work in fashion and ultimately at international fashion week. One makeup brand presented a clear pathway to that opportunity and it was MAC Cosmetics.

Nicole began work with MAC Cosmetics in 2005 and by 2009 was appointed to the Global Senior Artist team and the role of brand ambassador for the company in Australia. Nicole's creative flair and personality without pretense become a signature of her work. Soon she was a regular at Paris, London, Milan and New York fashion weeks, while also becoming sought after in Australia whether it be on the catwalk or in print. Affectionately known as 'Pinky', Nicole was recognized as the Australian Makeup Artist of the Year in 2014.

Nicole's artistry has graced the pages of magazines such as Harper's Bazaar and Vogue, and catwalk shows that include Moschino, Balmain, Romance was Born and Vivienne Westwood. Nicole has collaborated with some of the world's best photographers and worked with a long list of celebrities that range from Kate Hudson to Dame Edna Everage.

'Pinky' has used her growing profile to support causes such as the MAC AIDS Fund and the Sydney Children's Hospital. Nicole still lives in Sydney with her husband Adam and daughter Frenchie Mae.

First published in 2018 by New Holland Publishers
London • Sydney • Auckland

131-151 Great Titchfield Street, London W1W 5BB, United Kingdom
1/66 Gibbes Street, Chatswood, NSW 2067, Australia
5/39 Woodside Ave, Northcote, Auckland 0627, New Zealand
newhollandpublishers.com

Copyright © 2018 New Holland Publishers
Copyright © 2018 in text: Nicole Thompson
Copyright © 2018 in images: Steven Popovich

All rights reserved. No part of this publication may be reproduced, stored in a retrieval system or transmitted, in any form or by any means, electronic, mechanical, photocopying, recording or otherwise, without the prior written permission of the publishers and copyright holders.

A record of this book is held at the British Library and the National Library of Australia.
ISBN 9781921024993

Group Managing Director: Fiona Schultz
Publisher: Monique Butterworth
Project Editor: Liz Hardy
Designer: Sara Lindberg
Production Director: James Mills-Hicks
Printer: Toppan Leefung Printing Limited

10 9 8 7 6 5 4 3 2 1

Keep up with New Holland Publishers on Facebook
facebook.com/NewHollandPublishers